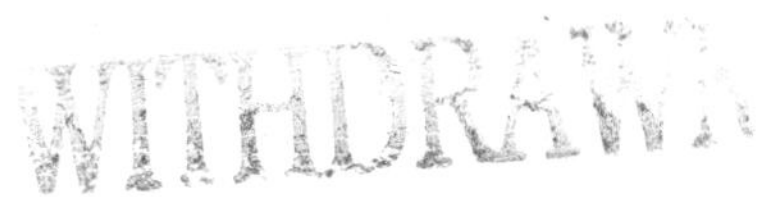

Aromatherapy: Therapeutic Use of Essential Oils for Esthetics

JIMM HARRISON

Aromatherapy: Therapeutic Use of Essential Oils for Esthetics
Jimm Harrison

President, Milady:
Dawn Gerrain

Director of Editorial:
John Fedor

Managing Editor:
Robert Serenka

Acquisitions Editor:
Martine Edwards

Product Manager:
Jessica Burns

Editorial Assistant:
Michael Spring

Director of Content and Media Production:
Wendy A. Troeger

Content Project Manager:
Nina Tucciarelli

Composition:
Pre-Press PMG

Director of Marketing:
Wendy Mapstone

Director of Industry Relations:
Sandra Bruce

Marketing Coordinator:
Nicole Riggi

Printed in United States
1 2 3 4 5 XXX 11 10 09 08 07

For more information contact
Cengage Learning, Inc.
5 Maxwell Drive,
CLIFTON PARK, NY 12065-2919
at http://www.milady.com

Library of Congress Cataloging-in-Publication Data

Harrison, Jimm.
Aromatherapy : therapeutic use of essential oils for esthetics / Jimm Harrison.
p. cm.
Includes bibliographical references.
ISBN-13: 978-1-4018-9895-3
ISBN-10: 1-4018-9895-5
1. Aromatherapy. 2. Essences and essential oils—Therapeutic use. I. Title.
RM666.A68H376 2008
615'.3219--dc22

2007037198

NOTICE TO THE READER

Publisher does not warrant or guarantee any of the products described herein or perform any independent analysis in connection with any of the product information contained herein. Publisher does not assume, and expressly disclaims, any obligation to obtain and include information other than that provided to it by the manufacturer.

The reader is expressly warned to consider and adopt all safety precautions that might be indicated by the activities herein and to avoid all potential hazards. By following the instructions contained herein, the reader willingly assumes all risks in connection with such instructions.

The publisher makes no representation or warranties of any kind, including but not limited to, the warranties of fitness for particular purpose or merchantability, nor are any such representations implied with respect to the material set forth herein, and the publisher takes no responsibility with respect to such material. The publisher shall not be liable for any special, consequential, or exemplary damages resulting, in whole or part, from the readers' use of, or reliance upon, this material.

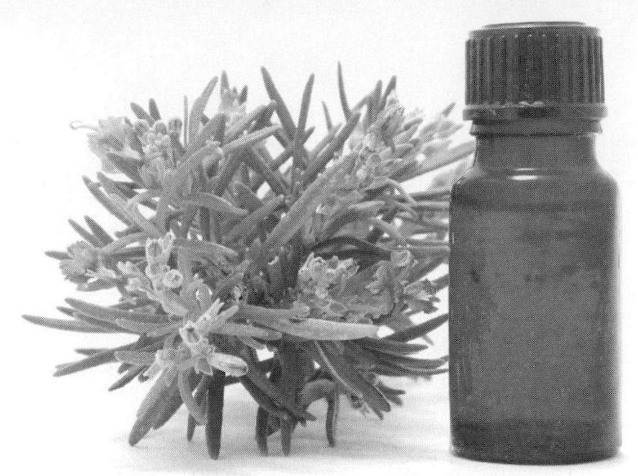

Contents

Foreword

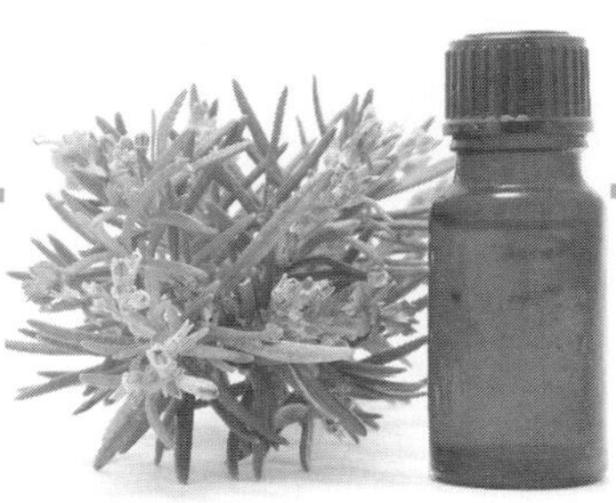

KURT SCHNAUBELT, PH.D.

When a nascent modern aromatherapy first made its way from its francophonic origins to the English speaking parts of the world, the field of cosmetics was among the first to embrace the new modality. As it is, the field of cosmetics—or the beauty industry (sic!) as it is often referred to in our commerce driven society—appears as one which is quick to embrace ever new promises of extended youth or miraculous and timeless preservation of physical beauty. It is in line with the current belief system of human domination over nature that these new promises for the most part are advances in one technology or another. Given the dominance of such technology driven innovations the integration of aromatherapy with its plant derived essential oils into many aspects of cosmetology was almost an anomaly. But alas, much of the new development of cosmetic uses of essential oils was driven by the enterprising energy of individual estheticians rather than having been magnanimously launched by corporate purveyors. In cosmetics as well as in many other areas of life in technological society nature is an impediment to the corporate need to mechanize, synthesize and industrialize. Not surprisingly it did not take too long before the budding essential oil trend in cosmetics was supplanted by the next wave of hyped innovation, if I remember correctly liposomes were the next guarantor of eternal beauty.

While the therapeutic use of essential oils and aromatherapy have continuously made inroads into many diverse healing arts, their integration into mainstream skin care has been curiously lagging after the first burst of interest in the mid 1980s dissipated. The extraordinary regenerative powers of essential oils have practically been ignored by a field, which does nothing but sell regeneration. If this is due to the understandable lack of corporate interest, rescue is now at hand in the form of Jimm Harrison's extremely well researched book: *Aromatherapy: Therapeutic Use of Essential Oils for Esthetics.*

It starts by setting its ambitions distinctly apart from the claims of the makers of exquisitely expensive cream pots, which often boldly insinuate gratification for all instincts, if one only were to acquire the latest breakthrough in regenerative technology. To the contrary Harrison claims that beauty and health are the currency of a larger unifying good, that what we perceive as beauty has its roots in traits we acquired through the course of biological evolution and that real beauty is a display of health and reproductive promise!

Aromatherapy: Therapeutic Use of Essential Oils for Esthetics goes on to give the reader a thoroughly holistic understanding of the composition, purpose and overall nature of essential oils. It expands this holistic approach to include and shape the notions of beauty of the reader beyond the often uncanny acceptance of the scars and ridiculously tight skin of the typical botched Las Vegas facelift.

Staying with the holistic theme *Aromatherapy: Therapeutic Use of Essential Oils for Esthetics* also elaborates on the many and varied ways in which our emotions reflect in our outward appearance and introduces the ways in which essential oils can perform the dual goal of supporting the regeneration of tissue as well as an easing of the mind. Harrison writes that early on he was influenced by a piece he read on aromatherapy that likened some of its phenomena to riding the crest of a wave. It appears to this writer that this book could well, after a long period of shallow surf, nurture some big swells of renewed fascination of the skin care and beauty field with the regenerative power of essential oils. Its great appeal lies with the precise language it uses to appeal to all those who feel attracted to holistic processes, but are averse to the often nebulous jargon of a superficial esotericism. Harrison leads us through a very insightful survey of the main protagonists of the field of aromatherapy to exactly where the field is today, taking us on an exhilarating ride from the botany of essential oil plants to the relation of essential oil components to neuropeptides and hormones. He makes it clear that not the "ditzy New Age sitcom blonde" but a modern and fact based approach to a holistic skin therapy holds the biggest promise to cultivate outward beauty as an almost casual by-product of maintaining emotional and physical health through the wise use of the powers of nature as they are so splendidly given to us in the form of essential oils.

About the Author

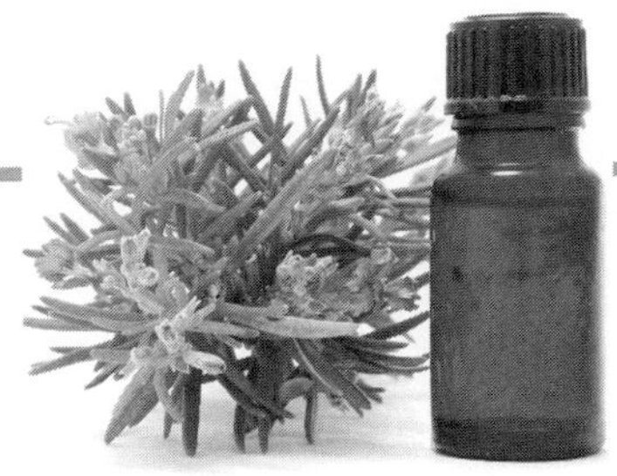

Jimm Harrison is an innovative educator and consultant with over 20 years experience in the beauty industry. His unique approach to beauty is the culmination of years of in-depth research on natural and nutritional beauty principles, apprenticing some of world's leading educators and researchers in the field of essential oils. He is a licensed cosmetologist, former salon owner and Certified Aromatherapist.

Jimm has been conducting certification programs in essential oil therapy for accredited massage, spa therapy, cosmetology and medical institutions across the country since 1993. In 1995 he founded the Phytotherapy Institute to advance increased education in essential oil and plant therapy. He is best known for his work on *Global Healthy Aging*, a unique beauty program that blends physiological, biological, psychological and sociological principles.

Jimm has written numerous articles on the subject of essential oil therapy, healthy aging, beauty and cosmetic safety. He is the co-founder of Spirit of Beauty Nutritional Skin Care and OHA Bio-Active Skin Care, products based on the healthy aging of the skin using organic botanicals, nutrients and essential oils. Jimm is the lead contributor and consultant for http://www.essentialoilresearch.com.

Acknowledgments

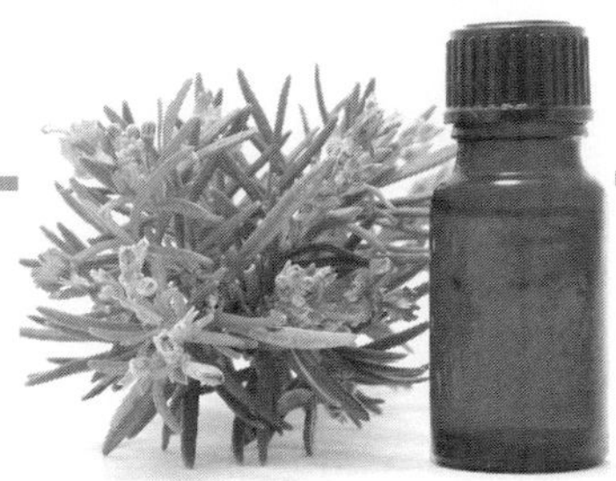

There's a lot more to aromatherapy than a study of essential oils. What I have developed as a practice of aromatherapy incorporates the many lessons I've learned from the many people I have met, befriended, loved, studied with, and worked with in my life. I wish to thank a lifetime of friends, family, partners, teachers, students, clients, and associates who were influential and supportive and provided the stepping-stones to writing this book.

This book is dedicated to my closest friend and brother, Bill, who has for my entire life given his support, love, and friendship; and also to my mother, Lillian. My children, Bowie and Jessica, and their mother Gail, deserve a special thanks for being willing clinical trial participants during my formative aromatherapy years.

My thanks, love, and a special dedication go to Martha, for helping to provide the environment and assistance that allowed me the opportunity to fully develop the skills and time to write this book. My thanks and appreciation also go to her children, Drea and Ryan.

I also thank my very best friend and aromatherapy mentor, Kurt Schnaubelt. May he forever rock the aromatherapy world with his aromatic, academic, political, and philosophical astuteness.

In the process of writing this book I have made a new friend, Christianne Vink, who read through the early chapters and provided me with valuable input and corrected information.

My personal editor, Sarah Dehart, I thank for finally convincing me that I needed an editor and that she was the right person.

I thank Janet D'Angelo for introducing me to Milady, making the publishing of this book possible.

My thanks to the Milady–Thomson Delmar Learning staff, especially Martine Edwards and Jessica Burns, for their splendid work in creating a successful outcome to this book.

Reviewers:

The author and publisher would like to thank the following professionals who have reviewed this text and devoted their time and expertise throughout the development process. We are grateful for your invaluable feedback.

- Helen Bickmore, LMT, CPE, AEA, Albany, NY
- Jeff Bockoven, Iowa Massage Institute, Des Moines, IA
- Felicia Brown, Balance Inc., High Point, NC
- Larkin Busby, Essential oil technician/instructor, Center for Aromatherapy Research and Education, MO
- Julie Green, The Sanctuary, Kiawah Island, SC
- Catherine Novak, Beads N Botanicals, Hoopeston, IL
- Carrie E. Pierce; Pierce Consulting Services (PCS) Int'l Educator/Port Townsend, WA
- David Stewart, Ph.D., Director, Center for Aromatherapy Research and Education, MO
- Wauneta Elaine Strobel C.C.I., The Body…Works, MI
- Barbara Vissers, JC Health Essentials, MI
- Leslie Vornholt, LCSW, CCI
- Michele A. Williams, RPh, Aroma Rx Inc, Los Alamos, CA

Photography Credits:

Cover photo of rosemary oil: Shutterstock, Daniel Hughes
Figure 1-1 A – Shutterstock, Eric Isselée
Figure 1-1 B – Shutterstock, Marcus Brown
Figures 1-3 and 1-4 courtesy of Dermnet.com/ Interactive Medical Media LLC, All rights reserved.
Figure 2-1 Shutterstock, Gina Smith
Figure 2-2, The Associated Press (http://apimages.ap.org)
Figure 3-1, Delmar Learning
Figures 4-1, 4-4a, 4-4b, 7-1, 7-3, and Plates 6, 7, 8, 9, 10, 11, 13, 14, 15, 16, 17, 21, 22 & 23– Courtesy of Pacific Institute of Aromatherapy
Figure 4-2 and Plate 24– Courtesy of Christopher McMahon, White Lotus Aromatics

Figure 4-3 – Photo courtesy of Jack Chaitman/Scents of Knowing Inc.
Figures 5-12, 5-21, 5-22, 5-23, 5-24, 8-1, 8-2, 8-3 and Plates 1-3, 28 & 29– Courtesy of Jimm Harrison
Figures 7-2, 7-4 and Plates 25, 26 & 27– Courtesy of Down Under Enterprises, Inc.
Plates 4, 5, 18, 19, 20 & 30: Courtesy of S&D Aroma LTD.
Plate 12, photo of Angel Lavender Farms in Sequim, WA by www.bestUSAphotographers.com
Illustrations compiled by Pre-Press PMG.

Introduction

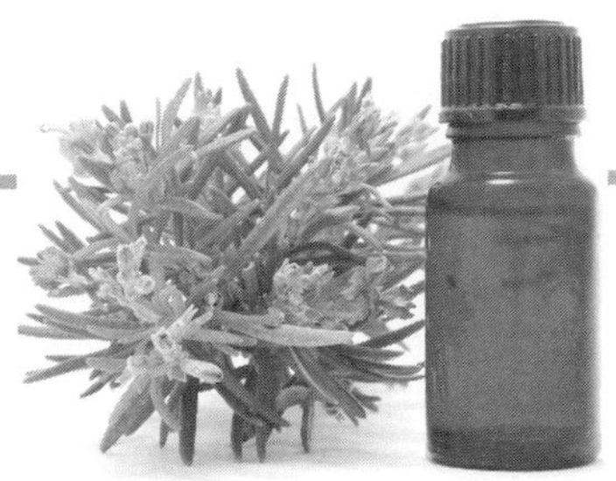

Aromatherapy is limited by popular perception. It's a practice that is much more expansive than a sniff of lavender to soothe the nerves, a drop of peppermint to stimulate a weary mind, or a dab of eucalyptus to clear congested lungs. Though these are valued and important properties, they represent only the most basic uses of the essential oils in aromatherapy. Much more can be expected of essential oils. There's also a wider range of oils from which to choose, offering an array of treatments and exotic fragrances. But even with the common oils of lavender, peppermint, and eucalyptus, extraordinarily diverse healing and therapeutic potential exists.

It doesn't take much effort to make use of the many properties available from essential oils. It's really rather simple. Buy some oils and use them. You would think, with more than 400 pages following this introduction, that there must be more to aromatherapy. It's true that this book contains a vast amount of information relating to the use of essential oils. Still, without any more knowledge than you have right now, you are capable of unleashing the therapy within aromatherapy.

Although you may be capable of using essential oils now, your potential will grow with the knowledge offered in the following chapters. Within this book are definitions, guidelines, and studies that will increase your abilities and the wisdom that allows you to develop an intelligent and well directed use of essential oils.

Aromatherapy is as simple a practice as it is complex. The beauty of essential oil therapy is in its simplicity. A drop, a sniff, or a rub of essential oils is all it takes to let loose their curative abilities. Their power unfolds from the complexities nature has provided, made evident in the study that follows.

An understanding of their molecular structures and intricate biological interactions enables specific application similar to pharmaceuticals.

Aromatherapy is both art and science. The science explains, as much as is possible at this time, the why and how of the therapeutic results of essential oils, such as their antiseptic, anti-inflammatory and wound healing properties. The art is the creative freedom to test the science and to take aromatherapy beyond the limits of academic understanding. Both the creative aspect and the intellectual understanding are developed over time. This time frame appears infinite, because there is always something new to be learned about essential oils and aromatherapy.

The therapeutic use of essential oils is a creative, versatile, and powerfully effective esthetic treatment. The intent of this book is to create an aromatherapy text and reference book that will supply the esthetician, cosmetology student, and clinical therapist with the tools and knowledge necessary to completely understand the complexities of essential oil therapy and confidently use its healing potential.

Although this book is directed toward the beauty, esthetic, and spa professional, it may also be used by anyone interested in essential oils. Aromatherapy is far too encompassing to limit its knowledge to the skin only. Besides, limiting essential oil study to its effects on the skin isn't the most sensible or comprehensive means of caring for the skin. Beauty comes from health. To achieve beauty and healthy skin, the entire health of the body—holistic health—must be considered. Using a holistic model of health is necessary when treating conditions of the skin. Aromatherapy is a holistic practice, as explained in Chapter 1 of this book. The ability to work with essential oils holistically is the most effective approach in providing maintenance or treatment for the skin. Therefore, this text contains information that addresses many functions of the body.

Within this book, you will find information regarding the use of essential oils that may appear to be medical in context. This in-depth material does not mean that you should use essential oils outside of your professional or licensed capabilities. The information is presented to promote deeper understanding and more effective use of the oils within your own practice. It is provided to assist you to be a better holistic practitioner. The practitioner or student interested in essential oil therapy may become as versed in the practice as he or she desires. This book is designed to enable the casual user to gain and use the information necessary to apply essential oils safely and effectively and to gather the knowledge to respond to the educated consumer. The book allows the reader to reference information as desired for limited or extensive essential oil use. Aromatherapy enthusiasts and clinical therapists will benefit from the book's in-depth and up-to-date coverage of scientific research, chemistry, and biology. This book incorporates areas of knowledge included in the standard aromatherapy certification courses offered across the United States and internationally.

Aromatherapy as a holistic practice is understood, and more fully developed, when psychology, philosophy, alternative health, diet, nutrition, and lifestyle are incorporated. Different aspects of life, and their possible influence on health and beauty, are studied in relation to the therapeutic properties of the essential oils. This information is then translated into a method of consultation and treatment, expanding beyond symptom-related treatment, and provides the student with a truly holistic process, or whole body focus, for applying essential oils.

This aromatherapy text and reference book includes detailed information about 33 essential oils, highlighted for their value in skin care and spa therapy. This information will assist the practitioner and student in creating a complete collection of versatile essential oils for immediate use in building an aromatherapy practice. Of course, complete and easy-to-follow application instructions and formulas are included.

Some areas of study included in this text may appear advanced and difficult for the beginning aromatherapy student. These areas are best approached using your particular level of education or comfort. The challenging subjects, primarily the chemistry, are a necessary aspect of essential oil use. This book includes a foundation of basic organic chemistry, molecular structures, and atoms. The information is included to help you comprehend essential oil structure and activity. To provide a thorough holistic model, the text discusses or briefly reviews many scientific subjects to augment your overall knowledge of health, healing, biology, and nature. These subjects are not for everyone. Skip those that may not interest you or that confuse you and come back to them at a later time.

The importance of understanding the chemical structure of essential oils is presented and explained using the Structure-Effect Diagram. This format enables those with little to no chemistry background to understand essential oil activity and safety by outlining the chemical properties that produce the aromatherapy result. This approach empowers the practitioner in essential oil selection and consultation, breaking away from the limits of essential oil knowledge based on a "this oil for that condition" approach to aromatherapy. Relevant human and plant biology and physiology are included to add dimension to your understanding of essential oil effectiveness and use.

The complex nature of essential oils is evident when comparing the sometimes confusing and contradictory information found within the array of aromatherapy sources. Why is lemon oil considered calming in one text and energizing in another? Are essential oils as safe or as dangerous as conflicting sources state? A main goal in writing this text is to explain these contradictions through a comprehensive overview of the many variables involved in essential oil activity. The reader benefits from a clearer understanding of why results from essential oil studies would conflict. These conflicts are periodically addressed to give the aromatherapy student and practitioner a more complete awareness and knowledge base from which to work and an ability to address issues arising from conflicting information.

Uncertainty is an underlying characteristic of nature and the human mind. Accepting unknowns as part of life has a benefit. Once accepted, the discomfort that surrounds uncertainty may be alleviated. The student may develop a beneficial openmindedness toward the study of essential oils by allowing this acceptance.

Though the following information is presented or perceived as fact, the element of uncertainty remains. This uncertainty could be the very aspect of aromatherapy that keeps one from becoming jaded. Essential oils continue to surprise and astonish. Even when their healing results are expected, there is often surprise that they actually worked. Every application of essential oils is novel. Each experience is unique, because each person who uses them is unique.

Aromatherapy is a simple practice. Pick an oil and smell it, dab it, or rub it in. Contrarily, the complexity of aromatherapy is apparent in the ongoing challenge of grasping the many variables that influence the outcome of essential oil application. The challenge is an attempt to understand confusion, create agreement in contradiction, order chaos, and clarify uncertainty. This is an impossible task, but an interesting and fulfilling journey.

Holistic Beauty and Skin Care

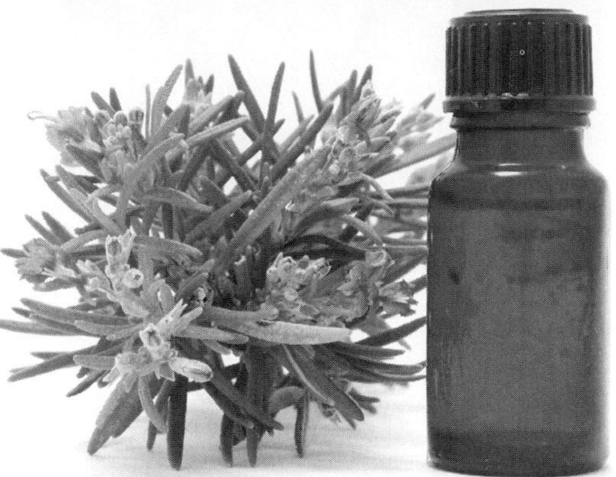

CHAPTER 1

One objective characteristic of beauty is that to a considerable extent, beauty is the expression of health. A well and harmoniously developed body, tense muscles, an elastic and finely toned skin, bright eyes, grace and animation of carriage—all these things which are essential to beauty are the conditions of health.

—Havelock Ellis

LEARNING OBJECTIVES

1. Develop a clear definition of holistic beauty and health, using measurable criteria.
2. Discuss the benefits of clearly defined holistic beauty goals.
3. Identify and describe the uses of essential oils, and other botanicals, as tools to achieve a holistic therapeutic result.
4. Define the role of a holistic practitioner that benefits both the practitioner and the client.

BEAUTY AS HEALTH

What is beauty? Like most people, you probably know it when you see it, but may be challenged when asked to describe or define it. To understand beauty, to be beautiful, or to define beauty, it is helpful to understand its relationship to health. Beauty has its basis in evolutionary biology and is a barometer of reproductive health and a sign of strong genes and immunity.[1] The peacock with the brightest feathers, the baboon with the brightest and most colorful posterior, and the strongest male of the pack are the ones who attract and get the mate. Extravagant spectacles of color and aggressive strength display health and reproductive promise. These traits show that the potential mate is not infested with parasites and has the vitality of healthy genetic material. Beauty's function, from a biological perspective, is to stimulate reproduction and enhance the endurance of living beings.

Aversion to Ill Health

The opposite of attraction is aversion. What is a typical response to "ugliness" or disease? Aversion appears to be a preprogrammed response to ill health. The once shiny and thick coat of a dog that has become parasite ridden or diseased is no longer beautiful but repulsive (Figure 1-1). Everything in nature

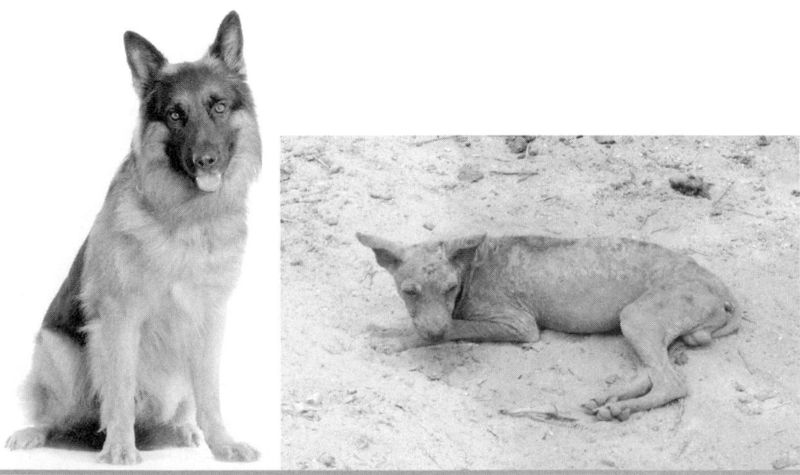

Figure 1-1 When looking at a diseased and healthy animal it becomes obvious that health and beauty are synonymous.

displays beauty when it is healthy. A lush, growing field is beautiful. When the land is abused, polluted, or clear-cut, it becomes ugly. Nature, when healthy, is beautiful. When disease is present, humans, other animals, and nature become unattractive.

Healthy Skin Is Beautiful Skin

If one accepts that health and beauty are intertwined, then it's logical to assume that any personal beauty ambition, whether it's glowing youthful skin, clear sensuous eyes, or firm, cellulite-free thighs and buttocks, will rely on a healthful, well balanced, and nutritionally nourished body and mind. Logic suggests that skin impurities and damage are signals that disease, toxicity, or systemic imbalance is present within the body. The skin condition is a symptom of disease or ill-health. Health must be regained to eliminate and correct a skin condition, to gain youthful vibrant skin, and to achieve overall beauty.

HOLISTIC HEALTH

Healthful beauty is more than just treating the symptom or skin condition. Much more than symptomatic relief is required to fully achieve health. Achieving **holistic health** means taking care of the whole person, rather than merely treating the symptom. Holistic health is based on **holism**, the understanding that the parts make up a unified whole. The parts are no longer viewed as individual units but are analyzed in relationship with the whole organism. In holistic health all parts of the person, cells, organs, body systems, and emotions affect each other as well as the whole person. No part or system can be diseased or damaged without it affecting, or causing disease or damage to, the remaining whole.

For example, stress and tension can cause proteins to be released from cells. These proteins, elements of the immune system, cause allergic reaction that results in symptoms of atopic dermatitis (Figure 1-2).[2] A connection also exists between dermatitis and a deficiency of essential dietary fats.[3] This fat deficiency is also thought to produce anxiety.[4] With a holistic model of health, symptoms are not treated in isolation; a symptom in one part of the body, such as the skin, is addressed by treating multiple systems or related causes. The body is quite complex, so holistic analysis rarely is a simple task.

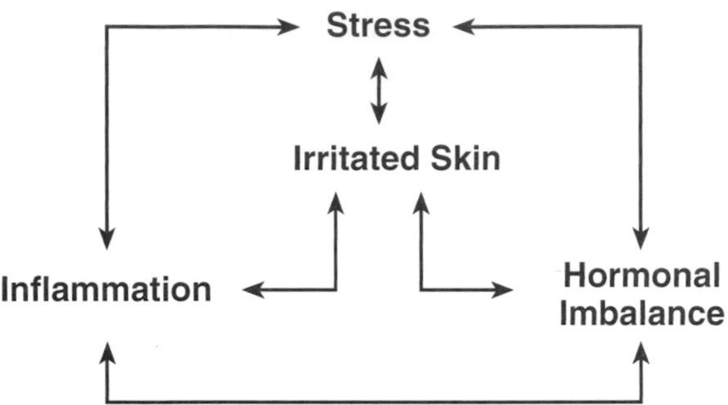

Figure 1-2 The cause of a skin condition can be difficult to trace as this diagram demonstrates there is a cause and effect loop that is common in many skin conditions. Stress may be the cause of hormonal imbalance that then results in irritated skin which causes stress causing inflammation causing hormonal imbalance and on and on.

HOLISTIC BEAUTY

Holistic beauty consists of inner and outer beauty and requires beauty maintenance throughout the aging process. Inner beauty not only relates to the internal body systems but also includes personality and mental health. Outer beauty concerns most of us and is inspired by our daily visits with a mirror. Beauty maintenance is largely affected by healthy regeneration of cells and resistance to environmental stress and free radical damage.

HOLISTIC UNDERSTANDING OF ESSENTIAL OILS

Essential oils have holistic, multi-therapeutic functions: They work by correcting or regulating many imbalances simultaneously. A holistic health and beauty program that includes the therapeutic use of essential oils addresses skin problems as well as the imbalance that may be causing the condition. Let's use **eczema** as a simplified model of the holistic benefits of essential oils (Figure 1-3).

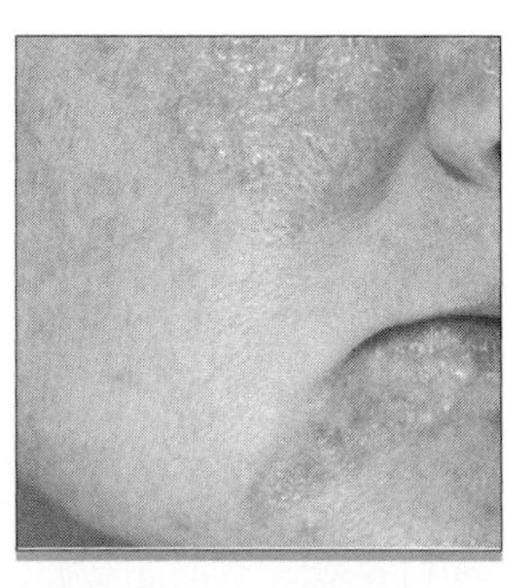

Figure 1-3 Atopic dermatitis or eczema is a difficult skin condition to treat as it has many possible causes.

The first step is to identify the symptoms and possible causes of the condition. These symptoms and causes may include:

- inflammation
- dry and dehydrated skin or lipid barrier deficiency
- allergies or immune response
- sensitivity

A holistic perspective unwraps each symptom and its cause. Inflammation may be caused by diet or environmental factors; the skin's lipid barrier can be compromised by stress or harsh detergents; skin sensitivities include several possible causes and may be increased by hormonal imbalance.

At times, this task may seem overwhelming and well beyond your expertise or clinical focus. Fortunately, the properties of essential oils may address several conditions at once and make it possible to treat holistically without full knowledge of the condition or its cause. This potential does not mean you are working blindly. It simply means that essential oils contain holistic capabilities that may exceed understanding. This possibility exists with almost anything that interacts with the body, such as topical skin applications, environmental toxins, or pharmaceuticals. The effects of any interaction with the body are holistic. The activity of any substance on cells, bodily functions, or body systems has a counter-effect, or holistic rection, through out the body. The results may be positive, negative, or neutral to the body. In all cases, they are reactions that you may not always anticipate. Studying and incorporating the information contained in this book will ensure a positive holistic healing benefit each time you use essential oils, even though some results may not be anticipated.

Introduction to Holistic Essential Oil Formulas

This example introduces you to the holistic value of essential oils (EOs). It also introduces some of the concepts of aromatherapy you will learn in this text, such as the common names (in bold) and the botanical names (italicized) of essential oils, principles of choosing oils for their known healing properties, and characteristics of the carrier oils used to dilute essential oils. For eczema, the following essential oils are selected as a holistic aromatherapy remedy designed to address both the symptoms and known and unknown causes:

everlasting (*Helichrysum italicum*) is chosen for its anti-inflammatory and cell regenerative properties.

German chamomile (*Matricaria recutita)* is chosen for its anti-allergic properties.

lavender (*Lavandula angustifolia*) is chosen for stress reduction and skin soothing properties.

neroli (*Citrus auranthium*) is chosen for stress reduction and sensitivity.

Aromatherapy treatments generally include a **carrier oil** (a vegetable, nut, or fruit oil) in which the essential oils are diluted. Carrier oils are also selected for their therapeutic and healing properties (see Chapter 9). Carrier oils are especially beneficial in supporting the lipid barrier function of the skin. In treating eczema, the following carrier oils may be recommended:

evening primrose oil (*Oenothera biennis*)
olive oil (*Olea europea*)
Rose hip seed oil (*Rosa rubiginosa*)

The essential oil blend in the carrier oil base shapes a holistic treatment that addresses the symptomatic and suspected causes related to eczema. Each essential oil contains more properties and therapeutic activity than those listed. As you expand your study of essential oils, you will learn the healing properties of individual essential oils and build upon the science and understanding of their holistic healing properties.

This simple example does not consider the effects of diet, emotional health, and lifestyle. These factors also influence the condition of the skin. Though these issues may be beyond the scope of your esthetic practice, they still may have an effect on the outcome of your work. This point is important! A client who is smoking and eating fast foods, or one who had recently appeared in court over a difficult divorce two days after a parent died, may not be successfully treated even with your best formulations and holistic intentions. As we delve deeper into the study of aromatherapy, you will see how these other factors are integrated into the holistic use of essential oils.

ESTABLISHING AN OUTCOME: THE HOLISTIC GOAL

For a treatment to be successful, a well-defined therapeutic goal—the desired outcome of treatment—must be established. The goal can be simple to define, such as wanting to reduce wrinkles or moisturize dry skin, and is commonly expressed in a proper skin consultation. A successful skin care treatment becomes more difficult for a practitioner in the beauty and wellness industry when the client's request is vague. A request to be "more beautiful" is certainly vague and would require some investigation to determine the client's true meaning. An accurately defined goal is necessary to establish a treatment protocol.

The importance of a well-defined goal becomes more evident in holistic beauty. A goal that is superficial and vague, such as "to correct dry skin," must be defined from a holistic perspective. Our proposal that beauty is health means that the goal, or outcome of hydrated skin, would require a holistic analysis to determine what health issue is causing the skin to be dry. The resulting goal would reflect the determined cause. Suppose the health issue is a compromised lipid barrier function that results in dehydrated skin. The goal can now be clearly defined to include regeneration of the lipid barrier function, a more holistic and complete goal than moisturizing dry skin. Holistically, this goal could be extended to include reducing nervous tension, which may be causing the compromise in lipid barrier function.[5] A goal focusing on total holistic health will be the most beneficial in generating beauty corrections that include reducing wrinkles and rehydrating dry skin.[6]

Creating a Holistic Beauty Goal

A holistic beauty program benefits from the incorporation of a beauty goal. This goal calls for the practitioner and client to acknowledge, and share in, an understanding and definition of beauty. Beauty, as ambiguous or individual as it may be, is the underlying goal of any skin care treatment. We have described beauty as a reflection of health that is used in nature to attract a mate. This description is not common to those who aspire to be more beautiful. The basic premise is correct in that a desire for beauty is a desire to be attractive. This desire is represented in a request for a youthful complexion, firmer skin tone, or fewer wrinkles, all of which are signs of health and vitality. The relationship between health and beauty must be acknowledged when developing a beauty goal. To meet the goal of youthful and vital wrinkle free skin the overall health of the individual, a holistic model, is considered within the treatment.

Defining a Beauty Goal

Defining the goal helps you gather information that will enlighten you when determining what the client really is looking for as an end result of treatment. You need to know what beauty looks like to the client, especially how they describe their own appearance and its relationship to their ideal of beauty. This knowledge will guide you to a more precise identification of the skin conditions that will be the focus of treatment. A well developed goal and definition of beauty also help to clearly identify a realistic outcome. Your client may have a unique definition of beauty, tied into anticipated results that may be impossible to achieve. What constitutes a realistic outcome depends on the client's desires, what she or he expects from you regarding attractive results, and what you can accomplish using your experience and trust in the chosen treatment methods.

DEFINING BEAUTY

Defining beauty is an elusive endeavor. It may be defined by individual experience or cultural influence. Definitions of beauty are often expressed through the words of poets, prophets, and philosophers, whose descriptions often include beauty's effect on us emotionally, physically, and spiritually. Recent studies and research offer scientific definitions by explaining beauty in terms of symmetry [7] and function.

The response to beauty is both biologically driven and triggered by cultural and social programming. In creating a definition and goal for beauty, you may find it helpful to understand the biological aspect of beauty along with the learned patterns associated with it.

For Your Information

The Definition of Beauty

beauty (byoo'te) *n.* 1. The quality of objects, sounds, ideas, etc., that pleases and gratifies as by their harmony, pattern, excellence or truth. 2. One who or that which is beautiful, esp. a woman.

–Funk & Wagnall's Standard Desk Dictionary

The Reproductive Nature of Beauty

The response to beauty is deep seated and has its roots in biologic evolution. The sense, or awareness, of beauty is a mysterious program embedded well below logic and intellect. It plays an obvious role in reproduction, where beauty and the attractiveness of fitness are barometers of reproductive health. Beauty, as in the vibrant coloring of the male peacock's feathers, shows that the potential mate has a strong immune system and healthy genetic material. The beauty of a healthy display of feathers says to the potential mate that this peacock will produce the strongest offspring. Beauty's function, from a biological perspective, is to stimulate reproduction and enhance the endurance of future generations. But for modern humans, beauty seems to signify much more than reproductive fitness.

A Pre-Programmed Beauty Ideal

Humans judge and analyze faces and find common dislikes in features such as a nose that appears crooked, lips that are too thin, and ears that are too large or too small. Too large, too small, and too thin compared to what? Where do we come up with the model or ideal whereby we judge beauty? Dr. Nancy Etcoff, in her book *Survival of the Prettiest,* examines this question along with scientific evidence linking biological standards to a beautiful face.[8]

A biological standard of beauty is supported by Dr. Stephen Marquardt, a former plastic surgeon, who says that beauty is a mechanism to ensure that humans recognize and are attracted to other humans. He says, "The most beautiful faces are the ones that are the most easily recognizable as human. Beauty is really just humanness." Dr. Marquardt used a formula to create a beauty mask based on the Golden Ratio, the mathematical number Phi(1.6183399…). The mask fit fairly well when placed over the faces of several famous beauties. He says, "The mask radiates, it advertises and screams: 'human, human, human'."[9] We discern whether a face is obviously human by unconsciously comparing it to an ideal face that lurks in the unreachable recesses of the psyche.

An accumulation of evidence points to a biological ideal of beauty. Still, one is challenged to find two people who agree on the beauty of a certain face. This difference in opinions about beauty may be influenced by learned and cultural beauty criteria. Humans may override a biological pre-programmed ideal of beauty in favor of an individual or cultural preference. This tendency adds to the complexity of defining beauty and makes it necessary to create beauty goals that incorporate your client's individual preferences.

DEFINING BEAUTY AS HEALTH AND VITALITY

Extreme beauty is not the norm, and very few faces fit perfectly into Dr. Marquardt's beauty mask. In reaching a personal definition of beauty, using biological parameters as a guide, rather than the "ideal" beauty presented by fashion magazines and Hollywood films, may be more reasonable. Ultra-thin, anorexic models who starve themselves into a Twiggy-like body shape are rarely healthy and, therefore, are not as biologically attractive.[10] A healthy body and a vital appearance override beauty ideals[11] created by the media.

VICTIM CONSCIOUSNESS

Social, emotional, and scientific explanations of beauty abound. The final individual definitions, goals, and concerns for beauty are left to the individual. Avoid the belief that we are victims of bad genes that give us big noses, hopeless thighs, or whatever else the mirror (or the mind) has portrayed all these years. Social conditions, fashion, the media, and cosmetic advertising heavily influence our perceptions of beauty and contribute to a victim consciousness. Simply, or not so simply, accept what can and cannot be changed. Assist your client (or yourself) in becoming armed with a realistic goal, a definition, and a beauty program that coincides with the amount of time, money and the motivation one is willing to invest. Defining a clear beauty goal, and understanding the effort involved in achieving the goal, are the first steps in creating a successful holistic beauty program.

EXPECTED OUTCOME

Many times, especially in the use of essential oils and other natural therapies, the expected outcome may not be immediately accomplished, even though healing has occurred. A common experience when treating acneic skin using a detoxifying herbal is that the treatment initially causes more flare-ups. Detoxifying impurities from the skin is a healing treatment that may cause more eruptions during the initial cleansing of impurities from within the tissue, a process that helps to prevent acne from reoccurring. If the request for treatment was to "make my acne go away," this initial stage could result in misunderstanding between client and clinician. The treatment does not make the acneic condition go away immediately and initially makes it worse. The therapist knows that to clear the skin, impurities must be extracted. Partial extraction is accomplished within the treatment. Removing debris that is trapped deeper in the follicle or tissue requires a process that happens gradually and naturally, with the support of detoxifying herbs, oils, or other skin preparations. This example demonstrates the importance of clearly defining a goal and outcome. If the goal is to "make my acne go away," and the result is immediate flare-ups, the client will interpret the treatment as a failure. If the goal states that to clear the skin, a healing or detoxifying phase is required, then no misunderstanding can arise between client and clinician. Acne is caused by clogged pores, inflammation, and bacterial infection. The goal for the clinician, after mechanical extraction, is to detoxify the skin and treat the origin of the problem in hopes of not only eliminating the acneic condition but also preventing reoccurrence and alleviating the cause of the condition. If this is the defined goal and final outcome, the client will consider treatment successful, despite initial flare-ups following the treatment.

Using Skill and Experience to Define the Outcome

Your skills and expertise will help guide you to create realistic and well defined goals. These goals will help you achieve mutually satisfying treatment results with your clients. You will learn through further study of aromatherapy how to create realistic beauty goals, using the predictable healing properties and the application techniques of essential oils.

AUTHOR'S **NOTE**

BEAUTY AS A GOAL

In practice, I chose to focus on hair. I was a highly regarded hair therapist, commonly known as a hairdresser. (Because I come from Boston, I would be further defined as a "hai'ehdressah.") I had the passion and knowledge for skin care, but not the desire to practice full time as an esthetician. I also had a zeal for study in holistic health, physiology, alternative healing, herbology, and nutrition. This knowledge extended into a personal and professional philosophy that pieced together aspects of quantum physics, Taoism, other Eastern and Earth philosophies, and tidbits of New Age spiri-tual self-help. I rounded off this philosophy with the practices of meditation, yoga, and good old Americanized fitness training. My truest obsession and pursuit became essential oils.

For me, being a hair therapist was not only the skill of artfully framing the face or of producing statements of individuality and fashion. Hair was part of a total holistic beauty protocol. Because of my extended interests and holistic outlook, the discussions I had with my clients eventually contained very little talk about hairstyles. If this were a business book, I would have to augment it with a section on how to sell services without actually talking about them. The scope of my client conversations, which were my consultations, was wide ranging. I wanted to know as much as I could about them. Mostly, I wanted to know who they were, not who they thought they were. It was also important to know what they were made of, physically, from the food they ate, and emotionally, the feelings that result from lifestyles, beliefs, and philosophies. The stories that portray similarities between hairdressers and psychiatrists contain more than a grain of truth. It's amazing what people will discuss with you when they feel comfortable in the casual setting of a spa or salon. This openness often involved a great display of trust from the client, which I accepted with respect and appreciation.

Using my experience and training, I often offered recommendations for skin treatments. This advice would include diet, supplements, and lifestyle suggestions. These recommendations were based on health or emotional issues that were unveiled during our discussions. Essential oils were my primary remedy for almost everything. And right there, following a side-angled, wispy-banged bob, I would concoct a blend of essential oils and offer it to my client. My aromatherapy treatments almost always focused on health issues. The goal was to alleviate aggravation and stress-related sleepless nights or develop a formula that relieved digestive spasm. Such goals are not typical, coming from the same guy that just added some gel to give the crown a bit more lift.

On the client's next visit, I would inquire how the treatment worked. All too often, the response would be, "not well." When I asked how often my blend was used, the typical response was, "I kept forgetting to use it." I don't find it at all unusual that essential oils can be particularly ineffective when they're not being used!

I think I've developed enough flavor to get to the point of this story: the beauty goal. I was a seasoned beauty therapist and had long studied holistic healing. Though both were in my repertoire, and it appeared that I was practicing both simultaneously, I was not presenting the two together and maintained a separation between beauty and health. Following my reading of Nancy Etcoff's *Survival of the Prettiest*, I had my great "Aha!" moment: Beauty and health are synonymous. From then on, when I blended my oils for a health condition I believed my client would gain both beauty and health from, I introduced it with a redefined goal. I offered the essential oil blends to my clients with a new goal by saying, "This will make you more beautiful." Amazingly, the formula would be used almost every time, and with positive results in both their beauty and their health.

WHY CLIENTS SEEK BEAUTY TREATMENT

Noting why a client seeks beauty treatment is important. This information guides the clinician in selecting products and techniques. Relevant information derived from a holistic client consultation, explored in Chapter 12, is used to address the social, lifestyle situations or emotional motivation that may affect skin conditions and thus must be attended to as a part of the treatment.

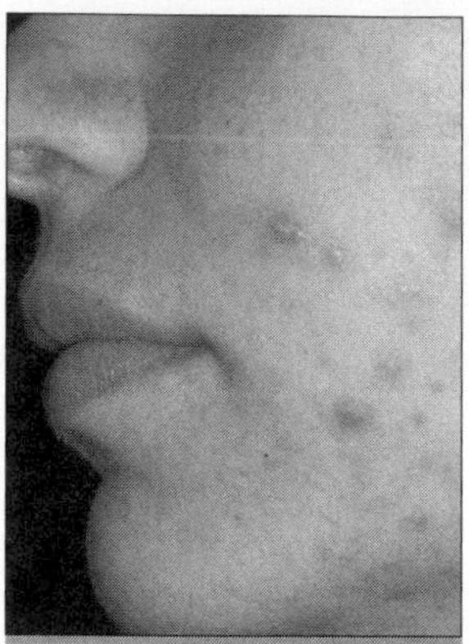

Figure 1-4 Emotional stress often results in stressed or irritated skin.

The Role of Emotions

Emotional motivation may be a key factor in selecting an appropriate and effective treatment. Beauty has a historic connection to self-esteem. A client's self-image and self-esteem have a direct effect on their emotions, which, in turn, affect the condition of the skin and the overall beauty of the person. Your practice and licensing likely does not include psychiatric or psychological evaluation and treatment. That means that emotional motivation, self-esteem, and self-image, considered to be in the realm of psychology, are not within your treatment protocol. But the skin is! To successfully treat the skin, psychological issues cannot, and must not, be avoided. Those who are licensed for psychological evaluation have a powerful tool at their disposal in analyzing and treating emotionally charged skin ailments. For those without proper credentials, nothing specific can be recommended for diagnosing the emotional aspect of skin care and beauty. In a holistic treatment, emotional issues relating to the skin are addressed according to your expertise as part of a complete beauty program. Through your aromatherapy studies, you will achieve the ability to select essential oils that address emotional issues. See Figure 1-4 to see the effect that stress has on the skin.

BECOMING A HOLISTIC PRACTITIONER

This entire text is based on the methods incorporated in holistic health and beauty. As you proceed through this book, you'll develop your own role as a holistic practitioner. Your holistic function and acceptance in the workplace depends on your field of practice, employers, coworkers, government regulations, and clientele. Your confidence level is also a key factor in how you will proceed as a holistic beauty practitioner. Table 1-1 defines the holistic practitioner and client.

THE ROLE OF THE HOLISTIC PRACTITIONER

Treating holistically requires understanding, training, and study of the treatment methods and philosophy underlying whole-body therapy and skin care. As a holistic practitioner, your role is to develop holistic skills. These skills

Table 1-1 Defining The Holistic Practitioner and Client
The Holistic Practitioner
• Keeps the responsibility of health and healing with the client.
• Is fully informed in the many areas that affect health and beauty, including diet and nutrition, emotional issues, exercise, lifestyle, medical concerns, environment, and allergies.
• Treats the whole person, not just the symptoms.
• Educates, informs, and makes relevant suggestions for beauty and health.
• Uses the least invasive and most effective techniques and tools available and continues to seek these out for clinical use.
• Is compassionate and supportive.
• Keeps appropriate professional and personal boundaries within the client relationship.
• Is professional and ethical at all times.
• Follows all of the guidelines of their profession including government licensing and regulations.
The Holistic Client
• Maintains full responsibility for their health and beauty.
• Attempts to understand the many aspects of holistic health through reading and personal research.
• Asks questions regarding any treatments or product recommendations given by a practitioner.
• Is aware of all the issues that affect health and beauty, especially those that are affecting their own health and beauty, as diagnosed by an appropriately qualified practitioner.
• Is active and involved in any treatments.
• Understands that health, healing, and beauty are processes, and that no "quick fixes" or "magic bullets" exist.
• Understands what to expect from the professional they have chosen.

complement your clinical qualifications gained through your training, licensing, abilities, and confidence. The training you receive in this text will cover skills that relate to essential oil use. Be careful not to recommend any treatments or make any suggestions that may violate government licensing or regulatory requirements (see Chapter 13). Through training and use of holistic aromatherapy, you will be capable of fulfilling the role of a holistic practitioner.

Self Responsibility

In holistic healing, the practitioner takes on the role of a team player. A vital characteristic of this role is handing responsibility for the treatment over to the client. Often, especially in the traditional medical setting, the client gives full responsibility for healing to the practitioner. The expectation is to receive a "cure" in the form of a pill, topical ointment, surgery, or service that will clear the condition without any effort on the part of the client.

As a team player, the holistic practitioner gives professional advice and treatment. Unlike the all too common professional/client relationship, in which professionals are the experts, and their opinion should go unquestioned, this role allows clients to add their requirements, needs, and knowledge to the treatment protocol. This role is self-empowering for the client. Healing potential is increased when the client is no longer an ostensibly helpless victim of his or her own condition. The practitioner is still responsible for expert opinion, proper diagnosis, treatment services, and product or take-home treatment recommendations. The client is responsible for self-treatment, as recommended by the practitioner. The client is also responsible for eating a healthful diet, proper nutritional supplementation, good lifestyle habits, regular exercise, and emotional stability. These aspects are all elements of self-responsibility and self-care. Table 1-2 outlines the roles of the holistic practitioner and client.

Support As Therapy

Support and encouragement are elements provided by the holistic practitioner. Providing them does not require any special licensing or training, and there are no government regulations to worry about. This is a skill that occurs naturally and is effective in gaining positive healing results. Support and encouragement work within any holistic practice, along with clear intention, thoughtfulness, and a positive attitude, as functional healing tools. Investigate some of the books available regarding the science of healing touch, distance healing,

Table 1-2 Roles of the Holistic Practitioner and Client

The Holistic Practitioner is responsible for:
• expert opinion
• proper diagnosis (dependent upon qualifications and licensing)
• treatment services (dependent upon qualifications and licensing)
• product and home-treatment recommendations
The Holistic Client is responsible for:
• responsibility of self-care
• healthy diet and nutrition
• healthy lifestyle
• regular exercise
• emotional health

and quantum healing to better understand the effects of consciousness (thought)- and energy-focused healing therapies. Intention acts as a guide and becomes the attitude by which you work. If your intentions are supportive of the client, and supportive of the established beauty goal, you are adding an element that contributes more than can be perceived. A negative attitude or unsupportive practitioner/client relationship can have an equally negative effect on the beauty result. For a positive outcome, the client must be self-supportive by having a positive perception of the chosen treatment and be in confident agreement with it. This requirement includes a favorable perception of you, the practitioner.

AROMATHERAPY FOR HOLISTIC BEAUTY AND SKIN CARE

Essential oils are holistic by nature. One essential oil may provide properties that address many biological functions and physical health issues. When essential oils are combined in aromatherapy blends, their holistic effects become wide-ranging. This expansion was demonstrated in the sample formula for eczema, in which a combination of essential oils is used holistically to treat many causes of this disorder. Used topically, whole plant substances, such as essential oils, influence other

For Your Information

Mechanical Manipulation and Isolated Chemical Treatments

It is important to understand how isolated chemical treatments, such as alpha hydroxy acids (AHAs) used in chemical peels and Botox, and mechanical manipulations including laser, plastic surgery, and microdermabrasion, fit into the context of this text and holistic beauty therapy. Mechanical and chemical treatments are quick-fix therapies that encourage a "magic bullet" or "cure" mentality for both the client and the practitioner. Though these kinds of treatments have their successes, effectiveness, and appropriate places in beauty care, they are not tools of holistic therapy as defined here. Mechanical and chemical treatments are one-dimensional and symptom-focused tools, unlike the multidimensional, causal-focus therapies required by holistic health and beauty care. Such treatments are aggressive and may damage tissue, causing inflammation and free radical damage to the cells. Such invasive treatments contradict the principle of using the least invasive treatments in holistic therapy.

These types of treatments do not encourage client responsibility or self-care and tend to make the client dependent upon the practitioner, rather than sharing in the treatment.

body systems as well as the skin. Topical application of the essential oil of Cape chamomile (*Eriocephalus punctulatus*) soothes and reduces an inflamed skin condition. It will also reduce irritation and activation of nerve pathways and alleviate emotional stresses that may be the direct cause of the inflamed skin condition.

HOLISTIC BEAUTY PROGRAM

By now, you understand that a holistic beauty treatment is one that incorporates total body health, emotional balance, mental health, and a healthy lifestyle.[12] This regimen includes self-treatment and personal responsibility for well-being and control over the health and healing process. A fully developed holistic beauty program is one that understands the importance of healthy aging or healthy regeneration of cells in the body.[13] This is not an anti-aging concept. Healthy aging begins at birth.[14] From this time on, cells are in a constant

AUTHOR'S **NOTE**

HOLISTIC EVALUATION IS NOT ALWAYS EASY

In 2005, I gave a presentation on the holistic treatment of difficult skin disorders. The talk addressed such conditions as psoriasis, atopic dermatitis, and acne, conditions that are often difficult when trying to pinpoint the direct cause. In this talk I introduced full spectrum methods using essential oils and botanicals that would best address these kinds of skin conditions and included holistic formulations containing a very wide spectrum of activity. The idea was to develop formulations that would address hidden, unknown causes of difficult skin conditions.

A woman came up to me following my talk to ask if I had any recommendations for a skin rash that had been present on her leg for the past year. She is a naturopathic doctor, so she was very knowledgeable about holism and the use of alternative therapies. I recommended a product and asked if she would call me to let me know how successful this recommendation was. She later emailed me to let me know that the product had alleviated the symptoms temporarily, but not permanently. I interviewed her and also asked her to send me detailed information regarding all the results from any tests she had had and any other treatments she had tried. I then sent her an aromatherapy blend designed according to the information she provided. Again, the results were minor and temporary.

My response (and hers) to this frustrating situation is that we were not aware of the true cause of her skin rash. It seemed parasitic, but tests did not detect any microorganisms in the infected area. I could have continued to try essential oil formulations one after another, which may have eventually addressed the origin of the rash.

When working in this manner, one need not allow ego to enter. I didn't have to feel that I had failed or that essential oils aren't the effective treatment I believe them to be. A precise holistic diagnosis, as with any medical diagnosis, is sometimes very difficult to find. The true cause can remain hidden, as was the case here, and the condition marches onward no matter what you do.

Almost six months later, the naturopathic doctor emailed me again. She wanted me to know that she recently visited her dentist who told her she had a low-level gum infection that may have been present, but undetected, for over a year. Following treatment for this infection, her rash disappeared. The rash had obviously been a remote effect of the gum infection.

I tell this story for two reasons. The first is to help you to fully understand the holistic balance that occurs in the body. The skin can be affected by the most unsuspected and seemingly unrelated causes. The second reason is that the cause of a skin condition can remain hidden and continue no matter how intensive the holistic consultation may be or how effective you believe your holistic full-spectrum treatment to be. I accept this reality and continue to do the best I can when presented with these challenges.

process of regeneration. The goal is to protect cells from damage and supply them with the vitamins and nutrients necessary for healthy regeneration. Damage to cells at an early age begins a process that may develop into disease at later stages of development. Sun damage in your teens may manifest into wrinkles, loss of elasticity, or melanoma at age 40. The concept underlying holistic, healthy aging is to protect and maintain cell health, which results in beauty.[15] By removing obstacles to healthy cell regeneration, such as free radical damage and inflammation, and by providing the cells with essential nutrients through whole foods and supplements, one enables the body to repair itself and continue to form and reform healthy cells. In a holistic framework, healthy cells are the beginnings of a healthy body, a healthy mind, and healthy skin that result in overall beauty.

The holistic beauty and healthy aging program within this text includes essential oils in conjunction with other methods of holistic therapy. Essential oils work holistically to treat and correct imbalances. Their antioxidant and anti-inflammatory properties provide protection to the cells. Protection is enhanced by the antibacterial, antifungal, and antiviral properties of essential oils. The benefits of essential oil use are directly affected by the total health, or ill health, of the body. This interconnection is the reason that our holistic beauty program includes the following as areas of concern for healthy aging and beauty:[16]

- diet
- supplementation
- emotional balance
- lifestyle
- exercise
- a natural skin and body care regimen
- environmental concerns

All of these concerns involve self-treatment and individual responsibility along with professional advice, guidance, and clinical services. The holistic beauty and healthy aging concept is also guided by psychology, philosophy, biology, sociology, physics, and advanced scientific study and theory.[17]

In this program, we will incorporate the wholeness found in botanical and other naturally derived ingredients and will limit the use of one-dimensional synthetic chemicals. A practice and philosophy of holism incorporated into cosmetic skin care formulation and ingredient selection is considered best for a whole body skin therapy program. Aromatherapy products used in a holistic program are formulated using essential oils in conjunction with other whole plant and natural substances to create a blend of healing properties that address many symptomatic causes of skin problems. This blend results in a more complete and effective treatment than is generally possible through most commercial products. Each chapter of this book builds upon these concepts of using essential oils to promote holistic beauty and healthy aging in concert with other holistic therapies used for the purposes of health and beauty.

CHAPTER SUMMARY

Beauty is directly linked to the health of the individual. For a person to achieve beauty, the whole body must be in a condition of health. Skin disorders, or other physical conditions that may compromise beauty, are a sign of disease or systemic imbalance. To establish a complete and effective beauty program, it is wise to incorporate the philosophy and practice of holistic health. Holistic health treats the whole person, not just a symptom, such as a skin disorder. Holistic beauty is the term used to describe the practice of beauty through holistic health. Essential oils, because of their naturally holistic function, are ideal for treating the skin in a holistic beauty program.

The clinician takes on the role of a holistic practitioner. This role takes into consideration all aspects of health and beauty including diet, emotions, lifestyle, and the environment when selecting essential oils to develop beauty treatments for clients. To incorporate holistic beauty treatments into your practice, creating well defined beauty goals is important. Doing so helps to identify a shared outcome between practitioner and client and can also identify possible causes of skin disorders.

REVIEW QUESTIONS

1. What is holistic health and holistic beauty?
2. Why are essential oils considered a holistic therapy?
3. What is a holistic beauty goal?
4. Why is a well defined goal helpful in selecting methods of treatment?
5. What is the role of a holistic practitioner?
6. What areas of health and well-being affect the skin and beauty?

CHAPTER REFERENCES

1. Etcoff, N. (1999). *Survival of the Prettiest*. New York: Anchor Books.
2. National Institute of Arthritis and Musculoskeletal and Skin Diseases. (1999). *Handout on Health: Atopic Dermatitis*. Washington, DC: National Institutes of Health.
3. Perricone, N. (2002). *The Perricone Prescription*. New York: Harper Collins.
4. Yehuda, S., Rabinovitz, S. & Mostofsky, D. I. (2005). "Mixture of essential fatty acids lowers test anxiety." *Nutritional Neuroscience 8* (4); 265–267.
5. Denda, M., Tsuchiya, T., Elias, P. M. & Feingold, K. R. (2000). "Stress alters cutaneous barrier homeostasis." *American Journal of Physiology – Regulatory, Integrative and Comparative Physiology 278* (2); R367–R372.
6. Harrison, J. (2005). *Foundations of Aromatherapy*. Bellevue, WA: Phytotherapy Institute.
7. Etcoff, N. (1999). *Survival of the Prettiest*. New York: Anchor Books.
8. Etcoff, N. (1999). *Survival of the Prettiest*. New York: Anchor Books.
9. Discovery Communications. (2005). *Human Face*. Accessed on July 27, 2007 at http://tlc.discovery.com.
10. Berger, G. (2004). *The Lure of Beauty*. Accessed on July 27, 2007 at http:// www.nyu.edu.
11. Harrison, J. (2001). *The Essentials for Beauty and Skin*. Bellevue, WA: Phytotherapy Institute.
12. Harrison, J. (2004). *Global Healthy Aging*. Bellevue, WA: Phytotherapy Institute.
13. Harrison, J. (2005). *Foundations of Aromatherapy*. Bellevue, WA: Phytotherapy Institute.
14. Harrison, J. (2006). *OHA Bio-Active Skin Care*. Bellevue, WA: Phytotherapy Institute.
15. Harrison, J. (2004). *Global Healthy Aging*. Bellevue, WA: Phytotherapy Institute.
16. Harrison, J. (2004). *Global Healthy Aging*. Bellevue, WA: Phytotherapy Institute.
17. Harrison, J. (2004). *Global Healthy Aging*. Bellevue, WA: Phytotherapy Institute.

Essential Oils and Aromatherapy

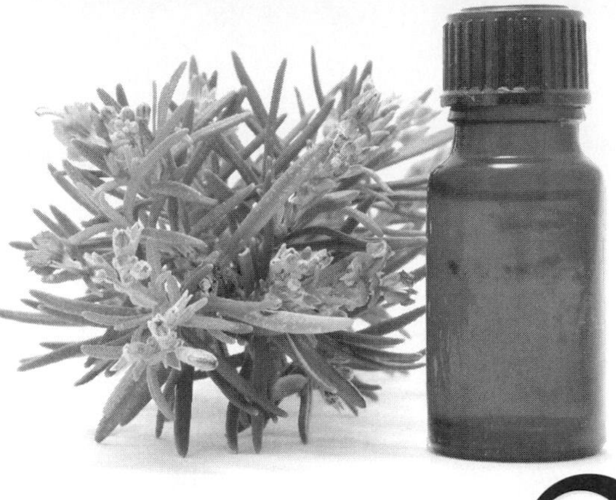

CHAPTER 2

Call it psychosomatic, but they do make us feel better...

– Robert Tissrand

LEARNING OBJECTIVES

1. Define essential oils according to the ISO specifications.
2. Define and describe the practice of aromatherapy.
3. Recount a brief history of aromatics and the people who shaped modern aromatherapy.
4. Describe the place of essential oils in spa and clinical environments.

AROMATHERAPY

Aromatherapy is the art and science of using essential oils derived from plants, flowers, fruits, seeds, and woods for the health and wellness of the body, mind, and spirit. Aromatherapy does not have a standardized definition. This fact has led many practitioners to use the term "essential oil therapy" when describing their use of essential oils for health and healing. For our purposes we will use the terms aromatherapy, therapeutic aromatherapy, and essential oil therapy to describe a therapeutic practice that uses essential oils as defined by the International Organization for Standardization (ISO).

ESSENTIAL OILS

The International Organization for Standardization defines an **essential oil** as a product made by **distillation** with either water or steam, or by mechanical process of citrus rinds, or by dry distillation of natural materials.[1] Dry distillation, utilizing heat without water or steam, is a method used primarily for fragrance compounds extracted from fossil amber or fragrant woods when a burned or toasted odor is desired. Following water and/or steam distillation, the essential oil is physically separated from the water phase.

COMPARING AROMATHERAPY MARKETING AND PRACTICE

To develop a foundation of knowledge about essential oils (EOs), it is important to understand the differences between pure therapeutic EOs and the substances marketed as "essential oils" that are found in most perfumes, shampoos, and massage oils (Figure 2-1).

To establish your practice of essential oil use, you must make a clear distinction between therapeutic use of essential oils in aromatherapy practice and the term "aromatherapy" as it is commonly used for marketing purposes. Aromatherapy marketing colors the perceptions of essential oil use. Through the study of essential oils, you will be capable of separating the fact from the fiction and marketing from the truth.

Defining Essential Oils

The distinction between therapeutic aromatherapy and aromatherapy marketing begins with a clear definition of essential oils. The only materials that are accepted by the aromatherapy community for therapeutic use are those that meet ISO standards as defined in the ISO Vocabulary of Raw Materials. Because there are no legal standards in place, any fragrant material can be called an essential oil, whether or not it has been produced through distillation or mechanical processing of fruit rinds. Since the beginning of the twentieth century, commercial fragrance houses have spent millions of dollars developing synthetic fragrance compounds. These compounds, which over the years have replaced naturally derived fragrances, are the main components in today's perfumes, processed foods, household goods and, now, aromatherapy products. This circumstance is most unfortunate, and one of your roles as an aromatherapist will be to identify synthetic versus natural fragrances as well as to educate your clients of this situation.

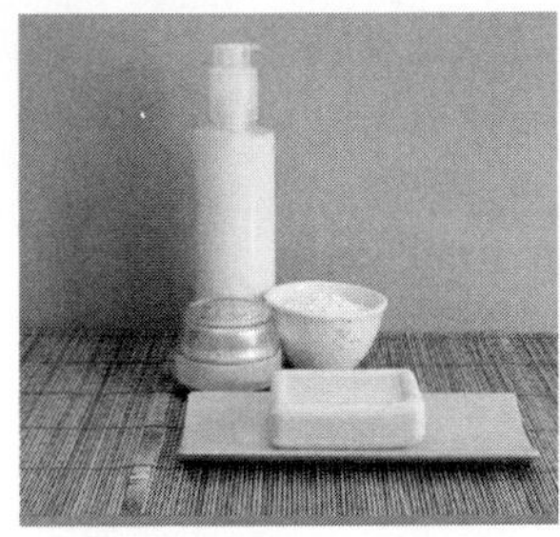

Figure 2-1 It is difficult to know which of these products contain the true essential oils used in aromatherapy or if they are synthetically fragranced, using the word aromatherapy for marketing purposes.

The Plant Essence

Before the oil is distilled, the substance within the plant is called the **essence.** The essence is an oily substance contained within pockets or cells of the plant. The essential oil is an easily evaporated, or **volatile,** portion of the plant essence. If the essence is not extracted through distillation or mechanically processing the rind (Table 2-1), it is not called an essential oil. By definition the term essential oil is used only to describe those essences extracted according to the guidelines set by the ISO. This does not diminish the use of essences extracted by other means as you will see in Chapter 4.

Table 2-1

Essential oils are products extracted from natural materials by:
• water, steam, or dry distillation
• mechanical process of fruit rind

WHAT IS ESSENTIAL OIL THERAPY?

A **therapy** is healing and curative treatment intended to remedy a disorder or undesirable condition. Aromatherapy is the use of aromas, specifically those in essential oils, for a therapeutic goal. This practice implies that essential oils have healing and curative properties. The use of essential oils in aromatherapy provides effective treatment for many physical and emotional illnesses as well as imbalances. Table 2-2 lists therapeutic uses of essential oils, ordered from most to least effective. Scientific documentation that includes clinical studies and **empirical evidence** (documentation derived from direct experience or observation) is used to identify these therapeutic results.

Essential oils are most effective against bacterial, viral, and fungal infections: They can restore balance to the autonomic nervous system and central nervous system and affect conditions of stress, depression, and anxiety. The oils have been used extensively, with great success, in the treatment of **civilization diseases:** ills that result from lifestyle or from a poor relationship with the environment, such as cancers, asthma, and autoimmune diseases. Essential oils also have a profound healing benefit for the skin and are used to heal wounds, regenerate skin cells, and strengthen skin tissue.

BEGINNINGS OF AROMATHERAPY

Aromatherapy is often portrayed as having a long history of use through ancient civilizations. Although this is true,

Table 2-2 Therapeutic Uses of Essential Oils
• infections: viral, bacterial, fungal
• regeneration of skin cells and wound healing
• immune system support
• nervous system imbalance
• emotional and psychological issues
• hormonal imbalance
• auto-immune disorders

the use of essential oils as practiced today is markedly different from ancient use and has a relatively recent history. A review of both the ancient and recent history of aromatherapy is useful to provide a framework for its natural ability to heal human beings, its safety, and its scientific validity.

The Historic Use of Aromatic Plants

Aromatic plants are those that contain a fragrance or aroma. Most plants have some aroma radiating from the essence contained within them. Through time, humans have discovered and learned about the healing properties and aromatic uses of plants (Figure 2-2). Aromatic and healing plants have a rich history that is well documented in many ancient texts, including the Chinese *Yellow Emperor Book of Internal Medicine* and The Bible. Evidence, such as herbal remedies found in a 60,000-year-old Neanderthal burial site, demonstrates a natural human tendency toward using plants for healing.[2] The history of using plants for their aromatic qualities includes medicines, rituals, aphrodisiacs, environmental fragrances, mummification, and perfuming. The essential oil use of today is based on the history of our relationship with aromatic plants, validated by modern, scientific research and clinical practice.

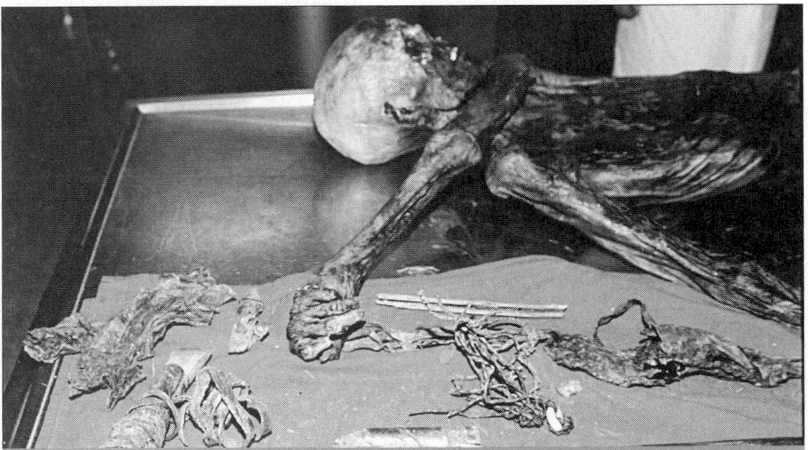

Figure 2-2 The "Iceman," a 5,300 year old prehistoric body discovered frozen in the Italian Alps in 1991. Mushrooms containing agaric acid, an oily substance toxic to bacteria and intestinal parasites, were found on autopsy. It is believed he used mushrooms to treat a parasitic digestive infection.[3]

To understand modern aromatherapy, it is useful to review the evolution of aromatic plant use. What has been mistakenly called the History of Aromatherapy in many books is actually a history of the use of aromatic and medicinal plants. The aromatics used by the Greeks, Egyptians, and Romans were not essential oils. These aromatics and medicines were unguents, resins, incenses, teas, macerations, decoctions, infusions, and other preparations. The first description of the distillation process didn't appear until around the first century A.D., though evidence exists that some sort of distillation process had been used as early as 3,000 B.C. Even so, distilled essential oils were rare until the advent of perfumery in the 16th century. Common use of essential oils did not begin until much later, at the start of the twentieth century. Until the 1900s, aromatics, as described in the mainstream aromatherapy literature, and later essential oils, were predominantly available only to royalty, alchemists, scholars, perfumers, and scientists.

Traditional Knowledge to Modern Aromatherapy

Intuitive and traditional knowledge of plants and aromatics, often called **folk medicine,** has been passed down from generations of use. This history is important to understand the development of modern aromatherapy and today's use of essential oils. The traditional knowledge, along with further perfection and artistry of essential oil distillation and perfumery, created the foundation on which modern aromatherapy stands.

From Folk Medicine to Chemistry

During the Middle Ages, perfumers and others whose work involved the use of essential oils and aromatics were known to survive the plague because of the antiseptic properties of the oils. This success propelled awareness that essential oils had potential therapeutic and antimicrobial activity. Since the Middle Ages, several texts have been written about the therapeutic use of herbs, such as Joseph Miller's *Herbal* (1722), William Whitla's *Materia Medica* (1882), and Joseph E. Meyer's *The Herbalist* (1918), all of which include a few descriptions of essences.

MODERN AROMATHERAPY

At the end of the 19th century, chemists and scientists began to research the antiseptic properties of essential oils. In 1928, the science of chemistry gave birth to aromatherapy by way of a perfume chemist, René-Maurice Gattefossé.

The "Father" of Modern Aromatherapy

René-Maurice Gattefossé coined the term "aromatherapy" in 1928. His personal experience with the healing power of essential oils has become aromatic legend. Gattefossé was a perfume chemist working in the family business. He, along with other scientists, had an established interest in the medicinal qualities and properties of essential oils. He had acquired a collection of papers, theses, and observations gathered since 1907. His interest blossomed after he burned his hand in a small explosion in his lab. The story is that he dipped his hand in a vat of pure lavender oil. The lavender relieved the pain, and the burn healed very quickly, with no infection and no scarring. This experience triggered further research into properties of essential oils.

Gattefossé first used the term aromatherapy when he wrote "Dermatological therapy would, thus, develop into 'Aromatherapy,' or a therapy employing aromatics in a sphere of research opening enormous vistas to those who have started exploring it."[4] His book, *Aromathérapie: Les Huiles essentielles hormones végétales,* was the first study of essential oils to explore their use as medicines. Gattefossé's approach was scientific and based upon specific chemical properties of the oils. Gattefossé acknowledged the individual chemical properties of EOs and expressed the importance of using the whole oil to achieve the healing results found in clinical research.

The Branching of Modern Aromatherapy

Many people assisted in the early and current development of aromatherapy. This text focuses on those who have had the most influence on modern aromatherapy. Admittedly, this is a simplified history, and the people mentioned here are those who have had the most popular influence.

Gattefossé represents the birth of modern aromatherapy. Following in his footsteps were Dr. Jean Valnet, who expanded the medicinal use of essential oils and brought it to the attention of European doctors, and Marguerite Maury, a biochemist responsible for introducing essential oils used in topical application and massage. The work of Valnet and Maury helped to develop two distinctly different methods of essential oil use, creating two schools of practice. Maury expanded her work in England and influenced what is now considered "British aromatherapy" while Valnet led the development of "French aromatherapy."

British and French Aromatherapy

British aromatherapy is known for topical application of essential oils, primarily used in massage, and is considered the more cautious approach, in which large amounts, undiluted use, and internal use are discouraged. French aromatherapy, or *aromamedicine,* incorporates massage and topical use but differs from the British school in its internal and undiluted use, and higher dosages. The French method may at times resemble the pharmaceutical approach of Western **allopathic medicine** practice. Allopathic medicine is a system of treating a disease by producing a reaction that is antagonistic to the disease and is the system used by most Western educated physicians.[5]

The style and philosophy of essential oil use cannot be so easily divided into French and British. Intentions and beliefs of aromatherapy practice vary through the mixing and blending of the two schools and also incorporating Chinese, Ayurvedic, anthroposophic or other medical, spiritual, and scientific methods of practice and thought. Aromatherapy practitioners, no matter which school of thought they study, eventually develop their own unique manner of practice. Understanding that the British and the French approaches differ is helpful, but not necessary to become expert in essential oil use. The road to expert use is a complete scientific and holistic study that discounts the propaganda of any "school."

People Who Helped to Define Modern Aromatherapy

René Maurice Gattefossé, a perfume chemist in France, coined the word aromatherapy in 1928. He was the first to explore the chemical composition of essential oils in relation to their therapeutic properties. Aromatherapy, as a scientific practice, originated with the publication of his book *Aromathérapie* in 1937.

Dr. Jean Valnet used essential oils as a doctor during the Indo-China war and wrote the landmark book *Aromatherapy: The Treatment of Illness With the Essence of Plants* in 1964. As a result, the medicinal use of essential oils was accepted as a medical practice in France, though it was not widely used and remained little known outside of Europe.

Robert Tisserand translated Valnet's book, *The Practice of Aromatherapy,* into English in 1976. In 1977 he published his own book, *The Art of Aromatherapy.* He is largely responsible for the popularity of modern aromatherapy.

Pierre Franchomme is a leader in essential oil research. He introduced the Structure-Effect diagram used to measure the electromagnetic frequency and polarity of aromatic molecules. In 1990 he cowrote, with Dr. Daniel Pénoël, *L 'Aromathérapie Exactement,* considered *the* medical aromatherapy text. Pierre Franchomme assisted in formulating the *Origins* line for Estee Lauder and has produced valuable essential oil data as a research scientist for that company. His research into the effects of essential oils at the cellular level continues to advance the practice of aromatherapy.

Paul Belaiche did extensive laboratory and clinical studies that document the effectiveness of essential oils against microorganisms. The result is the *aromatogram,* a testing system that enabled him to examine the effectiveness of essential oils against specific microorganisms. Belaiche is the author of a three-volume set, *Traité de Phytothérapie et d'Aromathérapie,* which describes the basic aspects of treatment with essential oils. His work represents thousands of tests and clinical cases used to investigate the effectiveness of essential oils in treating a wide range of conditions.

Dr. Daniel Pénoël has been using essential oils in his practice since the mid-1970s. His clinical research and documentation has created a valuable path of advancement in the medical and clinical uses of aromatherapy. His clinical studies and treatments are documented in *L'Aromathérapie Exactement.*

Dr. Kurt Schnaubelt is a chemist who continues to legitimize the medicinal value and everyday use of essential oils. He has established the importance of a scientific and molecular understanding of essential oils, while at the same time acknowledging the holistic nature of the oils. Dr. Schnaubelt has expanded the development of his aromatherapy concepts based on biology, traditional Chinese medicine, and an astute evaluation of the evolution of essential oils. His concepts are presented through his school, the Pacific Institute of Aromatherapy, and his books *Advanced Aromatherapy, Medical Aromatherapy,* and the *PIA Masters* series.

Jane Buckle, Ph.D., author of *Clinical Aromatherapy: Essential Oils in Practice,* is an advocate of essential oil use in nursing and medical settings. Her efforts have brought aromatherapy into mainstream hospital settings.

Progress in Modern Aromatherapy

The use of essential oils has continued to expand since the time of Gattefossé. Today aromatherapy is well known, though widely misunderstood outside of the ranks of those who practice and study it. Anything—from a candle with synthetic aroma to academic studies of **isoprenoids** (the main chemical structure of essential oil compounds)—is called "aromatherapy." Professional organizations, aromatherapy practitioners, and producers of essential oils have attempted to create industry standards. Unfortunately, marketing practices and goals of profit often derail the progress of aromatherapy as a true, well defined, healing practice.

Many scientific and clinical researchers continue to extend the therapeutic knowledge of essential oils. Several international aromatherapy conferences also assist in moving the use and scientific knowledge of essential oils forward. Aromatherapy is expected to evolve and expand into a well-respected holistic therapy for use both in clinical situations and for personal use by the layperson. This is an exciting and challenging time to be involved with essential oils and aromatherapy.

THE PRACTICE OF AROMATHERAPY IN CLINICAL AND PERSONAL HEALTH CARE

For the past few decades, aromatherapy has been used primarily by massage therapists and aromatherapists. Others who have incorporated essential oils into practice are naturopathic doctors, a variety of alternative practitioners, estheticians, and spa therapists. The nursing community, with the support

AUTHOR'S **NOTE**

ON THE CREST OF A WAVE

I was sitting in my first aromatherapy class reading through the handout. There was an article titled, *On the Crest of a Wave.* The article discussed how students of aromatherapy, once introduced to the discipline, become obsessed with essential oils. That was the moment I realized, "This may be the thing for me; I'm pretty good at obsessions." The article continued to describe aromatherapy as a blossoming field, the ultimate healing tool, the rising star of alternative medicine, the next big thing! And it said that, as students of aromatherapy, we were riding the crest of this wave. I felt this. I was excited, I was motivated, and I intuitively sensed the importance and the potential impact contained within the use of essential oils. I was ready to ride that wave.

It's been more than twenty years since that class. Aromatherapy is still cresting; the wave builds, but never quite breaks. The aromatherapy industry is growing, thanks to advances and extended research, important discoveries, and an increase in the availability and variety of therapeutic essential oils. Yet aromatherapy still hovers around the perimeter of serious alternative medicine.

In some ways this marginal presence is an expression of the power of aromatherapy. Its simplicity allows it to be presented as feel-good bath salts and gift shop items. It becomes difficult for us to accept that the same essential oil used as an air freshener contains compounds that have tumor reducing properties, demonstrated in academic studies. Herbs, homeopathy, and other botanical and alternative therapies appear much more serious in their context. They would give the ditzy New Age sit-com blonde much too much intellectual prowess, unlike the simple-minded effect of a punch line using aromatherapy. Wouldn't Phoebe on Friends appear far too smart, and not nearly as funny, if she was concocting herbal tinctures instead of sniffing lavender? How intelligent does the "hippie-chick" Meat is Murder volunteer, Experience, appear as she lights a candle, explaining "it's geranium" for her nerves, as she and her cohort run from killer sheep in the 2006 movie Black Sheep? The intricacies of herbal preparations or the needling in acupuncture are far too difficult to work into a

Continued

quick one-liner. The simple, no-brainer sniff of aromatherapy is easily utilized to develop humorous dim-witted situations. It then becomes a challenge to accept aromatherapy as a valid healing science, or intellectual study, within these media portrayals.

The beauty of aromatherapy is its simplicity. Its true magnificence is in the hidden complexity and potential of the essential oils. It seems, however, that only those who ride the crest of the wave see this point.

The wave builds. It continues to grow wider, higher, and stronger. I don't feel that a moment will come when the wave breaks, like a tsunami flooding the plains of alternative health. I don't anticipate a sudden impact from essential oil use. Aromatherapy, in a subtle and nurturing way, will infiltrate the soil and infuse into the health of the world through its roots. It will become ever-present, used for simple functions but creating deeper, holistic effects. As a student of aromatherapy, you are now riding an ever-cresting wave.

of Jane Buckle, Ph.D., has recently been expanding the use of essential oils in the hospital setting. This development has been slow because of the insurance and financial issues of the medical mainstream.

Estheticians and spa therapists are in place to have the most impact with essential oil use. This is not to say that other therapists recommending essential oils don't also have an important role. The unique quality of skin care is that it is something familiar to, and used by, most people. People are accustomed to applying, and generally are already using, skin and body care preparations. Essential oils can be added to skin care formulas for holistic therapeutic purposes without having the user change or add anything new, such as taking capsules or massaging a lotion, to their daily ritual. Therapeutic aromatherapy can be applied without prescription and thus does not step over boundaries created by insurance coverage and legal practice issues.

CHAPTER SUMMARY

A foundation for your practice is developed with clear definitions of essential oils and aromatherapy. The history of aromatherapy is often confused with the history of ancient use of aromatic plants. Though these plants, and the products made from them, were not essential oils, they were still the first step in the development and history of modern aromatherapy. The advent of modern aromatherapy is marked by the work of perfume chemist René-Maurice Gattefossé, who coined the word *aromatherapy.* Many influential people made contributions in developing early and current aromatherapy. For the past few decades, aromatherapy has been used primarily by massage therapists and practicing aromatherapists.

REVIEW QUESTIONS

1. Define essential oils.
2. Define aromatherapy.
3. How would you describe essential oil therapy?
4. How did the historical use of aromatic plants influence the modern use of essential oils?
5. Who is the "father" of modern aromatherapy?
6. Where is the practice of aromatherapy heading in the clinical setting?

CHAPTER REFERENCES

1. Technical committee 54, ISO Standards. (1997). Vocabulary of Aromatic *Natural Raw Materials* (ISO/DIS 9235:1997). Geneva, Switzerland: The International Organization for Standardization.
2. Challem, J. (2000). "Why Herbs Work." *The Nutrition Reporter.* Accessed on July 25, 2007 at http://www.thenutritionreporter.com.
3. Johnston, B. A. (1999). "Iceman's Medicine Kit." *Herbalgram 46*; 17. Austin, TX: American Botanical Council.
4. Gattefossé, R-M. (1937). *Aromathérapie: Les Huiles essentielles hormones végétales.* Paris, France: Librairie des Sciences Girardot.
5. Venes, D. (ed.) (1997). *Tabor's Cyclopedic Medical Dictionary* (18th edition). Philadelphia, PA: F. A. Davis Company.

The Olfactory System and Essential Oil Effects on Emotions

CHAPTER 3

We think we smell with our noses, [but] this is a little like saying that we hear with our ear lobes.

– Gordon Shepard, professor of neuroscience, Yale University

LEARNING OBJECTIVES

1. Recount the important relationship between the olfactory system and daily human life.
2. Describe the physiology and functions of olfaction (sense of smell).
3. Discover how essential oils affect emotions, memory, and hormone release.
4. Explain how human behavior is affected by scents and fragrances.
5. Learn important psycho-aromatherapy essential oil protocols that address human emotions, such as nervousness or lack of calmness.

INHALING ESSENTIAL OILS

Essential oils can have a profound effect on emotions and memory. By inhaling the aromas emitted by essential oils, the emotions may be calmed, soothed, or uplifted. Their effects on the **autonomic nervous system** can be influential and may restore the body to a balanced state.[1]

How can an inhaled substance have a therapeutic effect? Having a basic knowledge of the structure and function of the olfactory system is important to understand how the "scent" of essential oils works, especially in relation to their effect on emotions.

THE OLFACTORY SYSTEM AND THE SENSE OF SMELL

The sense of smell is a subtle sense, and its importance is largely underestimated. Its influence on human behavior generally goes unrecognized, as each of us responds to olfactory stimulation throughout our daily lives. Even now, there is a scent that is affecting your mood and behavior. Your memory is triggered, and your sense of ease or discomfort is manipulated, by the sense of smell and the odor molecules in your environment.

Smell, and taste, evolved from the phenomenon of **chemotaxis**, the first sense mechanism of single-celled organisms. Chemotaxis is the ability of cells to sense and move (taxis) toward or away from chemicals (chemo) in the environment. Think about how this same activity of moving toward or away from a smell, a response caused by a chemical that activates our olfactory nerves, is a function within our daily lives. Just like early humans, we rely on the sense of smell for survival. It warns of dangers such as fire or poisons in the air, to which we respond by moving away from the odor. It was, and still is, a key sense in mating and reproduction. The fragrance of attraction is just that: we are attracted by scent and therefore move toward a potential mate. The sense of smell was of primary use to our human ancestors and still is with other animals, to track food, medicines, and water. Using the sense of smell for attraction, aversion, eating, and drinking remains a function of modern humans, though within our modern culture we have become more visually dominant and less dependent on smell.

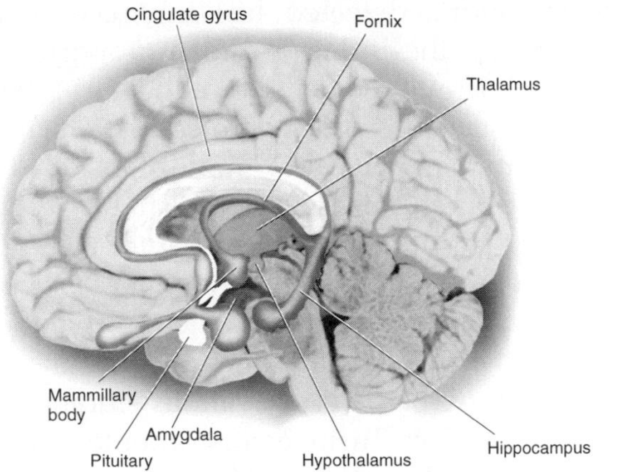

Figure 3-1 The limbic system of the brain

The Limbic System

Olfaction is one of the earliest distance senses, seeing and hearing would be our other distance senses, to arise in evolution and interacts with one of the most primitive parts of the human brain, the **limbic system**. The limbic system is within the midbrain, or limbic brain, just above the brain stem. The limbic system is often referred to as the "emotional brain," because it is the seat of the emotions and memory (Figure 3-1).

The system comprises the hypothalamus, thalamus, amygdala, and hippocampus. Through the limbic system, smell has powerful affect on human emotion and memory and plays an important role in identification and communication. It also influences the **endocrine system,** a network of glands that secrete hormones into blood or lymph, and the autonomic motor systems. The effects of olfaction are wide ranging because of its interaction with the **hypothalamus.** The hypothalamus is known to play a predominant role in the production and release of hormone-like substances that control hunger, thirst, body temperature, and other body functions related to **homeostasis** (physiological equilibrium).

How We Smell What We Smell

The sense of smell is fully developed at birth. Babies are born with the ability to detect the scent of their mothers and identify the smell of breast milk.[2] The exact mechanism for processing

For Your Information

Anosmia

Anosmia, loss of the sense of smell, is a devastating disease that demonstrates the importance of olfaction. People with anosmia lack a quality of life supplied by the sense of smell. They may experience anxiety, loss of appetite, and libido. Many dangers also accompany anosmia, such as not being able to detect smoke or rotten food.

odor, the way odor is detected, has only recently become understood. The hypothesis that has been supported by scientific academia and perfume chemists since the mid 1900s was based on the shape or structure of odor molecules. The nerve endings were believed to react with odor molecules in a lock-and-key fashion. According to this theory, the shape of the odor molecule (the "key"), as it fits into the receptor cell (the "lock") of the olfactory nerve, triggers perception of a particular odor, related to the signal sent by the molecule through the nerve ending. The shape theory has been challenged by an alternate odor detection hypothesis based on vibration. Vibration was studied and promoted by Luca Turin, as documented in the book *The Emperor of Scent*. His hypothesis states that smell is determined by frequency of the electromagnetic vibration of the odor molecule.[3] In 2004, Richard Axel and Linda B. Buck were voted Nobel Laureates in Physiology and Medicine for their studies clarifying the workings of the olfactory system.[4] They discovered a large family of odor receptor genes related to odorants, receptor cells, and the response to specific odorants. Mysteries still abound when it comes to the way we detect odors.

Smell detection, identifying and recognizing odors, is an area of study that is quite different from that of the therapeutic response to essential oils through inhalation. For aromatherapy purposes, it is not important *why* we detect odor, although shape, vibration, and genes must certainly play a role in the trigger mechanisms sent to the brain. It is important, though, to understand that essential oil molecules attach to olfactory nerve endings. To understand the therapeutic effects created by inhaling essential oils, we need to go deeper than the detection mechanisms. Other responses to smell are triggered with the use of essential oils that do not involve the ability to detect odor. People with **anosmia**, an inability to detect odor, still respond to the effects of essential oils, though this response may be caused by absorption of the molecules into the blood stream rather than an olfactory response.[5]

PHYSIOLOGY OF THE OLFACTORY SYSTEM AND LIMBIC SYSTEM

The sense of smell begins in the **epithelium**, a mucous layered area at the top of the nostrils, containing approximately 10 million olfactory nerve endings, called **odor receptor neurons**

(ORN). Unlike other neuronal cells of the human nervous system, the olfactory neurons regenerate and replace dead neurons every 60 days. In the epithelium, odor molecules are transferred to the ORN. The nerve impulses are amplified by the olfactory bulb, the section of the olfactory system that receives the signals from the ORN, and relays them to the limbic system, the hypothalamus, and the endocrine system. From here, a complex series of interactions occurs, giving the overall effects of the sense of smell, including physical and emotional responses.

AROMACOLOGY AND THE STUDY OF FRAGRANCE'S EFFECTS ON EMOTIONS AND BEHAVIOR

In 1982, the Olfactory Research Fund began a scientific study of smell, named **aromacology**. Aromacology primarily investigates the emotional and behavioral effects of odors. Aromacology has provided research into the effects of all odors, including those of essential oils. It has also provided insight into understanding the ability of essential oils to provoke emotional and behavioral outcomes. In creating a clear definition of aromatherapy, you should draw a distinction between these two areas of study. Aromacology is the study of the emotional and behavioral response to *all* odors. Aromatherapy, which may include aspects of aromacology, is limited to the therapeutic effects of essential oils.

For Your Information

Olfactory Activation in the Brain

The parts of the brain that are activated by olfaction in electroencephalographic (EEG) studies are the orbitofrontal and primary olfactory cortices, the cingulate gyrus, lateral temporal cortex, cerebellum, and the parietal and occipital lobes.[6]

AUTHOR'S **NOTE**

RECONNECTING WITH THE SENSE OF SMELL

Early in my aromatherapy practice, I was talking with a potential client about the wonders of essential oils. He gave me one of those doubting looks as I was explaining the calming effects of the oils. I can almost guarantee as you pursue aromatherapy that this look will be passed your way when speaking with hard core non-believers in botanical medicine. In a tone that people use when confronted with a subject they find to contain elements of absurdity, this man said to me, "How can anything you smell make you feel anything?"

Continued

This is a question that is saturated with a high level of disconnect. It only takes a moment of thought to realize how we are constantly altered by our sense of smell. This question demonstrates a disconnect from nature and the effects that a fragrant floral garden or a pine-scented forest have on your mood. Far too many people have this disconnect between their own biological functions and the moods that develop from their senses. How cranky do you get when the constant slam of a jackhammer persistently assaults your eardrums? Does sitting on a slimy slip of mildew-coated plastic make you feel comfortable and relaxed? The influence of smell is not always as obvious, though you may notice that the stench of a garage truck on a hot humid day does readjust your outlook on life, at least for the moment.

This wasn't the first time I had been confronted with doubt. I generally try to dislodge doubt with simple explanations of the olfactory system and examples of how we are powerfully affected by the sense of smell. The standard example of the connection between smell and memory is recalling a time when you were instantly brought back to your grandmother's house when the scent of a pie was in the air. This chapter contains slices of olfactory fact that can be used to explain how a scent can make you feel something.

Some people have a hard time understanding that a smell is a solid physical substance that causes a physical reaction in the body. The odor of an object comes from molecules emitted by the object. These molecules attach to the olfactory nerve. When you smell something, you are actually in contact with a piece of the object. I will sometimes punctuate this statement to a doubting audience by pointing out that the odor emanating from a sewage leak is actually a piece of this sewage stuck to the top of the nasal passage. This may not be a subtle example, but it can be very effective.

MEMORY, EMOTION, AND BEHAVIOR

The limbic system has either direct or short links with systems in the brain and with parts of the endocrine system. Within the limbic region, odors stimulate the release of **neuropeptides,** which are messenger molecules that distribute information throughout an organism. Peptides include **hormones** and **neurotransmitters** such as **serotonin,** an important hormone related to depression, and **endorphins,** chemicals that reduce pain and stimulate sexual arousal.

The odor message is analyzed by the **hippocampus** and **amygdala.** These are the brain's memory and emotional response centers. Recall a time when an odor created an instant and very vivid childhood memory. This connection happens because every memory has an odor association stored within the hippocampus and amygdala. During the act of smelling, the olfactory system activates odor-related emotions, memory, and behaviors.[7] This response bypasses the intellectual centers of the brain. You don't have the capacity to "think" about this memory and emotional response. Boom, there it is, a memory movie with a real emotion tied to it starts playing, without you being able to pre-analyze it or stop it.

Getting Tricky With Memory and Emotion

The memory and emotional response that occurs in the limbic system can create a tricky aspect to working with essential oils. The memory and emotional response is so genuine that an essential oil can trigger a very profound emotion that can be positive or discomforting. If the essential oil is related to a negative stored memory and emotion, the result may be anxiety, emotional discomfort, or even a rash.[8] It is possible, and more common, for the essential oil (or any odor molecule) to trigger only an emotion. If no memory response is present, detecting the emotional relationship of the odor is quite difficult. Detecting a negative feeling triggered by an odor is much easier if the odor also triggers a memory. It would not be surprising to hear someone say the fragrance of a rose makes him or her feel depressed because the memory association is of a dying grandmother who was last visited in a room filled with the flowers. Some people love the smell of gasoline because of the memory of family outings. These are examples of a recognized memory connected to the emotional response to the odor.

If you are working with essential oils when an emotional response occurs without a conscious memory, recognizing emotional variations may be difficult. You will need to be aware of emotional response to odor when presenting oils to a client. Positive results or responses are always accepted with ease. A negative reaction is cause for greater concern. Negative issues are individual and must be documented to avoid repeating them. The situation becomes very tricky when reaction to the scent results in a rash. You must question whether the response is a true physical, allergic response or an emotionally triggered response. This reaction may occur with an essential oil that has always produced only positive results. Physical emotional reactions, such as a rash, are uncommon or at least not commonly related to an emotional trigger. Most negative memory and emotional reactions are subtle or create a simple "I don't like that smell" reaction. You will become more proficient with essential oils by maintaining an attentive awareness of relationship between scent, emotions, and memory.

AUTHOR'S **NOTE**

ANXIETY FROM A ROSE?

I was hired by an aromatherapy company to present products to a spa. In my presentation, I told this story as an example of memory association and essential oils. I made this story up as an effective, though unlikely, example of the power of scent on memory and emotion.

The story depicts a person who, as a child, was often beaten with a stick by the mother who happened to wear real rose oil at the time of the beatings. Years later, as an adult, the person would react negatively when confronted with the fragrance of real rose. The smell of rose triggered the emotions of anxiety and fear associated with being beaten with a stick, but not the actual childhood memory of being beaten. Because the person did not remember the beatings, the anxiety caused by the scent of rose had no clear association and appeared to occur without any cause.

This story, though it is a good example of the scent-emotion connection, borders on absurdity. Rose is an oil of love and compassion, not anger. To me, it would be absurd to think that anyone wearing real rose oil could beat her child with a stick. I presented this anecdote as an extreme example of hidden and unanticipated olfactory effects that may occur with essential oil use, such as the unanticipated anxiety associated in this story to rose oil.

Many of the formulas I presented for the aromatherapy company contained rose oil. In one spa, there was a woman who would stand up and leave the room when anything containing rose approached her. This response went beyond a typical dislike of the rose odor, in which she would have simply refused the offered sniff of the product. She had an obvious anxiety that was attached to the fragrance of rose. I don't believe that this woman was beaten with a stick by a mother wearing rose oil. I stand by my association of rose with compassion and assume that this is an improbable scenario. What I do propose is that an anxiety related situation had occurred in this woman's life that was associated with the scent of rose, which later triggered anxiety whenever she smelled it.

The woman did not relate a memory association and only demonstrated the emotional discomfort of being within odor detection of rose. She didn't even recognize her unusual behavior toward the rose products, although she did express her dislike of rose oil. As I have said, her behavior was on the radical side of simply disliking an odor. We are often unaware of our actions that result from the effects of fragrance on emotions. If stress or anxiety had caused a rash in this woman, it may have been translated as an allergic reaction to rose essential oil.

Paying Attention to Scent

What if, without any awareness or connection to an odor trigger, a sudden unexpected emotion occurs? We make a connection between odor and emotion only when we are consciously aware of an odor and can acknowledge our response at the same time and attribute it to the odor. We don't often pay attention to emotion and smell simultaneously. A casual sniff of lavender in the market doesn't necessarily coincide with awareness that an emotional memory is being released. We don't really notice that the smell also relaxes us and releases tension in our muscles, or that the smell of a pesticide nearby causes an alert stance and a desire to avoid the odor. In aromatherapy, we are often asked to pay attention to how we "feel" while smelling the oil. It is a different awareness and takes some practice. What if the response is a negative emotion, when a positive response is anticipated? Smelling rose should be a euphoric experience. If a negative emotion is stored within the amygdala and hippocampus, rose can trigger anxiety or fear. This area of smell-awareness will change the way you respond to your olfactory environment and work with aromatherapy-related products and services.

Avoiding Manipulation by Odor

What does paying attention to "feeling" odors mean in your everyday life? If an emotional response is not predicted, so what? By understanding the emotional and memory effects of odor, one can guard oneself from being manipulated by emotional olfactory responses. Pay attention to random, uncomfortable feelings or bouts of anxiety that seem to arise for an unknown reason. Certain odor molecules within the atmosphere that are associated with the negative emotion may be the cause of the feelings. When working with essential oils, be aware of the feelings triggered by odor/memory association and how these feelings may influence the body and mind. The common viewpoint is that essential oils, because of their botanical origin, create positive feelings that link to memories of being in nature, at the park or in a flower garden.

However, odors are often used to manipulate consumerism. Popcorn emanating throughout the movie theatre or the fragrance filling a shoe store, which has been researched for its ability to increase sales, are just a couple of ways consumers are manipulated through their sense of smell to spend money.

THE SCENT OF ATTRACTION

Through the hypothalamus, smell effects eroticism and sexuality, including swelling of the genitalia and orgasm. The sexual and hormonal olfactory response of the hypothalamus and pituitary glands is called the "naso-genital alliance."[9] Fragrance has powerful links to sexuality. This fact has developed into a multi-billion dollar perfume industry that creates fragrances designed for attraction and aphrodisiac effects. Even in our visually dominant approach to mating, smell often overrides visual attraction. Imagine someone walking into a room, who you find visually appealing and sexually alluring. Their visual presentation may trigger sexual responses in your body. If this person steps into your smell space emitting an aromatic haze of rotting garbage, what do you think will happen to your physical responses to their visual image? They'll most likely be shut down, and the attraction will be replaced by aversion. The smell doesn't have to be as overpowering as rotting garbage for this response to occur. Odor may control attraction and aversion in very subtle, almost undetectable ways. Think of this situation in reverse. A person whom you find attractive, but not overwhelmingly so, steps into your smell space—and you suddenly feel Cupid's arrow pierce your heart. "Love at first sight" may very well be "Love at first smell!" Humans emit an individual odor, which is a result of genetics, immunity, diet, lifestyle, and health. This personalized odor, which may also include attractor hormones, strongly influences attraction and aversion.

Have you ever had a passionate relationship that was difficult emotionally or was socially incompatible? Have you been in a relationship that fit your emotional and lifestyle needs, though something just didn't "smell" right? These opposing examples illustrate how our limbic system can be at odds with our frontal lobe; that is, how our primitive responses can oppose our modern intellect and desires, our thinking responses.

Scent Attractors in Essential Oils

Many compounds found in essential oils are similar to odor molecules that are erogenous or anti-erogenous.[10] The oils that contain these compounds are generally considered aphrodisiacs and are useful to enhance romantic, euphoric, and sensual situations. Aphrodisiac oils include rose, frankincense, ylang-ylang, and the extracted essences of jasmine and tuberose.

The Perfect Scent for the Perfect Mate

The olfactory response relating to attraction is complex and not fully understood. Scent obviously plays an important biological role, with deep evolutionary roots in human sexual relationships and mating. The olfactory response has been linked to healthy reproduction.[13] Smell may be directly related to selecting a mate best suited for producing strong offspring. One's odor profile provides a scent map that leads to mate selection based on diversity of immunity and genetics. This diversity, along with odor detection of disease, leads to stronger offspring that have immunity acquired from both parents. This basis for attraction gives "love at first smell" a function in reproductive behavior. Studies have shown that smell, and its relationship to compatible genetics and immunity, may play a role in fertility issues. In one study, Swiss

For Your Information

Pheromones

The response to **pheromones**, the attractor hormones of insects and animals, is not connected with the human olfactory response to odor. There is an organ just behind the opening of the nose on the septum of humans, the **vomeronasal organ (VNO)**, whose function is mysterious but is thought to be the detection mechanism for pheromones.[11] Animals use the VNO to detect minute chemical compounds, to communicate subtley with members of the same species, to smell prey, and to detect pheromones.[12] Whether humans detect pheromones using the VNO is still uncertain.

For Your Information

The Scent of a Man's Man

Scientists at the Karolinska Institute in Stockholm, Sweden, discovered that gay men responded to the odor of male sweat in a way similar to the response of women.[14] When heterosexual men smelled EST (an estrogen derivative), it triggered activity in the hypothalamus, the area of the limbic system involved in sexual behavior. Heterosexual women and gay men, however, showed this activity when they smelled AND (a testosterone compound). A similar study by this same team of researchers demonstrated the reaction of lesbian women to estrogen-like steroid was identical to the response of EST in heterosexual men. These studies provide evidence that people are born, or are biologically prone, to be gay. It also demonstrates the extreme power of scent in sexual attraction.

researchers found that women on birth control were scent-attracted to men they normally would not have noticed and who were likely not genetically compatible. These couples experienced difficulty conceiving, which according to the research team "was not caused by infertility, but to an unfortunate combination of otherwise viable genes." This research demonstrates the importance of smell as a biological factor in reproductive relationships.

ESSENTIAL OILS AND EMOTIONS

Psycho-aromatherapy, a term coined by Robert Tisserand (see Chapter 2), refers to the use of essential oils to achieve and maintain emotional balance. Aromatherapy's popularity is largely based on the use of essential oils to calm and relax. This quality has become a selling point of many fragranced products, such as candles, that are sold as "aromatherapy." The ability of essential oils to reduce stress and depression is well documented. These findings are supported by clinical studies that analyze brain wave activity before and after inhaling essential oils. Electroencephalograms (EEGs), recordings of the electrical activity in the brain, have been used to demonstrate the effects of essential oils on brain waves. Essential oils such as lavender and rose have properties that increase alpha and theta brain wave activity. These brain waves relate to a calm, relaxed, meditative state. Beta and alpha waves are decreased after smelling rosemary or pepper. Both of these oils are known to increase mental alertness, which is related to the change of activity in the brain.[15]

Essential Oils and Neuropeptides

Relaxation is a function of aromatherapy that is valid and has been well researched.[16] For relaxation also, essential oils are linked to the limbic system and to release of neuropeptides, which affect the emotions. Aromatherapy literature and Internet sites often attribute the emotional effects of essential oils to their effects on serotonin and endorphins. You do not need to know which specific neuropeptides are being released with essential oil use, as long as you know that the calming and pain relieving oils influence serotonin, endorphin[17] and encephalin release in the body.

Endorphin Activity and Touch

Massage and touch therapy encourage endorphin activity. This response is an added benefit of the relaxing quality of an aromatherapy massage or facial. This combination is especially beneficial for pain-relief massage.

CREATING A NEW ODOR/MEMORY ASSOCIATION[18]

Essential oils can be used to alter memory and emotional response. This work is accomplished by directly changing a memory association or by introducing a new memory response to a particular odor. Doing so can be very beneficial for someone experiencing anxiety or anticipating a stressful situation. Spa therapy and facials provide an excellent environment for creating an effective relaxation and anti-stress odor/memory association.

The method used is as follows:

1. Select an essential oil or aromatherapy blend to use as the associated odor. An essential oil or a blend that triggers release of relaxing neuropeptide activity is most beneficial for anxiety and stress. Suggested oils include cardamom, cedarwood, clary sage, lavender, and ylang-ylang. Also select some more uncommon essential oils, such as Australian sandalwood, cape chamomile, rockrose, or St. John's wort. It is important that the oil or blend has a positive appeal to the user.
2. Use the oil *only* in a relaxing environment. This place or time can be a quiet meditation space or during a relaxing and quiet treatment, such as a massage or facial. The blend or single oil can be used as part of a service, such as massage, or as a meditative or room fragrance. The most effective approach is to make this oil the only blend or fragrance used. If other scented products such as cleanser or mask are used, the oil used to create the new

odor/memory association should be used at the end of the service, and ample relaxation time should follow.

3. Use the aromatherapy blend or oil in the relaxing environment exclusively for 2 to 3 weeks if used twice a week, or for 3 to 4 once-weekly sessions. Caution the person not to use the oil outside of this environment during this time. The purpose is to set the odor/memory association for this oil or blend with the relaxing environment.
4. Following the allotted period, the blend or single essential oil can be carried around and inhaled to recall the "feeling" of comfort established within the relaxing environment. This practice can be particularly useful at times of deep stress and in anxiety-producing situations.

ESSENTIAL OILS FOR PSYCHO-AROMATHERAPY

Essential oils may be easily used for their emotional balancing properties. Use Table 3-1 as a reference guide when selecting essential oils for use in psycho-aromatherapy.

Table 3-1 Emotional and Psychological Use of Essential Oils

Aphrodisiac
Used For: emotional coldness, shyness, impotence, frigidity; to enhance sexual pleasure.
Essential Oils: clary sage, hibiscus seed, jasmine, nutmeg, patchouli, rose, sandalwood, tuberose, ylang-ylang
Euphoric
Used For: depression, moodiness, lack of confidence.
Essential Oils: champaca (absolute), clary sage, jasmine, melissa, neroli, rose, tuberose
Sedative
Used For: anxiety, stress, hypertension, insomnia, anger, irritability.
Essential Oils: anise seed, cape chamomile, clary sage, bergamot, geranium, lavender, lemon verbena, melissa, mandarin, mandarin petitgrain, marjoram, neroli, orange, roman chamomile, rose, tarragon

Table 3-1 (continued)

Mental Stimulant
Used For: mental fatigue, concentration, poor memory.
Essential Oils: basil, peppermint, rosemary
Invigorating
Used For: fatigue, lethargy, immune deficiency, boredom.
Essential Oils: cedarwood, clove, cypress, fir, peppermint, pine, rosemary, spruce
Mood Regulating
Used For: anxiety with depression, mood swings, menstrual or menopausal imbalance.
Essential Oils: clary sage, geranium, lavender, roman chamomile, rose
Neurovegetative (Autonomic Nervous System) Regulating
Used For: high blood pressure, insomnia, "nervous stomach," migraine.
Essential Oils: angelica, anise seed, cedarwood, geranium, mandarin petitgrain, melissa, neroli, tarragon

CHAPTER SUMMARY

The sense of smell is a subtle sense, and its importance is largely underestimated. Its influence on human behavior generally goes unrecognized, even though each of us respond to olfactory stimulation throughout our daily lives. The limbic system, the oldest part of the brain, is triggered by olfaction, directly affecting our moods, regulatory systems, and sexuality. The interaction of odor with the hypothalamus plays a predominant role with substances that control hunger, thirst, body temperature, and other body functions. Essential oils are used in psycho-aromatherapy to help balance emotions and moods, invigorate the mind, and enhance sexual attraction.

REVIEW QUESTIONS

1. What influence does fragrance have on the mind?
2. What part of the brain is triggered by fragrance?

3. The limbic system has short or direct links to what system of the body?
4. What is the difference between aromacology and aromatherapy?
5. What effect does odor have on sexual attraction?
6. What is psycho-aromatherapy?

CHAPTER REFERENCES

1. Dayawansa, S., Umeno, K., Takakura, H., Tori, E., Tabuchi, E., Nagashima, Y., Oosu, H., Yada, Y., Suzuki, T., Ono, T., & Nishijo, H. (2003). "Autonomic responses during inhalation of natural fragrance of cedrol in humans." *Autonomic Neuroscience 108* (1–2); 79–86.
2. Children's Hospital Boston. (2005–2006). *Newborns: Senses*. Accessed on July 16, 2007 at http://www.childrenshospital.org.
3. Burns, C. (2002). *The Emperor of Scent*. New York, NY: Random House.
4. Press Release: The Nobel Prize in Physiology or Medicine. (October 4, 2004). Accessed on July 25, 2007 at http://nobelprize.org.
5. Snow, L.A., Hovanec, L., & Brandt, J. (2004). "A controlled trial of aromatherapy for agitation in nursing home patients with dementia." *Journal of Alternative and Complimentary Medicine 10* (3); 431–437.
6. Shiino, A., Morita, Y., Ito, R., Suzuki, M., Matsuda, M. & Handa, J. (1999). "Functional MRI of the human brain responses to olfactory stimulation." *No Shinekei Geka—Neurological Surgery 27* (12); 1105–1110.
7. Furlow, F.B. (1996). The Smell of Love. *Psychology Today*. Mar/Apr 1996. New York, NY: Sussex Publishers, LLC.
8. Harrison, J. (2005). *Reducing Stress with Aromatherapy*. Bellevue, WA: Phytotherapy Institute.
9. Stoddart, D.M. (1997). *Follow Your Nose*. Accessed on July 16, 2007 at http://partners.nytimes.com.
10. Schnaubelt, K. (1985). *The Aromatherapy Course*. San Rafael, CA: Pacific Institute of Aromatherapy.
11. Bernstein, J. (1999). *Sixth Sense: The Vemeronasal Organ*. Final Web Reports. Accessed on July 16, 2007 at http://serendip.brynmawr.edu.

12. Helmenstine, A.M. (2006). *Jacobson's Organ and the Sixth Sense*. Accessed on July 25, 2007 at http://chemistry.about.com.
13. Furlow, F.B. (1996)."The Smell of Love." *Psychology Today*.
14. Savic, I., et al. (2005). "Brain response to putative pheromones in homosexual men." *Proc Natl Acad Sci USA 17*; 102(20): 7356–7361.
15. Diego, M.A., Jones, N.A., Field, T., Hernandez-Reif, M., Schanberg, S., Kuhn, C., McAdam, V., Galamaga, R. & Galamaga, M. (1998). "Aromatherapy positively affects mood, EEG patterns of alertness and math computations." *International Journal of Neuroscience 96* (3–4); 217–224.
16. Shepard-Hanger, S. & Stokes, T. (1998). *Aromatherapy and Psychotherapy in Treatments of Behavior and Emotional Disorders*. 3rd Aromatherapy Conference: Science and Emotion. San Rafael, CA: Terra Linda Scent and Image.
17. Nie, H., Shen & Y.J. (2002). "Effect of essential oil of radix *Angelicae dahuricae* on beta-endorphin, ACTH, NO and proopiomelanocortin of pain model rats." *Zhongguo Zhong Yao Za Zhi 27* (9); 690–693.
18. Harrison, J. (2005). *Reducing Stress with Aromatherapy*. Bellevue, WA: Phytotherapy Institute.

Discovering Essential Oils

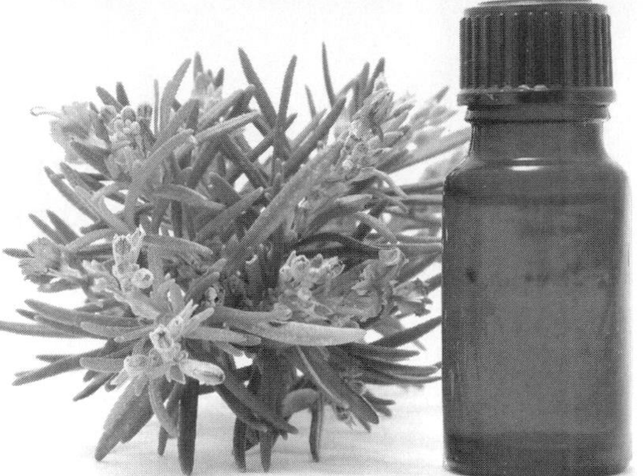

CHAPTER 4

Nature does nothing uselessly.
– Aristotle

LEARNING OBJECTIVES

1. Develop a deeper understanding of essential oils and of the quality necessary for aromatherapeutic purposes.
2. Learn about essential oil distillation and other methods of extracting the essence from a plant source.
3. Discover the importance of essential oil purity and authenticity.
4. Understand what adulterated essential oils are and why they should not be used in aromatherapy practice.
5. Acquire confidence in selecting essential oils for therapeutic function and quality.

ENSURING THAT ESSENTIAL OILS ARE ESSENTIAL OILS

To be successful in the art of aromatherapy, you must have a clear definition and understanding of the essential oils used for therapeutic purpose. To avoid complications and succeed with aromatherapy you have to be certain that the oils you are using are true aromatherapy-grade oils. You should also be able to recognize the many oils and fragrances that are synthetic or, if natural, have been altered from their original composition.

Many kinds of fragrant materials are bottled and sold as true essential oils. It is up to you to distinguish among synthetic or altered fragrances and the true essential oils that are appropriate for use in aromatherapy.

Growing Demand for True Essential Oils

Industrial customers, primarily those in the flavor and fragrance industries, have been the essential oil traders' main customers. These corporate buyers, being interested in the bottom line, attempt to drive prices below market value, making it impossible for producers to maintain a profit. The solution has been to stretch, by **adulteration,** the pure oils while maintaining the illusion of authenticity.[1] Adulteration is the practice of adding synthetics, isolated compounds that are common to the specific oil, or cheaper natural oils to the pure essential oil in order to lower the price. Adulteration is also done to produce a more "even" and consistent industrial fragrance. Adulterated essential oils have seeped into the aromatherapy market but are not of a quality that is suitable for aromatherapy purposes.

Since the mid 1970s, demand has been growing for essential oils used specifically for aromatherapy. The demand for quality essential oils has increased steadily. Currently, the global number of producers distilling "aromatherapy grade" essential oils is growing. This expansion is a good thing for the aromatherapist interested in finding oils suitable for therapeutic producing results.

Identifying True and Unadulterated Oils

Without standards or regulations regarding essential oil identity (see Chapter 2), the words "aromatherapy" and "essential oil" can be used as marketing terms to sell any product containing any fragrance compounds. This same lack of standards means that aromatherapy products and even single oils might contain adulterated essential oils or completely synthetic fragrance compounds. Because of these conditions, it becomes the responsibility of the individual practitioner to distinguish true therapeutic-quality essential oils from those oils produced mainly for flavor and fragrance. This duty is a challenge for even the most seasoned aromatherapist. The general rule to follow is "trust your supplier." Doing so is not a simple task. To generate this trust, you will need to develop a backbone of knowledge based on an understanding of essential oil production and quality. As always, experience will be your best guide in the search for quality essential oils. To help you develop and establish the skills and methods for purchasing therapeutic quality essential oils, this section reviews four categories of information:

- extraction methods
- quality of essential oils for therapeutic activity
- identifying the botanical plant source of the essential oil
- determining essential oil composition through GC/MS analysis and identifying adulteration

AUTHOR'S **NOTE**

HOW TO FIND THE RIGHT AND REAL ESSENTIAL OILS

When I began working with essential oils I, like everybody else, had difficulty judging their quality. I had doubts about the oils I was buying. My doubts were valid, because I now know that most of the oils I was buying were of an inferior grade, adulterated, and not even close to the quality I now purchase. At that time, it was much more difficult to find decent essential oils. I survived this stage of my aromatherapy life, and so did the people on whom I used the oils. I still use some of these oils: they make an ideal demonstration of poor quality oils in my classes.

My intention in constantly warning and cautioning about the abundance of poor oils and the many different ways you can be deceived or ripped off is to keep you aware and nudge you into finding those oils that are best for therapeutic

Continued

results. This persistence helps you, your clients, the reputable producers of quality oils, and the environment.

You may or you may not end up using questionable essential oils. As you develop a "nose" for quality oils, you will make good purchases and find reputable distributors of essential oils. The beginner is on the learning curve, so for now, just follow your nose.

EXTRACTING ESSENTIAL OILS

Essential oils are extracted from plants, seeds, fruits, wood, roots, bark, leaves, stems, peels, resins, and flowers. Several methods are used to extract the essence from the plant. Distillation and, in the case of citrus fruit peels, cold expression are the extraction methods used for those substances that the International Organization for Standardization (ISO) defines as essential oils (see Chapter 2).

Distillation

Distillation is a process that uses steam to extract the essence from plant materials. This text uses terms and basic descriptions of distillation that are common to aromatherapy and essential oils, leaving more accurate scientific terminology and descriptions of thermodynamics, chemistry, and the mechanics of distillation for your own research. The issues of most concern in producing a quality distilled essential oil are temperature, boiling points of the materials, pressure, and accurate timing of the distillation process. The art and skill of the producer, whether passed down from generations of practice or newly developed using scientific and high tech methods, will always be the determining factor in the quality of the oil produced. The developed and experienced aficionado has deep appreciation of an oil produced by a skilled distiller. The therapeutic activity required for aromatherapy purposes is present in essential oils distilled with care and artistic skill. See examples of stills used in distillation in Figures 4-1 and 4-2.

Three distillation methods are used to extract essential oils from plant material.

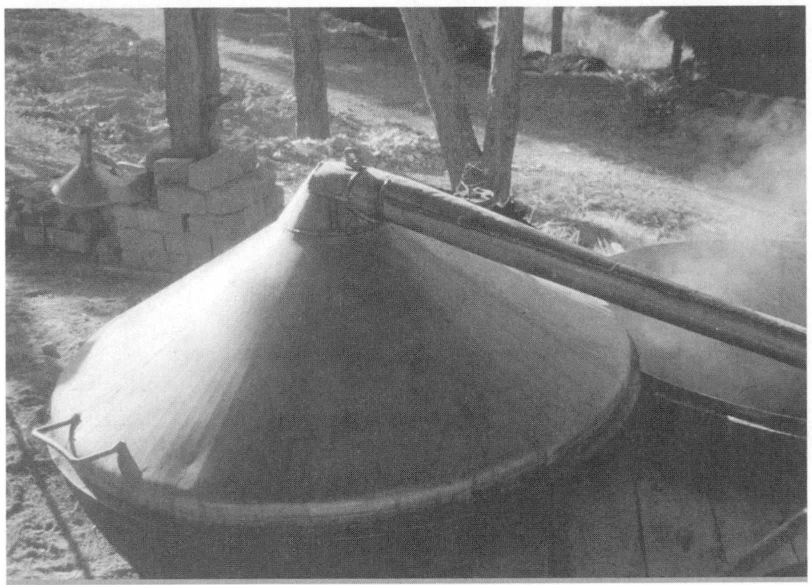

Figure 4-1 Distillation in Madagascar

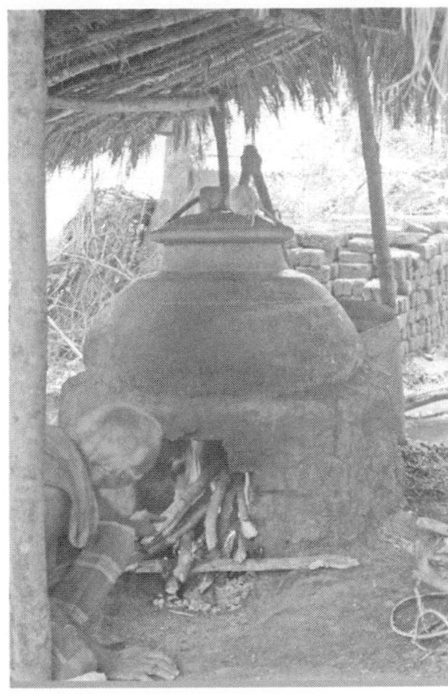

Figure 4-2 Traditional Indian distillation of golden champa

Steam Distillation: Dried plant material is placed on a grate inside a still. Steam is injected into the dry plant material. The essential oil is released from the plant and carried with the steam through a condensing tube. The now liquid combination of water and essential oil flows into a container. The oil naturally separates from the water. This method uses a very high temperature, which can compromise the essential oil components. Steam distilled oils are not the best for therapeutic use in aromatherapy.

Water/Steam Distillation: In this method, the plant material is placed in a still filled with heated water, unlike the dry container used for steam distillation. Steam is injected from a separate apparatus. Steam and oil follow the same pathway of condensation and separation as in steam distillation. A lower heat than that used for steam distillation makes this technique more suitable and most desirable for oils destined for therapeutic use.

Water Distillation: Plant material is placed in a still that is completely immersed in water. The water is heated, causing the oils to evaporate without the use of steam. This method is the most suitable for heat-sensitive oils. The lower temperature prevents the oil from decomposing and creates a finer grade, therapeutic essential oil. This process is also called **hydrodistillation.** See a still used for hydrodistillation in Figure 4-3.

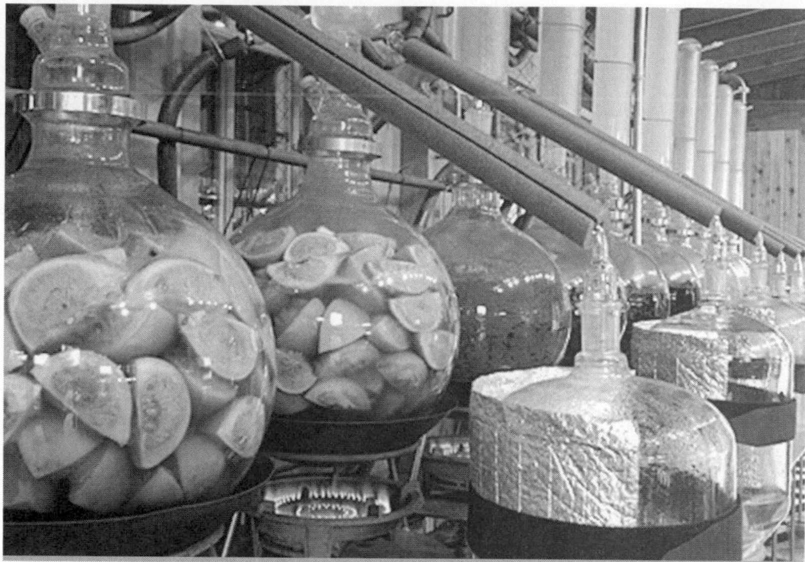

Figure 4-3 Alchemical hydro-distillation apparatus designed by Jack Chaitman of scents of knowing. Assisting the plants to release their soul into the oil using the ancient art form of alchemical distillation.

Hydrosols: By-Products of Essential Oil Distillation

At the end of the distillation process, where the water and oil have been condensed and become liquid, the essential oil is separated from the water and removed. The water remaining is considered a by-product of the distillation process. This by-product contains water soluble plant components along with some essential oil molecules. The by-product, called a **hydrosol** (also referred to as a **hydrolate**), is a therapeutic product with uses similar to those of the essential oils and also has properties unique to the hydrosol. Hydrosols can replace essential oils for a more subtle effect or when a less aggressive treatment is required. Hydrosols have beneficial properties and a therapeutic function in skin care and spa therapy.

Cold Expression

The process used to extract the essential oil from citrus peels is called **cold expression** or **scarification.** The peel is crushed, and the oil is extracted with **centrifugation,** a force created by spinning at high speeds. Organic citrus oils are best because of the potential pesticide contaminants that may be extracted from conventionally grown fruit. Pesticide residue is generally not carried over in steam or water distillation because of the density and higher boiling point of pesticide molecules, but they may easily be extracted with the oil during cold expression. The use of organic or wild plants is still preferred for both distilled and **cold pressed** oils.

Other Methods of Extracting the Essence from Plants

Some plants produce oil that is too delicate or not plentiful enough to be extracted using distillation.There is either not enough oil contained within the plant to be carried over in distillation or the distilled oil is destroyed by the heated process and no longer has a value as an essential oil. Other methods have been developed to extract these delicate essences from their plant source. Following is a list of alternate extraction methods. Keep in mind that these extracted essences are not technically considered essential oils.

Solvent extraction: Many of the finer floral oils, such as jasmine and tuberose, are too delicate to be distilled. The most common way of extracting these more delicate essences is to produce an **absolute.** The first step is to create a **concréte** from the plant material. To produce a concréte, the plant material is treated with hexane, a petrochemical solvent. The solvent is then evaporated, creating a salve-like substance, the concréte. The next step removes the waxes and chlorophyll from the concréte using alcohol at a temperature of 50° C. This extraction is then cooled to 5° C and filtered. The alcohol is removed through evaporation.[2] The remaining essence is called an absolute.

Enfleurage: This process is an ancient method of extracting the essence from plants and flowers. The plant material is placed in direct contact with an animal fat (beef or pig) or a vegetable oil. The fat absorbs the essence from the plant. The essence is then extracted from the fat using an alcohol. The alcohol is evaporated, resulting in the enfleurage essence. In today's market, one rarely finds oils extracted using this method.

Oleoresins: These compounds are oils that are extracted from the gums or resins of trees and plants. Oleoresins are extracted from the plant resins and gums with alcohol. The alcohol is evaporated to produce an oleoresin. Acetone is used instead of alcohol in some countries. Acetone-derived oleoresins should be avoided due to the poor quality and possible toxicity of these products.[3]

Modern Extraction Methods

Attempts and experiments have been made to create new methods of extracting oils from their plant source, especially those plants from which producing a useful extract by standard methods has proved too difficult. Two methods that have been successful are supercritical carbon dioxide extraction and florasol extraction.

Supercritical Carbon Dioxide (CO_2) Extraction: This process uses carbon dioxide in a supercritical state in which it exhibits both a liquid and a gas state, extracting the essence under high pressure and at a constant temperature (30° C). This method is much gentler than distillation and produces oils with fragrances truer to the natural fragrance within the plant. Compounds that are usually not extracted in the distillation process, such as the triterpenes, are found in supercritical CO_2 extracts. These compounds add a broader-spectrum therapeutic intensity[4] not found in distilled essential oils. An oil extracted using supercritical carbon dioxide may be labeled as such; for example, frankincense CO_2.

Florasol Extraction: This method is even gentler than CO_2 extraction. It employs the use of "non-CFCs" (non-chlorofluorocarbons) or florasols, a benign family of compounds that had been introduced to replace the environmentally hazardous chlorinated fluorocarbons, in a room temperature extraction, creating oils that are as close to their natural state as possible. Dr. Peter Wilde developed this process in the late 1980's. The resulting extracts, previously referred to as phytols, are now called florasols.

QUALITY OF ESSENTIAL OILS FOR THERAPEUTIC ACTIVITY

The word *quality* has been, and will continue to be, used throughout this text. Each time the word is used, its meaning must be clarified. The meaning of the phrase "quality essential oil" particularly should be well defined as a criterion for purchasing essential oils. Unfortunately, the words "quality," "therapeutic grade," "organic," and "natural" are used often as marketing terms that carry little meaning or truth. To overcome this commercial whitewashing of useful terminology, we must develop standards for describing the essential oils you will use for their therapeutic functions.

Pure, Natural, and Complete: Genuine and Authentic

Henri Viaud, a distiller of essential oils, expanded upon the importance of using the unaltered and natural composition of the whole oil. In 1983, he created a set of standards that have become the criteria for oils used therapeutically. These oils are often defined as *genuine and authentic,* though not all producers or distributors use this term. We use these criteria as our model and guide for the quality of essential oils used for therapeutic aromatherapy.

Buying Genuine & Authentic Oils

To select oils that are best suited for aromatherapy purposes, you will need to identify them as genuine and authentic. Genuine and authentic oils are (1) pure, natural, and complete; (2) not redistilled (rectified); and (3) grown and processed under conditions that assure maximum authenticity. They are produced using water or water/steam distillation. The distillation process uses lower temperature and pressure than others and is carried out slowly, thus preventing damage and preserving the molecular structure of the oil.

Genuine and authentic oils are:

- *Genuine,* meaning that nothing is added to the essential oil and that it is pure, natural, and complete.
- *Pure,* which specifies that no other essential oils or vegetable oils are present in the product. An oil diluted with a vegetable oil, like grapeseed or canola, is generally easy to detect by its texture and its inability to evaporate. Oftentimes, more expensive oils are stretched, or adulterated, using other oils. For example, bergamot (*Citrus bergamia*) may be stretched using lemon (*Citrus limon*), and lavender (*Lavandula angustifolia*) may be stretched with lavandin (*Lavandula x intermadia*).[5] This type of stretching is much harder for the inexperienced aromatherapist to detect.
- *Natural,* which means that no synthetic ingredients are added to the essential oil. Perfume oils, even so-called natural perfume oils, may be diluted with petrochemicals like

mineral oil, propylene glycol, phthalates, or other synthetics. This dodge should be easy enough to detect, but again, experience is important in the detection process.

- *Complete,* indicating that the oil has not been decolorized or deterpenized. The flavor and fragrance industry requires certain molecules (terpenes) and color to be extracted from natural oils. This practice, not used in aromatherapy, may cause the oils to have less activity or to become irritants.
- *Authentic* describes the source of the oil. An essential oil used in aromatherapy should be clearly defined as coming from one plant of an identified botanical source (see this chapter's section about Specified Botanical Origin). The distillation should be from one specified plant and not a mix of similar plants or plants that grow alongside the chosen plant.

DETERMINING THE SOURCE: SPECIFIED BOTANICAL ORIGIN

When purchasing essential oils, you should know their *specified botanical origin.* This criterion tells you which plant the oil was extracted from and is generally identified by the genus and the species of the plant (see Table 4-1, Genus and Species). An oil labeled "chamomile" could be from *Matricaria recutita, Anthemis nobilis,* or *Ormensis multicolis.* Each of these plants produces oils that have distinctly different properties. Several species of eucalyptus plants are distilled; each produces an essential oil that is unique to its specific eucalyptus species. You will avoid confusion and possible treatment contraindications by knowing the correct botanical designation of the essential oil.

One Name but More than One Origin

Most essential oils have a common name that relates to one specified plant origin. Some oils, however, such as eucalyptus and chamomile, may be derived from one of several different plants. Each plant species and genus produces a different oil with differing therapeutic uses and properties. The following essential oil descriptions may all have the common name

Table 4-1 Genus and Species

Plants are identified using categories of classification called genus and species. This text does not describe the science behind these classifications and uses them only to identify plants used in aromatherapy. The botanical names as a rule are written in italics, with the genus capitalized. Some examples are:

Common Name	Genus	Species
Lavender	Lavandula	angustifolia
Jasmine	Jasminum	grandiflorum
Blue gum (eucalyptus)	Eucalyptus	globulus
Eucalyptus	Eucalyptus	radiata
Lemon eucalyptus	Eucalyptus	citriodora
Peppermint	Mentha	piperita
Spearmint	Mentha	spicata
Tea tree	Melaleuca	alternafolia
MQV	Melaleuca	quinquenervia
Petitgrain	Citrus	aurantium
Bitter Orange	Citrus	aurantium
Neroli	Citrus	aurantium

You can see from this list that some oils are extracted from plants in the same genus but from a different species of that genus, such as tea tree and MQV. Eucalyptus oils are derived from several different species that are categorized under the same genus. In the case of the *Citrus aurantium,* the different common names actually identify the part of the plant from which the oil is derived. These three oils, petitgrain, bitter orange, and neroli, are from the sticks and leaves, peel, and flower blossoms, respectively, of the *Citrus aurantium*, or bitter orange tree. Very few plants are used this extensively to produce oils, however.

chamomile. You can see from their descriptions that they are not the same plant, with similar activity. These descriptions include essential oil compound names that are explained in Chapter 5.

Common Name: Chamomile

***Anthemis nobilis* (Roman chamomile)** This oil is the preferred oil for relaxation, stress, and anxiety and for soothing irritable children. Roman chamomile is high in ester compounds and is a relatively expensive essential oil.

***Eriocephalus punctulatus* (Cape chamomile)** Produced in South Africa, this essential oil has a nice balance of anti-inflammatory properties and relaxing esters. It also has a very pleasing and fruity fragrance.

***Matricaria recutita* (German chamomile)** The German chamomile is best for inflammatory conditions as a result of its high azulene (sesquiterpene) content. The essential oil of *Matricaria recutita* is sometimes called blue chamomile. This oil should not be confused with the oils extracted from *Ormensis multicolis* or *Tannacetum annuum.* These two oils are also high in azulene but contain other compounds, and properties, that are not similar to those of *Matricaria recutita*. *Ormensis multicolis* is referred to as chamomile Maroc (Moroccan chamomile), and *Tannacetum annuum* is called blue tansy but may also carry the name Moroccan chamomile. You can see from these examples that common names are inconsistent and may cause confusion. The identity of the species and genus clearly defines the plant source of the essential oil.

***Ormensis mixta* (chamomile mixta or Moroccan chamomile)** This oil is generally sold as a cheap replacement for Roman chamomile. It has relaxing qualities similar to those of the Roman chamomile but is therapeutically inferior. This oil is often used to adulterate or replace an oil labeled as Roman chamomile.

Common Name: Eucalyptus

The eucalyptus oils are generally referred to by their botanical names. In fact, the common names included are not commonly used.

***Eucalyptus citriodora* (lemon gum)** This eucalyptus is not the common eucalyptus found in the marketplace. The citriodora species has a distinct lemon fragrance and is used for relaxation and as an antiviral or antiseptic.

***Eucalyptus dives* (broad leaved peppermint)** The dives species contains a high amount of piperitone, a ketone, so it is used as a mucolytic and for cell regeneration in skin care. Ketone contraindications are observed, as described in Chapter 5.

***Eucalyptus globulus* (blue gum)** This is the oil that is used as common eucalyptus. It contains large amounts of the compound eucalyptol, giving it the familiar eucalyptus fragrance and the expectorant properties expected of eucalyptus. Eucalyptus globulus is often redistilled (rectified), reducing the leafy, fruity fragrance of the whole oil and depleting its therapeutic benefits.

***Eucalyptus polybractea* (blue mallee)** The polybractea species also contains large amounts of eucalyptol and is used as an expectorant.

***Eucalyptus radiata* (common peppermint)** Radiata is also rectified for commercial use as eucalyptus. When it is not redistilled, the composition of this oil produces a broad spectrum of activity and a pleasant fragrance.

More than one common name may be used to describe an essential oil extracted from the same plant, such as everlasting and immortelle, both of which are from the oil extracted from *Helichrysum italicum*. There are also times when more than one common name is used to differentiate essential oils extracted from the same plant. For example, MQV is the common name used for the essential oil extracted from the tree, *Melaleuca quinquenervia viridiflora*, grown and produced in Madagascar. The essential oil extracted from this same species from other areas, most commonly New Caledonia, is called niaouli. The reason the name MQV was given to the oil from Madagascar is due to the fact that this area produces a superior quality oil from this tree. This differentiation, like many other non-rules in aromatherapy, is not always used by sellers of essential oils.

DETERMINING ESSENTIAL OIL COMPOSITION: GC/MS ANALYSIS

In 1979, Karl-Heinz Kubeczka developed guidelines to determine the quality of essential oils for use in medicine. His guidelines are based on the complex synergy of essential oil compounds detected through a **gas chromatography/mass spectrometry analysis,** a method used to analyze the composition of essential oils and uncover falsifications and adulterations. He recently updated and revised these guidelines.

GC/MS is the most reliable method used to determine quality and structure of essential oils. Suppliers of quality oils will often state that their oils are GC or GC/MS tested. GC/MS analyzes the molecular structure of volatile substances, such as those in essential oils. The gas chromatograph (GC) vaporizes a sample of essential oil, then separates and analyzes the various components. Each component creates a characteristic spectrum that is recorded on a sheet of paper (a **chromatogram**) as a peak. The size of the peaks on the chromatogram is proportional to the quantity of the corresponding substance in the essential oil. For instance, a chromatogram for lavender will generally show the highest peaks of linalyl acetate and linalool, its two main compounds. See Figure 4-4a and 4-4b for an example of a GC/MS chromatogram of the essential oil extracted from rosemary.

Interpreting GC/MS Results

GC/MS displays the molecular composition of an essential oil. It is used to identify an oil's therapeutic structure and, now more commonly, to detect adulterations or additives in the essential oil tested. For aromatherapy purposes, the test is used to ensure the use of whole unadulterated oils. For pharmaceutical purposes, it may be used to ensure a standard of active isolated components. This is a valuable tool for quality assurance, but it is not foolproof. Testing for an expected concentration of one or more defined components does not necessarily determine that the oil does not contain added substances. In some cases, to meet the pharmacopeia requirements of some countries, a known component is added to an oil, such as eucalyptol in eucalyptus, to match the standard set by this requirement. Lavender has a naturally occurring concentration of 35 to 45 percent linalyl acetate. A GC/MS may show that it has the correct percentage of linalyl acetate and other compounds, but the oil could still be adulterated using synthetic or natural additives that would include the proper balance of the linalyl acetate. The proper peak proportion of a main constituent, such as linalyl acetate, on a GC/MS could well be an added compound. Therefore, Kubeczka developed a basis whereby essential oil quality must take into account an oil's secondary and trace constituents, not just the isolated main constituents. This is an important aspect of essential oil use. The synergistic activity of all the components of an oil are believed to give the oil its distinct and effective therapeutic properties. Determining the

Sample & lot: *Rosmarinus officinalis* ex Hvar, W.Corsica
Run: 010090101.D
Date: 10/9/02

RT	Component	Area % by GC/MS
13.38	tricyclene	0.36
14.10	alpha-pinene	26.57
15.37	alpha-fenchene	0.07
15.86	camphene	8.41
17.67	beta-pinene	1.59
18.48	thuja-2,4(10)-diene	1.11
19.61	delta-3-carene	0.20
20.06	beta-myrcene	0.97
20.49	alpha-phellandrene	0.46
21.28	alpha-terpinene	0.40
22.45	limonene	4.42
23.11	1,8-cineole	7.98
24.04	(Z)-beta-ocimene	0.06
25.05	gamma-terpinene	0.45
25.55	3-octanone	0.31
26.73	p-cymene	2.77
27.36	terpinolene	0.47
37.91	1-octen-3-ol	0.22
38.12	p-cymenene	0.11
45.93	camphor	9.20
46.04	linalool	1.96
47.76	iso-pinocamphone	0.26
50.30	bornyl acetate	11.74
51.81	terpinen-4-ol	1.20
57.00	cis-pinocarveol	0.26
58.40	alpha-humulene	0.12
59.14	(E)-verbenol	0.21
61.02	alpha-terpinoel	1.26
61.61	borneol	8.81
63.38	verbenone	5.57
75.92	geraniol	1.18

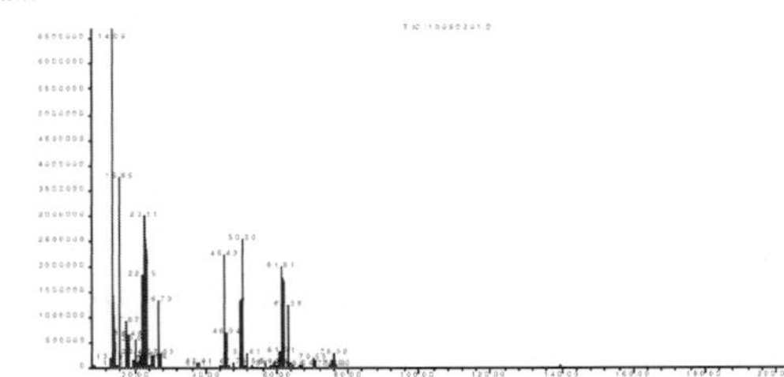

Sample & lot: Rosmarinus officinalis ex Hvar, Adriatic Sea
Run: 010090103.D
Date: 10/9/02

RT	Component	Area % by GC/MS
13.40	tricyclene	0.27
14.10	alpha-pinene	15.38
15.39	alpha-fenchene	0.10
15.90	camphene	7.07
17.77	beta-pinene	3.91
18.50	thuja-2,4(10)-diene	0.11
19.66	delta-3-carene	0.09
20.15	beta-myrcene	2.27
20.57	alpha-phellandrene	0.26
21.37	alpha-terpinene	0.77
22.73	limonene	3.38
23.58	1,8-cineole	30.82
24.14	(*Z*)-beta-ocimene	0.10
25.17	gamma-terpinene	1.32
25.63	3-octanone	0.52
26.79	*p*-cymene	1.62
27.42	terpinolene	0.56
37.91	1-octen-3-ol	0.11
39.44	*trans*-sabinene hydrate	0.05
41.50	alpha-ylangene	0.08
42.32	alpha-copaene	0.15
45.61	camphor	11.34
46.03	linalool	0.82
47.77	iso-pinocamphone	0.05
50.15	bornyl acetate	2.96
51.92	(*E*)-beta-caryophyllene	5.80
58.50	alpha-humulene	0.89
60.07	alpha-amorphene	0.12
61.07	alpha-terpineol	2.14
61.61	borneol	6.36
63.19	verbenone	0.15
66.79	delta-cadinene	0.14

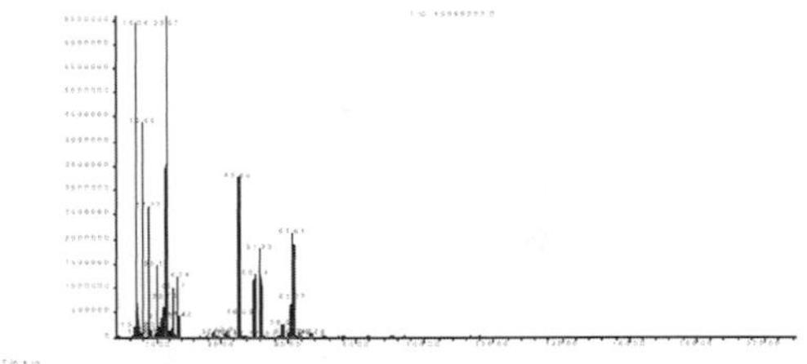

Figure 4-4a and 4b Using GC/MS it becomes apparent how the same plant (*Rosmarinus officinalis*) will produce different essential oil composition depending on where it was grown and distilled. Figure 4.4a is a Corsican distillation with higher peaks of alpha-pinene and bornyl acetate. The rosemary distilled in Hvar, figure 4.4b, shows higher peaks and related amounts of the compounds 1,8 cineole and camphor.

composition of the whole oil takes a skilled scientist performing GC/MS analysis and interpreting the results.

Using GC/MS to Deceive

Most suppliers you buy from will supply a GC/MS test result if you ask for it. This document does not guarantee a quality oil. A falsified GC/MS report may be used by disreputable distributors to support their talk of "high quality" essential oils. More and more, savvy suppliers are manipulating oils in ways that cannot always be detected by GC/MS. As good as GC/MS is for analyzing essential oil composition, it is a limited source of information for the end consumer who lacks the scientific understanding and ability to read the chromatogram. Still, GC/MS is one of the best methods available for determining the quality and authenticity of an oil.

ADULTERATION OF ESSENTIAL OILS

This section fully explains adulteration, the process of adding natural or synthetic compounds to "stretch" an essential oil or adjust its fragrance or color. For example, it has been previously stated that the main constituents in lavender are linalool and linalyl acetate, which give lavender the soothing and calming properties for which it is known. These compounds are generally used to extend lavender. Many oils are adulterated in a similar way, by adding isolated natural or synthetic compounds that are found in the pure oil. The adulterated essential oil, though it may contain natural compounds, does not have the same effects as an essential oil that has not been adulterated. Adulteration is often suspected to be the culprit that causes sensitivity and allergic reactions that people experience from essential oil use. The ingredients used in adulteration could have potential irritant qualities or other toxic effects.

"Stretching" French Population Lavender

French "population" lavender (*Lavandula angustifolia*) from Provence yields an oil commonly called *lavande fine.* It is distilled from plants that seed naturally and are not grown from cuttings or clones. Lavande fine from Provence is thought to be the best lavender essential oil. In the year 2000, the small exclusive group of distillers who produce and sell Provençal population lavender calculated the entire crop of this specialized product for that year. The total yield sold that year was 25 tons. The lavender was sold to buyers from around the world. In the United States alone, 250 tons of "lavande fine from Provence" was sold that year.[6] Do the math, and you will find a 225-ton discrepancy between the lavender produced and the lavender sold in the U.S. And that difference assumes that all the lavande fine produced in Provence that year was sold in the United States! The reality is, the oil bought from the French producers is adulterated by the addition of compounds similar to those found in the natural oil, which extends the amount of essential oil. A buyer purchases the lavender, then adds either lavandin (a cheaper variety of lavender) or isolated components similar to those found in lavender. The quantity of lavender may grow from 10 kilos to 20 kilos using this method of adulteration. Then it may be passed on to another distributor, who also extends the lavender. Soon, from a 25-ton yield, you have 250 tons of a so-called lavande fine essential oil. It is also very likely that much of what was sold in the United States in 2000 as French population lavender was oil that came from another source and was simply labeled as lavender fine.

Disrupting the Natural Balance

Essential oils have a natural structure that is in balance and harmony. When oils are adulterated, this natural balance no longer exists. This disruption can cause sensitivity issues. Oregano, for instance, contains a very active irritant compound but also contains a small amount of a compound with anti-inflammatory and cooling actions. An adulterated oregano oil may have the cooling compound reduced, enhancing the irritant qualities. Many other changes to essential oil activity occur because of adulteration. They include a loss of therapeutic activity that results from the effect that adulteration may have on the essential oil's therapeutic structure.

Detecting Adulteration

As already explained, GC/MS is one method designed to detect an adulterated or synthetic oil. This is an expensive test, however, and may not be the best way to discover adulteration for every oil you buy. Price is sometimes a good indication of the quality and possible adulteration of essential oils. A French lavender selling for $10 an ounce has an unrealistic price for an authentic, unadulterated essential oil of lavender. Lavender in the retail market would be more likely to cost $30 to $45 an ounce. Price does not always ensure quality. A seller may still offer a synthetic or adulterated oil for the higher price you expect to pay for quality essential oils.

Concerns Raised by Adulterated Essential Oils

In a 2003 presentation to the International Federation of Aromatherapists, Tony Burfield discussed the consequences of using adulterated essential oils.[7] His list of concerns included:

- toxicity of adulterants such as phthalates, traces of residual solvents (hexane and cyclohexane), and pesticides
- interference of adulterants with the expected physiological or psychophysiological effects of essential oils

Trusting Your Supplier, Becoming Knowledgeable

The ways to spot adulterations in oils are beyond the capabilities of the casual user or clinical practitioner because of the equipment required. Guarding against adulteration again comes down to trusting your supplier. The information gathered from this text will give you as much information as possible to help guide you in your pursuit of the best oils for effective therapeutic use. Experience will become your constant guide.

CHAPTER SUMMARY

The quality of essential oils you use determines the therapeutic outcome and value of your aromatherapy work. You must have a good working knowledge of all aspects of producing essential oils for therapeutic use. The steps taken to achieve this knowledge include: understanding extraction methods, developing a clear definition and understanding of the quality expected of essential oils for therapeutic activity, identifying the botanical plant source of the essential oil, determining essential oil composition through GC/MS analysis, and identifying adulteration.

REVIEW QUESTIONS

1. What is adulteration?
2. For an oil called an "essential oil," what extraction methods are used to derive the oil from the plant?
3. What is an absolute?

4. What are the guidelines for determining a "genuine and authentic" essential oil?
5. What is Specified Botanical Origin and how does it relate to eucalyptus?
6. What does Gas Chromatography/Mass Spectrometry (GC/MS) tell you about the essential oil?

CHAPTER REFERENCES

1. Burfield, T. (2003, October). *The Adulteration of Essential Oils.* Presented at the International Federation of Aromatherapists Annual General Meeting. London, England.
2. Schnaubelt, K. (1985). Aromatherapy Course. San Rafael, CA: Pacific Institute of Aromatherapy.
3. Newmark, T. M. & Schuluck, P. (2000). *Beyond Aspirin.* Prescott, AZ: Hohm Press.
4. Burfield, Tony, (2003, October). *The Adulteration of Essential Oils*. Presented at the International Federation of Aromatherapists Annual General Meeting. London, England.
5. Kubeczka, K. (2002). *Essential Oils: Analysis by Capillary Gas Chromatography and Carbon 13-NMR Spectroscopy.* West Sussex, England: Wiley & Sons.
6. Schnaubelt, K. (2001). *Aroma: Lavender*. San Rafael, CA: Terra Linda Image and Scent.
7. Burfield, Tony, (2003, October). *The Adulteration of Essential Oils*. Presented at the International Federation of Aromatherapists Annual General Meeting. London, England.

Essential Oil Biology and Chemistry

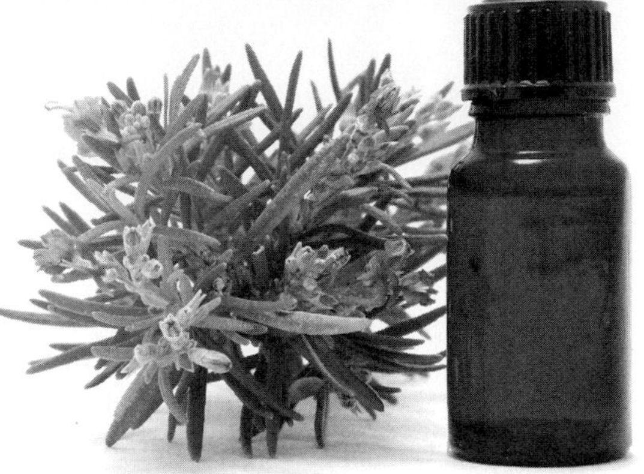

CHAPTER 5

We can give up on life by presuming to understand it – that is, by reducing it to the terms of our understanding and by treating it as predictable or mechanical.

From *Life is a Miracle* –*Wendell Berry*

LEARNING OBJECTIVES

1. Broaden your understanding of the chemistry and biology that underlie the functions and qualities of essential oils.
2. Learn how essential oil chemistry provides a scientific basis for the healing properties of essential oils and provides guidelines for therapeutic application.
3. Discover how the Structure-Effect Diagram and a description of the molecular groups provide valuable tools for the aromatherapist.
4. Obtain a deeper insight into the healing potential and properties of essential oils through the basics of plant biology.
5. Develop a better understanding of how humans and plants co-evolved.

SCIENCE AS A GUIDE, NOT A RULE

Life is mysterious. It remains elusive, and our understanding of it is not absolute. The sciences of chemistry and biology have created a foundation of knowledge and continue to unveil mysteries of life. A new mystery may lie beneath each discovery. These sciences are best used as guides to the mechanics of life. Chemistry provides knowledge of, and a language that is useful to describe, parts of the whole. Biology attempts to explain the interaction of these parts. Each year, with each new discovery, new interpretations of biological activity are developed that build upon or dismiss that which came before. The sciences assist in understanding essential oils and aromatherapy. If we understand the structure of essential oils, we can guide their activity and, at times, predict results. We must accept that aromatherapy has many unknown variables and learn to expect the unpredictable.

Scientific Understanding of Essential Oils

Chemistry is the science used for analysis and explanation in today's model of medicine and healing. Unraveling the chemistry of essential oils will satisfy the mind that desires or requires a scientific evaluation of essential oil activity. The science of chemistry is the accepted system to support any claims that are made, though there are clearly limits to chemical scrutiny alone. Beyond chemistry, essential oils and their interaction with human beings require the input of biology, physics, and alternative sciences to develop a comprehensive understanding of healing. A review and study of essential oil's chemical composition provides a foundation of knowledge that will further your therapeutic potential and accuracy in working with the oils. Knowledge of essential oil chemical activity and composition does not provide exact rules but instead acts as a guide to expand upon the craft, art, and accuracy of aromatherapy. The sciences can be employed to stimulate intuition in this art and escalate the promise of essential oil application.

Limits of Scientific Studies

Scientific research is a significant part of any medical system. It provides support, guidance, and a certain amount of legitimacy for use of healing substances. Many research methodologies and variations exist for scientific study. Studies can use animals or humans and can be performed in a lab or in a clinic. A number of variables that can potentially influence the outcome of a study must be accounted for. The obvious ones include the number of test subjects, conditions in which the test was performed, and acknowledgment of unknown, outside factors. This last condition is most challenging, because that which is unknown must become known to acknowledge its influence on the outcome.

The available research regarding essential oils is limited. Studies having to do with complex botanical substances, including those using essential oils, may not always hold up under scrutiny of the design and execution of the research.[1] Some flaws found in essential oil studies include studying an essential oil without properly identifying the oil's plant source, using animals that do not necessarily share similar reactions to essential oils as humans, and using essential oils that may have been tainted with other substances. Another consideration is that living organisms do not inevitably cooperate and behave according to scientific explanation. Life is exceedingly complex and, even with the advances made in scientific study, it still will challenge evaluation under the current research methodology.

Science as a Tool

We use science, primarily chemistry and biology, as a means to safely, effectively, and fully use the power of essential oils. This chapter contains an abundance of scientific information, though it is not the intent of this book to teach biochemistry. The following information is designed to develop a greater potential for accurate use of essential oils, based on their chemical composition and biology. Some sections may not appear to be crucial for expertise in aromatherapy. They are included to give a wider perspective of organic science and are beneficial for the expansion of aromatic consciousness.

This chapter should be approached for its primary intention: to develop a better working relationship with essential oils. The therapeutic activities of essential oils are primarily attributed to their chemical composition. A working knowledge of elements and chemical bonding should provide insight into this activity. The biological functions of the oils within the plants provide clues to their properties and to the intricacies of biological interaction and harmony they may have within the human body. For this reason, such diverse subjects as evolution and emerging properties are presented later in this chapter. If you have a scientific background, you may find the included information very basic and simplified. The novice may view the material as difficult and potentially overwhelming. In either case, translate this information to your own level of understanding to assist in the development of a complete holistic study of essential oils.

AUTHOR'S **NOTE**

DO I REALLY NEED TO KNOW THIS?

When teaching my classes I notice signs of apprehension, accompanied by a sampling of moans and groans, as I approach the science of essential oils. Sciences are considered a left-brain study and perceived as difficult by the right-brained audience who are the majority of my esthetics students.

When I was first exposed to the structural chemistry of essential oils, the information didn't exactly download like data into an MP3 player. I knew straight away this was not the instinctive or experiential side of aromatherapy. I was going to have to hear this a few times for the science to register and also do a little more reading on my own. I was motivated and began to re-examine first year chemistry. I blended this review with research into the available literature addressing the essential oil chemical composition. My review of basic chemical structures was supportive and helped me to form a solid foundation.

I include some beginning-level chemistry in the next few sections of this chapter, but I don't believe it's necessary that you absorb it completely. Sections regarding the properties of water, ions, and other sidebars of chemical knowledge are topics I include in my classes. These topics help my students develop an awareness of the intricacies and interesting formations that occur in nature. They provide depth to understanding the essential oil's chemistry and activity, and they also present information and language that may be encountered when reading through product marketing literature. In a live presentation, I can lighten these topics up by beginning with

"Dude, check this out," or, "OK, this is really weird." When you get to a section that seems overwhelming, unrelated to aromatherapy, or just too much science, mentally add one of these phrases and see if it doesn't help.

As a beginner, I intuitively sensed the value of a thorough grasp of the science; that is, I used my right brain influence to push my left brain activity. Even though it's possible to work with little understanding of the chemistry, this ignorance can hinder your work as an aromatherapist. This possibility will become more evident as you read through this chapter.

There is an art to the science. Thoughtful and creative therapeutic manipulation becomes possible when working with the chemical families identified in the Structure-Effect Diagram. I discovered this potential early on when a friend asked me to make a remedy for injuries incurred by falling off a bicycle. I wanted to test the value and use of the Structure-Effect Diagram. The formula I made used the properties associated with the chemical families. I matched the symptoms of pain, inflammation, and scrapes that resulted from the fall with the corresponding properties. Read on and you will see how this is done. To this day, that formula has been one of the best and most effective I have ever made. You'll find the recipe, called *Pain Remedy*, in the Appendix: Therapeutic Essential Oil Formulas.

ORGANIC CHEMISTRY

Atoms bond to form molecules, and molecules interact to build the simple and complex structures of all matter. This is chemistry. Our focus is on **organic chemistry,** the study of carbon based compounds. Organic chemistry is the chemistry of life. Life is expressed through an intricate construction of biological structures. These structures range from DNA of one-celled organisms to human beings.

THE ATOM

For our purposes we will examine the atom as the building block of all matter. The atom is composed of subatomic particles: **electrons** with a negative electric charge, **protons** with

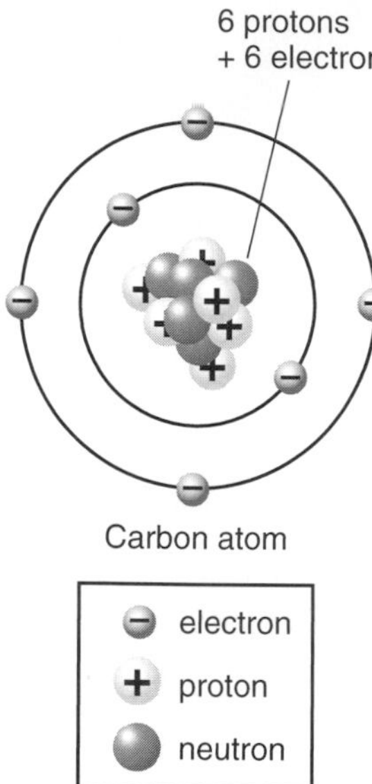

Figure 5-1 A carbon atom with 6 electrons and 6 protons.

a positive electric charge, and the **neutron** with neutral, or no, charge. Every atom contains a different number of these subatomic particles giving each a unique quality. The number of protons in an atom determines the identity of the atom; hydrogen with one proton, carbon with 6 (Figure 5-1), and nitrogen with 7 protons. Hydrogen contains one electron, one proton, and zero neutrons (Figure 5-2). An oxygen atom contains 8 electrons, 8 protons, and 8 neutrons. Atoms contain an equal number of protons and electrons and so are electrically neutral.

Elements are the primary substances that build all other objects and things. Elements include oxygen, carbon, hydrogen, silver, and zinc. More than 100 elements have been identified. **Atoms** are the smallest particle of an element that still retains its character. A small bit of the element gold consists of billions of gold atoms. The **Periodic Table** arranges the elements according to their atomic weight and atomic number (Table 5-1). In conventional notation, the number above the element's symbol represents the **atomic number** equal to the number of protons in the atom. The number below states the **atomic weight**, the sum of the neutrons and protons contained within the atom. One can calculate the number of neutrons in the atom by subtracting the top number from the bottom number.

Energy Levels and Electron Arrangement

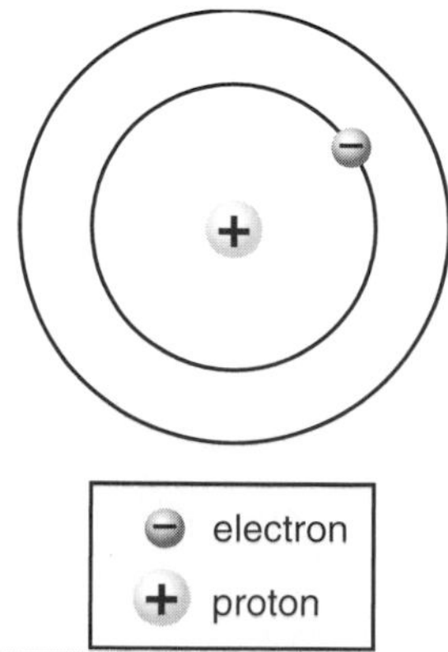

Figure 5-2 A hydrogen atom with 1 electron and 1 proton.

The positioning of electrons around the nucleus, made up of protons and neutrons, determines the chemical properties, or activity of the atom. Electrons are arranged in **energy levels** around the nucleus called the **electron arrangement.** Electrons are described as orbiting the nucleus. Orbits have a specific shape around the nucleus and contain a maximum of two electrons for each orbit. This arrangement is called electron pairing. The electrons in the energy level closest to the nucleus are in a lower energy state than the electrons in levels further away from the nucleus. A fixed number of electrons is allowed for each level; level 1 holds a maximum of two electrons, Level 2 has a maximum of eight electrons, and Level 3 has a maximum of 18 electrons. See Figure 5-3 for the energy arrangement of carbon. When stable, electrons occupy the lowest energy states. If excited by an outside source of energy, such as heat or light, an electron may "jump" to a higher energy level. At a higher,

Table 5-1 Periodic Table

Periodic Table of Elements

Key: Hydrogen — Element; 1 — Atomic Number; H — Symbol; 1.008 — Atomic Mass; State of Matter

○ Gas
Liquid
■ Solid
● Synthetic Elements

	1A 1	2A 2	3B 3	4B 4	5B 5	6B 6	7B 7	8B 8	9	10	11 1B	12 2B	13 3A	14 4A	15 5A	16 6A	17 7A	18 8A
1	Hydrogen 1 H 1.008																	Helium 2 He 4.003
2	Lithium 3 Li 6.941	Beryllium 4 Be 9.012											Boron 5 B 10.811	Carbon 6 C 12.011	Nitrogen 7 N 14.007	Oxygen 8 O 15.999	Fluorine 9 F 18.998	Neon 10 Ne 20.180
3	Sodium 11 Na 22.990	Magnesium 12 Mg 24.305											Aluminum 13 Al 26.982	Silicon 14 Si 28.086	Phosphorus 15 P 30.974	Sulfur 16 S 32.066	Chlorine 17 Cl 35.453	Argon 18 Ar 39.948
4	Potassium 19 K 39.098	Calcium 20 Ca 40.078	Scandium 21 Sc 44.956	Titanium 22 Ti 47.88	Vanadium 23 V 50.942	Chromium 24 Cr 51.996	Manganese 25 Mn 54.938	Iron 26 Fe 55.847	Cobalt 27 Co 58.933	Nickel 28 Ni 58.693	Copper 29 Cu 63.546	Zinc 30 Zn 65.39	Gallium 31 Ga 69.723	Germanium 32 Ge 72.61	Arsenic 33 As 74.922	Selenium 34 Se 78.96	Bromine 35 Br 79.904	Krypton 36 Kr 83.80
5	Rubidium 37 Rb 85.468	Strontium 38 Sr 87.62	Yttrium 39 Y 88.906	Zirconium 40 Zr 91.224	Niobium 41 Nb 92.906	Molybdenum 42 Mo 95.94	Technetium 43 Tc 97.907	Ruthenium 44 Ru 101.07	Rhodium 45 Rh 102.906	Palladium 46 Pd 106.42	Silver 47 Ag 107.868	Cadmium 48 Cd 112.411	Indium 49 In 114.82	Tin 50 Sn 118.710	Antimony 51 Sb 121.757	Tellurium 52 Te 127.60	Iodine 53 I 126.904	Xenon 54 Xe 131.290
6	Cesium 55 Cs 132.905	Barium 56 Ba 137.327	Lanthanum 57 La 138.906	Hafnium 72 Hf 178.49	Tantalum 73 Ta 180.948	Tungsten 74 W 183.84	Rhenium 75 Re 186.207	Osmium 76 Os 190.2	Iridium 77 Ir 192.22	Platinum 78 Pt 195.08	Gold 79 Au 196.967	Mercury 80 Hg 200.59	Thallium 81 Tl 204.383	Lead 82 Pb 207.2	Bismuth 83 Bi 208.980	Polonium 84 Po 208.982	Astatine 85 At 209.987	Radon 86 Rn 222.018
7	Francium 87 Fr 223.020	Radium 88 Ra 226.025	Actinium 89 Ac 227.028	Rutherfordium 104 Rf (261)	Dubnium 105 Db (262)	Seaborgium 106 Sg (263)	Bohrium 107 Bh (262)	Hassium 108 Hs (265)	Meitnerium 109 Mt (266)	Ununnilium *110 Uun 269	Unununium *111 Uuu 272	Unumbium *112 Uub 277		Ununquadium *114 Uug 285		Ununhexium 116 Uuh 289		Ununodium *118 Uuo 293

*Names not officially assigned. Discovery of elements 114, 116, and 118 recently reported. Further information not yet available

Series														
Lanthanide Series	Cerium 58 Ce 140.115	Praseodymium 59 Pr 140.908	Neodymium 60 Nd 144.24	Promethium 61 Pm 144.913	Samarium 62 Sm 150.36	Europium 63 Eu 151.965	Gadolinium 64 Gd 157.25	Terbium 65 Tb 158.925	Dysprosium 66 Dy 162.50	Holmium 67 Ho 164.930	Erbium 68 Er 167.26	Thulium 69 Tm 168.934	Ytterbium 70 Yb 173.04	Lutetium 71 Lu 174.967
Actinide Series	Thorium 90 Th 232.038	Protactinium 91 Pa 231.036	Uranium 92 U 238.029	Neptunium 93 Np 237.048	Plutonium 94 Pu 244.064	Americium 95 Am 243.061	Curium 96 Cm 247.070	Berkelium 97 Bk 247.070	Californium 98 Cf 251.080	Einsteinium 99 Es 252.083	Fermium 100 Fm 257.095	Mendelevium 101 Md 258.099	Nobelium 102 No 259.101	Lawrencium 103 Lr 260.105

excited state, the electrons are unstable. They drop back down to the lowest possible energy state. When an electron goes from a higher excited energy back down to a lower energy, it emits energy.

Free Radicals

Electron pairing is introduced to explain how free radicals are formed. Two electrons that spin and orbit in opposite directions around a nucleus join to form an **electron pair**. If an atom or molecule loses an electron, as they do in chemical reactions or when weak bonds are split, the result is an atom or molecule with an **unpaired electron**. A **free radical** is an atom or molecule with an unpaired electron. To regain the stability of an electron pair, the free radical steals electrons from other molecules. Free radicals are very unstable and have a short lifespan (1/1000000 to 1/10 of a second); they react quickly with other compounds. The free radical that steals an electron has been **reduced**, meaning that it has gained an electron. The molecule

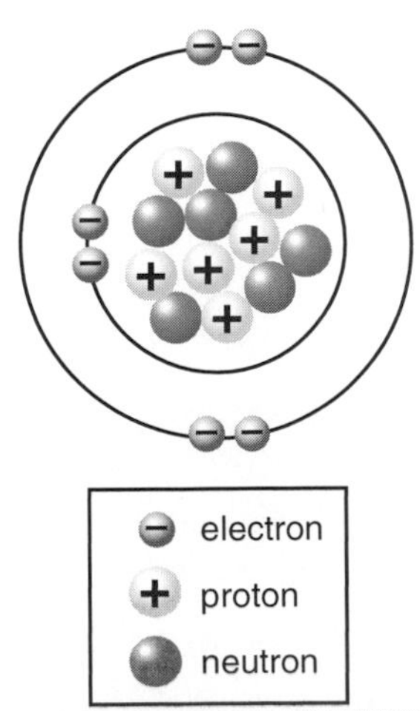

Figure 5-3 The energy arrangement of carbon.

that lost an electron has been **oxidized**, meaning that it has lost an electron. The oxidized molecule or atom may become a free radical with an unpaired electron. This process goes on in a continuous chain reaction. Free radicals in the human body are caused by inflammation and also arise during the body's normal metabolism. Environmental toxins, stress, diet, and cigarette smoke also produce free radicals.

The most likely targets of free radicals in the body are the **lipids**. Lipids are fats or fat-like substances. Cells become damaged when free radicals steal electrons from the lipid membranes and other parts of the cell. Free radical damage also occurs in proteins and the DNA structure. Free radical damage is believed to be a factor that causes many diseases and increases the rate of the aging process.

Antioxidants are the body's defense against free radical damage. Antioxidants are compounds that neutralize free radicals by donating an electron to the free radical's electron pair. The antioxidant can give up an electron and remain stable. Antioxidants are an important part of the diet, a fact that is commonly noted in the nutrition literature. Foods with color, such as dark green, red, and yellow vegetables, are often touted for their antioxidant activity. Supplementation with vitamins A, C, E, and other antioxidant nutrients is recommended to prevent free radical damage. Chapter 11 deals with this topic in greater depth.

The body has developed its own mechanisms to reduce free radical damage. The protection the body produces against free radicals includes superoxide dismutase and other enzymes produced by the cells, and antioxidants such as alpha lipoic acid, a protective compound that will be discussed in Chapter 11.

Valence Electrons

Valence electrons are the electrons that occupy the outer most energy level. The electron configuration at the outer most level will determine the chemical activity of the atom. Elements are listed in groups as you can see on the Periodic Table in Table 5-1. The group number identifies the amount of valence electrons in the atom.

Bonding and Compound Formation

Elements achieve stability by filling their outer shells. You have read that each energy level has a maximum number of electrons. The first energy level is stable with two electrons; the second is stable at eight electrons. Though the following energy levels can hold more, they are stable when they contain eight electrons. Once eight electrons occupy these outer energy levels, the next levels begin to fill. The tendency for atoms to adjust to eight valence electrons is called the **octet rule**. The noble, or inert, gases in Group VIII of the Periodic Table are stable, with eight valence electrons, with the exception of helium, which has only two electrons making its first energy level stable. Hydrogen is another exception to the octet rule. With one atom in its first level, it needs to gain or share one electron to create the stability of two electrons in its first energy level. Atoms create a balance of eight valence electrons by losing, gaining, or sharing electrons in their outer energy level.

Chemical Bonds: How Compounds Are Structured Atoms combine to create a balance in their outer energy levels. Carbon, the atom of most importance in essential oil chemistry, needs four electrons to become stable. To do this, it shares electrons with other atoms, creating **chemical bonds**. This bonding and sharing of electrons is how **compounds** are created.

Ions

Ions are atoms with an electrical charge and are created when the atom loses or gains an electron. Atoms have an equal number of protons and electrons, making them electrically neutral. When they lose or gain an electron, they become electrically charged ions. To form a stable outer energy level, metals lose electrons and become positive ions; nonmetals gain electrons and become negative ions.

Ion chemistry is useful to better understand surfactants used in cleansers and shampoo. Surfactants can be ionic, amphoteric, or nonionic. Ionic surfactants release cations or anions and are thought to be the more aggressive cleansers. Nonionic surfactants and amphoterics are used for their gentle cleansing action.

MOLECULES

Molecules, or compounds, are formed when atoms chemically bond to each other. Three types of chemical bonding occur: ionic bonds, covalent bonds (both polar and nonpolar), and hydrogen bonds.

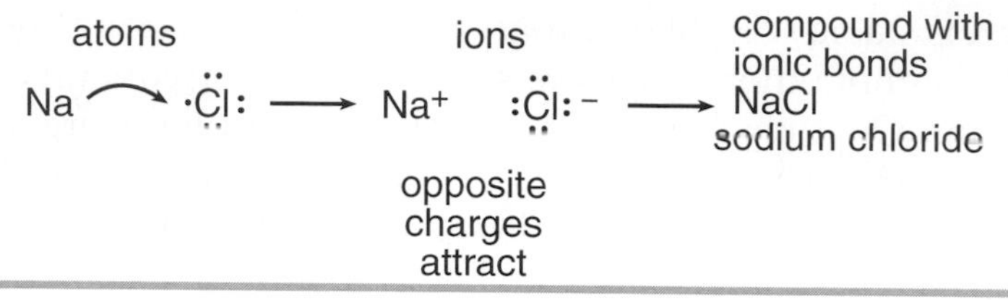

atoms | ions | compound with ionic bonds
Na ⁀ ·$\ddot{\underset{..}{Cl}}$: ⟶ Na^+ :$\ddot{\underset{..}{Cl}}$:$^-$ ⟶ NaCl sodium chloride
opposite charges attract

Figure 5-4 Ionic bonding of sodium chloride or table salt.

- **Ionic bonds** – Ionic bonds are formed when the electrons of metals are attracted to the nuclei of nonmetals. In this formation the metal loses an electron, this is called **oxidation**, and the nonmetal gains an electron, called **reduction**. This whole process is called the **redox reaction**. An example of an ionic bond to form common salt is shown in Figure 5-4.
- **Covalent bond** – Nonmetal elements form covalent bonds by sharing electrons. Nonmetals, with the exception of hydrogen, have four or more valence electrons. This is too many to lose, so instead, they bond by sharing electrons. See the covalent bonding of carbon and hydrogen in Figure 5-5.

  Carbon has four valence electrons in its outer energy level and requires four more to be a complete, or stable, octet. To accomplish this feat, carbon must share four electrons. Hydrogen requires just one more valence electron to become complete. In this figure, four hydrogen atoms bond with one carbon to make each stable and create the hydrocarbon compound methane.

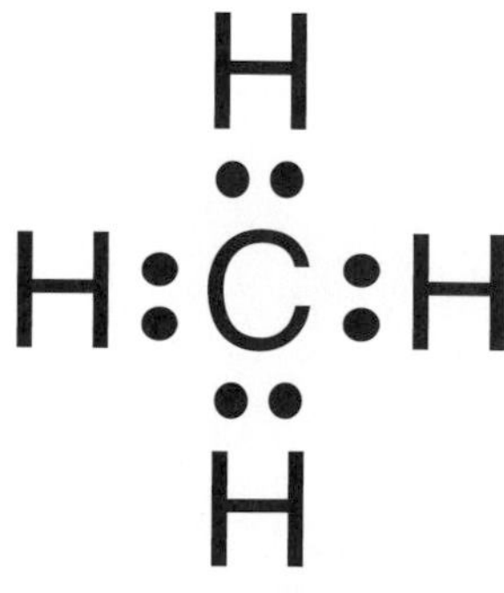

Figure 5-5 A covalent bond.

- **Nonpolar covalent bond** – The polarity, a type of attraction, of a covalent bond is determined by the distribution of electrical charges within a molecule. In a covalent bond, the shared electrons are pulled closer to the atom with the greatest electronegativity. **Electronegativity** is the tendency of an element to attract electrons in a bond. A nonpolar bond results when the bonding atoms have an equal distribution of electrical charges. Two hydrogen atoms have identical electronegativity. When they share electrons to form a covalent bond, the distribution of electrical charges in the resulting molecule is even. The hydrogen molecule (H_2) is a nonpolar molecule. See Figure 5-6.

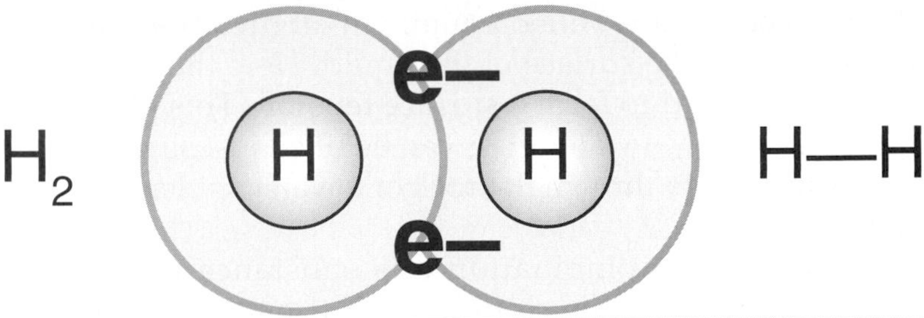

Figure 5-6 Two hydrogen atoms form a nonpolar covalent bond.

- **Polar covalent bonds** – A polar molecule occurs when two or more atoms of differing electronegativity, the electric charge, share electrons in a covalent bond. The shared electrons are pulled closer to the atoms with greatest electronegativity, resulting in an unequal distribution of electrical charges. Water is a polar molecule because the electrons of the two hydrogen atoms are pulled closer to the more electronegative oxygen atom. This configuration causes the water molecule (H_2O) to have a partial positive charge around the hydrogen atoms and a partial negative charge surrounding the oxygen. A polar molecule can be understood by comparing it to a magnet with a negative charge at one end and a positive charge on the other end.
- **Hydrogen bonds** – Hydrogen bonding is the force between water molecules and other interesting and important molecular arrangements that play an important role in the chemistry of life. The water molecule is a polar molecule. Oxygen is strongly electronegative and arranges itself towards the hydrogen end of another water molecule, which exhibits **electropositivity**. Hydrogen bonding is a weak force or bond that gives water its unique qualities.

Unique Properties of Water Molecules

The properties of water are a result of hydrogen bonding. Hydrogen bonds are not as strong as ionic or covalent bonds, and this difference results in the unique properties of water. Water has a high boiling point (100° C) and more energy is needed than would be expected to break the hydrogen bonds. Molecules of water at the freezing temperature are further apart than in the liquid state. This difference is the reason that ice, being less dense than the liquid, will float on water. Water

(H_2O) molecules are pulled equally in all directions as they bond, except at the surface of the liquid. Here the molecules are pulled inward to form a **surface tension**. This phenomenon explains why a water glass can be filled just slightly over the rim and why a thrown flat rock or a water spider can skim across the surface.

The chemical combination of a substance with water is called **hydration** (the saturation of tissue in the body is also called hydration). Salt dissolves in water when the negative chloride ions are pulled away from the sodium ions. The negative chloride ions are attracted to the positive hydrogen end of the molecule, while the positive sodium ions are attracted to the negative oxygen force. This arrangement weakens the ionic bond of the salt (NaCl), causing it to dissolve into the water. Substances with polar covalent bonds may also dissolve in water; for example, a sugar molecule's positive end is attracted to the negative oxygen end of the water molecule, and its negative end is attracted to the positive hydrogen end.

Water is important and necessary to life on this planet. It serves as a solvent for salts, gases, and other molecules necessary for biological activity. The hydrogen bonding of water is important to maintain the active structures of proteins and genetic substances in the body. Water carries molecules to functional areas of the body, penetrating membranes using a passive transport system called osmosis.

CARBON BONDING

Carbon is the backbone of organic molecules. Compounds containing carbon are called **organic compounds**. Carbon atoms are the most versatile building blocks. They have four valence electrons and form four chemical bonds to complete their outer layer. One of the unique qualities of carbon is its ability to bond with other carbon atoms to form chains of varied numbers and length. They can form straight chains, branched chains, or be arranged in closed rings (Figure 5-7). They also form covalent bonds with other elements, mainly with hydrogen, nitrogen, oxygen, and sulfur. When two carbon atoms bond to each other, they may share two or three electrons to fulfill the required valence electrons. When two

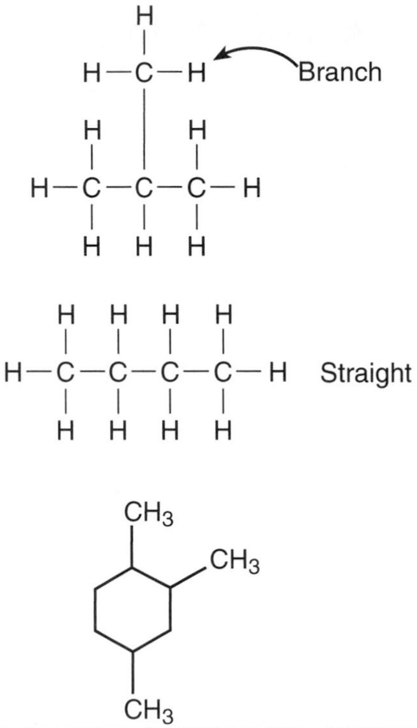

Figure 5-7 Straight chain, branched chain, and closed ring carbon structures.

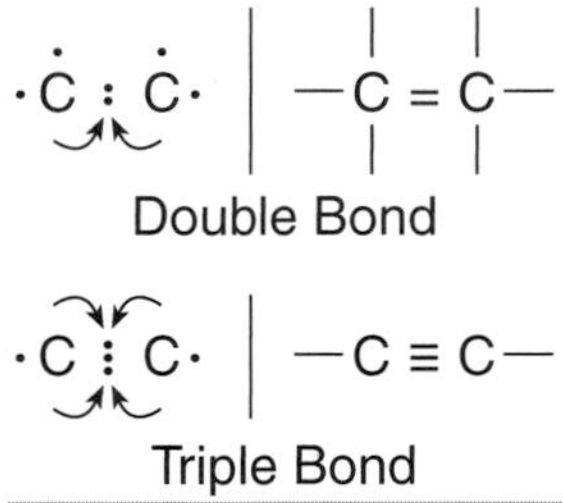

Figure 5-8 Carbons share electrons to form double and triple bonds.

Figure 5-9 Carbon dioxide.

carbon atoms share two electrons each they form a **double bond**, when they share three electrons each they form a **triple bond** (Figure 5-8). Carbon can also form double bonds with other elements, such as the two double bonds it forms with oxygen to form carbon dioxide (CO_2) (Figure 5-9). In Chapter 8, double bonds explain the meaning of saturated and unsaturated fats.

HYDROCARBONS

Hydrocarbons are the foundation of all essential oil compounds. Hydrocarbons are structures consisting of nothing more than hydrogen atoms bonded to carbon atoms. When carbon and hydrogen bond, they form very stable, nonpolar bonds.

For Your Information

Hydrocarbons as Fuel

The breakdown product that results from the decomposed remains of organisms that lived millions of years ago is composed mainly of hydrocarbons. After a refining process, this hydrocarbon product is called petroleum, the fossil fuel that lights up the living room and powers your transportation to work.

ISOMERS AND CHIRALITY

Variations occur in the three-dimensional arrangement of organic molecules because of carbon's ability to bond with itself, forming chains, branches, and ring shaped molecules. It has become important to know which variation, or structural arrangement, is being used in medicines and natural health. **Isomers** are molecules that have the same summary formula, meaning the number and type of atoms is the same, but a different structural arrangement of the atoms in the molecule. Your hands have the same summary formula, four fingers, a thumb, etc., but differ in their three-dimensional arrangement, which becomes obvious when you put one on top of the other. Isomers have different properties and activities from each other (Figure 5-10).

A special case of **structural isomers**, which have a variation in the covalent arrangement of the atoms, is called **enantiomers.** Enantiomers are molecules with almost identical formula and arrangement, their only difference being its symmetry. They are a mirror image of each other. Enantiomers, being mirror images, are like a right and left hand. Objects that cannot be superimposed on their mirror image, like hands, are called **chiral.** Enantiomers are two chiral molecules (Figure 5-11).

Synthetics and Chirality

Synthetic compounds are not always chirally correct. An example of chiral molecules is found in the common form of

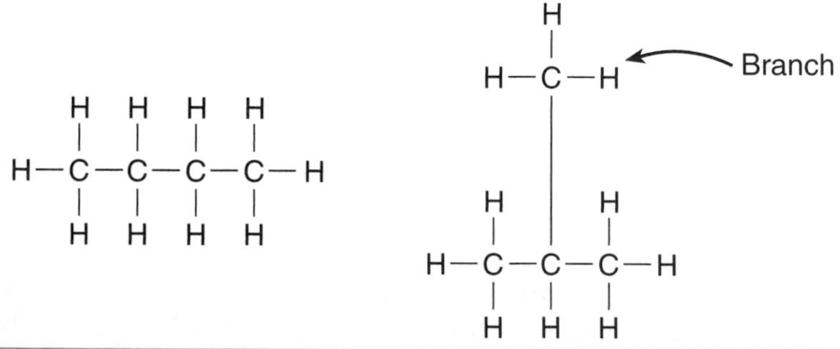

Figure 5-10 Two C_4H_{10} isomers. One is a straight chain and the other is a branched chain. Both compounds contain 4 carbon atoms and 10 hydrogen atoms, it is only their arrangement that is different.

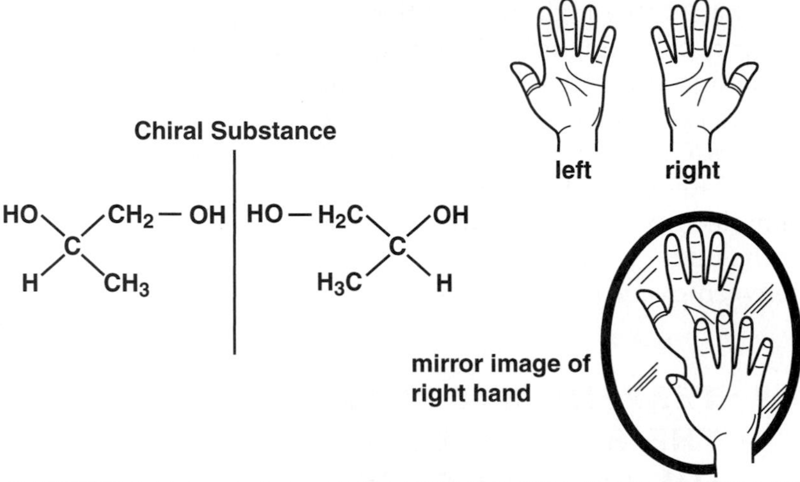

Figure 5-11 Molecules that are similar in every way but cannot be superimposed on each other are called enantiomers. This is the same as a right and left hand, which are constructed of the same elements but do not match when placed one on top of the other, and do match when facing each other as if they were a mirror image.

vitamin E used in many supplements and skin care. The vitamin E compound, alpha-tocopherol, can be derived from nature, and is the single enantiomer that is labeled as d-alpha-tocopherol. The synthetic vitamin E is a 50:50 mix of both enantiomers, labeled dl-alpha-tocopherol. The d- represents the right enantiomer and l- is the left. The term used for this 50:50 mixture is **racemic mix.** The natural d-enantiomer has better bioavailability and is more effective as a nutrient and antioxidant.

Pharmaceutical companies and cosmetic chemists are claiming to produce chirally correct molecules for use in drugs and skin care. Some compounds created in labs are meant to duplicate fragrant compounds in essential oils. These compounds are useful only to produce synthetic fragrances and have nothing to do with aromatherapy. From the perspective of holistic health and aromatherapy, substances should be used that are extracted from nature in the already chirally correct form.

Using a natural extract means that you are using the correct enantiomer. Using a synthetic version of chiral molecules usually means using the racemic mix not found in nature. The synthetic enantiomers can create side effects, such as irritation, or may have other toxic possibilities. An example of the possible dangers of mixing enantiomers is the drug Thalidomide, prescribed in the 1960s as a sleep aid and for morning sickness during pregnancy. The drug was a combination of two enantiomers. One enantiomer produced the sedative effect, but the other caused birth defects.[2] Common sense supports the use of molecules in their natural state for harmonious interaction in the body, which is a consequence of years of co-evolution between plants and humans.

TERPENE HYDROCARBONS: THE BACKBONE OF ESSENTIAL OIL COMPONENTS

Terpenoid compounds, or **terpene hydrocarbons**, are hydrocarbon compounds and the most abundant components in essential oils. These molecules are made up of multiples of a five carbon atom unit called an **isoprene unit**. A prefix is used to describe the size of the terpene molecule based on how many isoprene units the compound contains. The prefix *mono-* tells you that the molecule contains two isoprene units or 10 carbon atoms; a *sesqui-* prefix would mean the terpene compound contains 15 carbon atoms, or three isoprene units; the prefix *di-* comes before a terpene containing 20 carbon atoms; and *tri-* represents a compound with 30 carbon atoms (Table 5-2). Monoterpenes and sequiterpenes are the most abundant in essential oils. Because of their molecular weight, the diterpenes are found in only a few oils; an example is the sclareol compound found in clary sage. Triterpenes are not found in essential oils.

Table 5-2 Carbon Atoms in Terpene Compounds
• *Mono-* denotes a 10 carbon atom structure.
• *Sesqui-* denotes a 15 carbon atom structure.
• *Di-* denotes a 20 carbon atom structure.
• *Tri-* denotes a 30 carbon atom structure.

THE STRUCTURE-EFFECT DIAGRAM

Essential oils may have many, sometimes contradictory, therapeutic properties. This variation is caused, in part, by the complexity of essential oil composition, biological phenomena, and the intricacies of human physiology. This variation is also the reason that identifying individual components, and their activity, within an essential oil is useful. The **Structure-Effect Diagram** (Figure 5-12) is a chart that connects essential oil components to pharmacological effects. The diagram offers guidance to the therapeutic selection of essential oils by visually sorting benefits, activity, and functions of the chemical families, or groupings, of essential oil components. This diagram is a functional tool to classify essential oils according to their chemical composition and physical properties. One advantage of the Structure-Effect Diagram is that it is not necessary to be a chemist to use it. Use the Structure-Effect Diagram as your individual interests or understanding dictates. This chart can be used as a visual tool that uses common language, such as positive, dry, or calming, or for a study of the sciences on which it is based. Remember that the Structure-Effect Diagram is limited by its reductionist methodology and that essential oil use tends to be much broader and less predictable in practice.

Positive and Negative Charge

The Structure-Effect Diagram, largely introduced by Pierre Franchomme and Daniel Pénoël in their book *l'aromathérapie exactement*,[3] organizes the compounds contained in essential oils according to their ability to donate electrons (nucleophilic and negative force) or attract electrons (electrophilic and positive force). Franchomme discovered that essential oils and their isolated components give off an electrical charge that corresponds to their ability to either donate an electron or uptake an electron. The action of giving up or donating an electron affects the surrounding area and molecules.[4] This influence is then translated into the calming, energizing, or other properties of essential oils.

Polarity

The horizontal axis of the diagram represents polarity; that determines the degree that the molecule is hydrophilic (wet)

Table 5-3 Structure-Effects of Essential Oil Compounds

• Positive charge	– energizing, yang quality
• Negative charge	– calming, yin quality
• Lipophilic polarity	– dry, strongly repels water, non polar
• Hydrophilic polarity	– wet, more harmony with water, weakly non polar

or lipophilic (dry). Polarity describes the degree of attraction or aversion oils have to water. The hydrophilic essential oils and compounds do not mix with water. They have an affinity with water, seen by the way they spread out across the surface when dropped into water. The lipophilic oils have a tendency to bead up, with more resistance to water.

Positive and negative charge and polarity all influence the effects of essential oil compounds, as summarized in Table 5-3.

The Yin and Yang of It

Using terminology from traditional Chinese medicine, the positive charge may be portrayed as *yang*, with the qualities of aggressive, energizing, hot, and stimulating; or *yin*, which has the qualities of calm, soothing, cool, and relaxing.

Like the Eastern yin and yang, other interesting and metaphoric interpretations have been used along with the Structure-Effect Diagram. These interpretations include associating Hippocratic temperaments or the Ayurvedic doshas to the structure effects of essential oils.

READING THE STRUCTURE-EFFECT DIAGRAM

The electric charge and polarity of the essential oil compounds determine much of their character. They can be electropositive and polar; electronegative and polar; electropositive and non polar; electronegative and non polar; or neutral. The compound's electric current and polarity combine to create a specific therapeutic activity that is illustrated within the parameters of the Structure-Effect Diagram. Knowing what

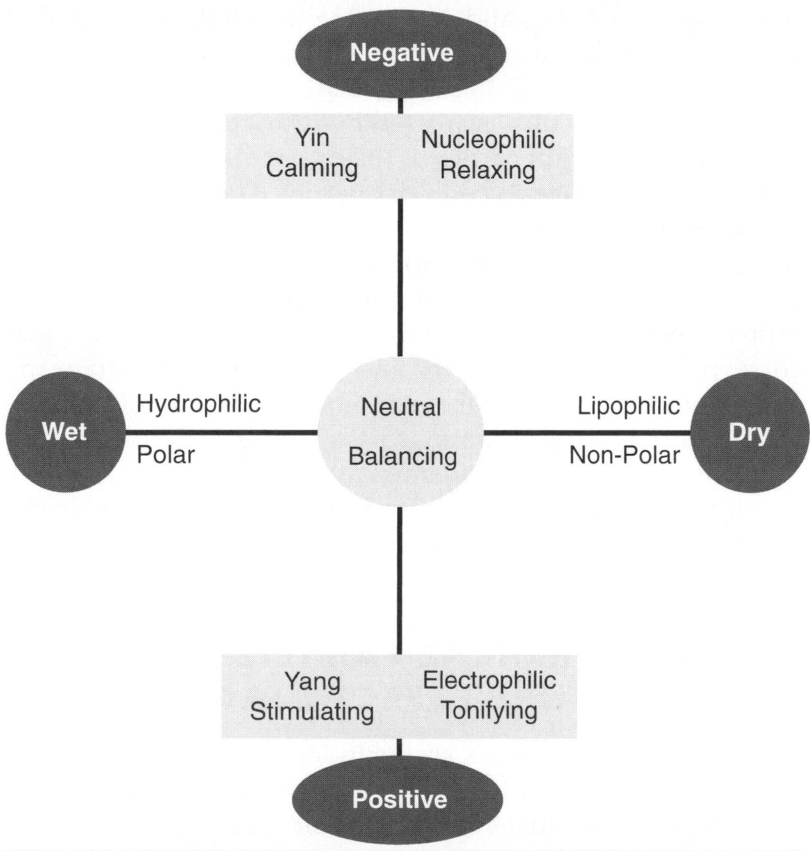

Figure 5-12 The Structure-Effect Diagram organizes the essential oil chemical family groupings by their electropositive or electronegative force (shown by their vertical position) as well as their polarity (shown by their horizontal position).

combinations of activity are contained within the oil will guide you to its use in aromatherapy (Figure 5-12).

The Color Connection

The features established in the diagram can be coded by color. An electropositive compound has an energizing, stimulating, and warming pharmacological effect on the body. The associated color is red. A compound with an electronegative charge is calming, soothing, and cooling. Blue is the color that best represents these qualities. These characteristics can be built into a usable model for selecting oils. If the symptom is hot and irritated, such as inflammation, the obvious remedy would be a soothing and cooling compound. A compound that has electronegative cooling effects is a good choice for inflammation.

A rainbow of color is created by drawing a line from the lower, hot/wet, right corner of the diagram through the neutral center to the upper, cool/dry corner. The rainbow begins as a deep red to orange and changes to green just beyond the neutral center; it ends at the upper right corner as blue. This is how nature provides assistance to help us identify the properties of essential oils. Some essential oils are the color that corresponds to their activity and position on the diagram. A blue oil, such as German chamomile, contains compounds that give it an anti-inflammatory, cooling activity. The red hued oils (oregano and cinnamon are good examples) are hot, irritating, and contain compounds associated with the lower left, hot, and irritating side of the diagram (Plate 1).

THE CHEMICAL FAMILIES ON THE STRUCTURE-EFFECT DIAGRAM

Twelve chemical families are included on the diagram. The structure of a molecular compound determines the family it belongs to. Essential oils contain hundreds of known compounds. Most of these compounds can be categorized into a particular grouping on the Structure-Effect Diagram. For instance, pinene and limonene are two differing compounds common to essential oils. Limonene and pinene are members of the monoterpene hydrocarbon grouping, because they have a related structure that defines the composition of this group. This method of grouping compounds is similar to the way an orange and an apple are categorized as fruits by the features that define members of the fruit family. See Plate 2 to see where the chemical groups are positioned on the Structure-Effect Diagram.

Functional Groups

—OH

Figure 5-13 The structure unit OH, called the hydroxyl group. When this functional group is attached to a terpene compound it is defined as an alcohol.

Functional groups are structure elements, an atom or groups of atoms usually containing oxygen or nitrogen, that bond to hydrocarbons. See Figure 5-13 for an example of a structure element. Functional groups cause changes in the hydrocarbons, making them more chemically reactive. Most of the chemical activity of the compound occurs at the site of the functional group. Many of the molecular groupings in the Structure-Effect Diagram are compounds that have a functional group attached. The benefits derived from these compounds stem in large part from the activity of the functional group.

Naming Chemical Groups

Nomenclature, the naming of the chemical, describes the structure and sometimes other features of the chemical compound. Knowing why a group or component is so named is not entirely necessary. For most aromatherapists, knowing the chemical families, where they are on the diagram, and the properties associated with them is enough to accommodate an accurate understanding of the chemical compounds and enable selection of essential oils for therapeutic results.

USING THE DIAGRAM

This system permits a more symptom specific selection of essential oils. A dry cough requires a different compound and essential oil than a cough that contains mucous. As the properties for each family are described, one can see how a selection for a dry cough includes compounds from the hydrophilic side of the diagram. A symptom such as the dry cough can be incorporated onto the chart. If the dry cough is associated with an inflamed condition, it would be associated with the lower right, positive/dry side of the chart. A selection of oils that include compounds in a family positioned on the opposite side would most likely alleviate the symptoms.

This is a very simplified instruction for using the Structure-Effect Diagram. You will ultimately find that there are variations for this method. This simplified method provides a starting point for use of the Structure-Effect Diagram. See how symptoms and conditions of the skin relate to the diagram in Plate 3.

ESSENTIAL OILS AND THE STRUCTURE-EFFECT DIAGRAM

Essential oils contain many compounds. Some essential oils are simple, containing a few family types that are easily defined and found on the diagram. Other essential oils contain a vast amount of compounds from several chemical families. Essential oils also contain compounds that are unknown or are categorized in a different way than that found on the diagram. Most of an essential oil's activity comes from its most prevalent compounds. The oils described in Chapter 7 include their most predominant compounds. Remember that the composition of an essential oil is a synergistic blend of many compounds, and you should not limit the activity and properties to individual compounds. Secondary and trace compounds within the essential oil may not be identified on the Structure-Effect Diagram but may still offer profound therapeutic activity.

The concept underlying the diagram is to guide you to a more accurate use of essential oils in aromatherapy and to also alert you to contraindications. The diagram can also help you choose alternate oils that contain similar compounds or contain a wider variety of compounds for more holistic therapeutic action.

THE CHEMICAL FAMILIES

The descriptions of the chemical families includes essential oils that contain high amounts of each family as well as the physiological activity and psychological properties of the compounds. Some examples of specific compounds are also included in the description of a chemical family.

The compounds within a chemical family are often identified by a suffix added to their name. This suffix helps further define and associate a single essential oil component with a chemical group. The endings do not specify whether the compound has 10 carbon atoms, 15, or more, identified by the prefixes mono, sesqui, and di (see Table 5.2). A compound from the monoterpene and the sesquiterpene group will both end in *-ene*. The suffix will not alert you to the size, sesqui or mono, of the terpene hydrocarbon.

This list and the Structure-Effect Diagram are a limited representation of the compounds found in essential oils. Many compounds found in essential oils are not included in the text or noted on the diagram.

Monoterpene Hydrocarbons

The **monoterpene hydrocarbon** is the most basic essential oil molecule, and it is found in most essential oils. This molecule

is a terpene hydrocarbon containing 10 carbon atoms, which may be written as C-10 hydrocarbon. It is found in the highest concentrations in citrus and needle oils. The suffix *-ene* defines the terpene hydrocarbons. Two examples are the monoterpene hydrocarbons pinene and limonene (Figure 5-14).
Essential oils: needle tree oils, such as cypress, pine and spruce; citrus oils such as grapefruit, lemon and orange; frankincense
Properties: stimulating, tonic, diuretic, anti-viral

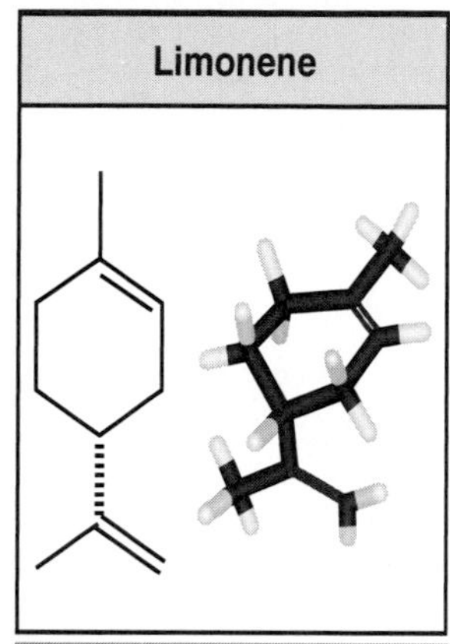

Figure 5-14
The monoterpene (C-10) hydrocarbon limonene.

Sesquiterpene Hydrocarbons

The 15 carbon (C-15) sesquiterpene molecules are compounds that, in general, make up about 10–20 percent of the total composition of the essential oils that contain them. The sesquiterpene is a larger molecule with a higher viscosity and lower **volatility,** or evaporation rate, than monoterpenes. Essential oils containing high amounts of sesquiterpenes tend to be dark in color, such as the blue color of azulene, and are also thicker or more viscous than oils composed mostly of monoterpenes. The sesquiterpenes, being terpene hydrocarbons, also end in *-ene.* Two examples are caryophyllene and chamazulene.
Essential oils: German chamomile, *Helichrysum italicum* (everlasting)
Properties: anti-inflammatory, anti-allergic, cooling

FUNCTIONAL GROUPS

The following list of chemical families contains bonded functional groups. The functional groups form some of the most versatile and useful properties in aromatherapy. Each chemical family is named for their functional group.

Monoterpene Alcohols

These components are considered the most beneficial and safest of the essential oil compounds. **Monoterpene alcohols** are defined by a hydroxy group, an oxygen and hydrogen combination (-OH), bonded to a C-10, monoterpene hydrocarbon (Figure 5-15). Essential oils high in monoterpene (C-10) alcohols are effective antiseptics. Because of their low toxicity, they

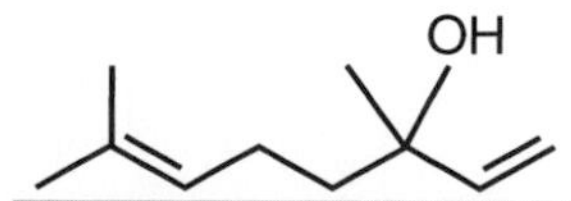

Figure 5-15
A monoterpene alcohol compound, linalool.

can be used every day in skin care and as a general tonic. One of the features of these molecules is the pleasant fragrance they contribute to an essential oil. Monoterpene alcohols are identified by the suffix *-ol* in their names. Linalol, menthol, and geraniol are monoterpene alcohols.
Essential oils: Lavender, MQV, palmarosa, peppermint, rosemary, tea tree, ylang-ylang
Properties: Antiseptic, immune stimulant, bactericidal, energizing (except linalol, a sedative in lavender and others), **tonic** (strengthening, or toning, to the body or to a specific area or organ), low toxicity

Sesquiterpene Alcohols

When a hydroxy group (-OH) bonds to a C-15, sesquiterpene hydrocarbon, the resulting molecule is called a **sesquiterpene (C-15) alcohol.** These molecules are an interesting, diverse, and beneficial group in aromatherapy. Their properties are similar to those of the monoterpene alcohols, although each individual C-15 alcohol has unique properties. Because of the size of these compounds, they tend to be more viscous. This quality creates a beneficial character for skin care by slowing down evaporation and absorption of the oils, allowing a topical application to sit longer on the skin and provide a kind of time release for the therapeutic properties. Sesquiterpene alcohols, with an *-ol* ending, include cedrol and santalol.
Essential oils: sandalwood, cedarwood, frankincense, ginger, patchouli
Properties: Properties vary according to the oil. General properties include: liver support and glandular stimulant, anti-inflammatory, tonic for the muscles and nerves, and general skin care (especially mature and dry skin conditions)

Diterpene Alcohols

When a free hydroxy group (-OH) is attached to a diterpene alcohol, the resulting compound is a diterpene alcohol, also called a diterpenol. The structure of the diterpene alcohol resembles human steroids (hormones). Though these compounds may resemble human hormones it is not certain that they are accepted in the same way by the chemoreceptors of the cells. The most popular diol is sclareol, found in clary

sage. Clary sage is recognized as one of the best essential oils for hormone, specifically estrogen, imbalance.
Essential oils: clary sage
Properties: Best known for hormone and menstrual cycle balance

Monoterpene Aldehydes

A monoterpene (C-10) **aldehyde** has an oxygen atom attached by a double bond to a carbon, a **carbonyl group,** at the end of a hydrocarbon chain, along with a hydrogen atom attached to one side of the same carbon atom (Figure 5-16). Citral and citronellal are C-10 aldehydes, which are responsible for the lemon fragrance common to many essential oils including lemon, melissa, and lemongrass. Aldehydes are often used in perfumery and fragrance. The main properties of the C-10 aldehydes are their sedative and anti-inflammatory activities. Low concentrations have demonstrated the most profound of these effects, and studies have shown that sedative and anti-inflammatory effects are decreased at higher concentrations.[5] Increased irritant effects may also occur at higher concentrations. Aldehydes end in *-al,* as in citral and neral.
Essential oils: lemon verbena, melissa, citronella, *Eucalyptus citriodora*
Properties: antiseptic, anti-inflammatory, anti-viral, hypotensive, sedative
Contraindications: Can be a skin irritant when used undiluted or in high concentrations.

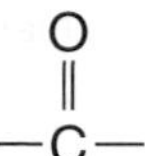

A: Carbonyl group

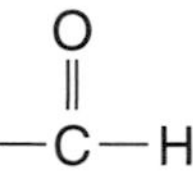

B: Aldehyde group

C: Geranial

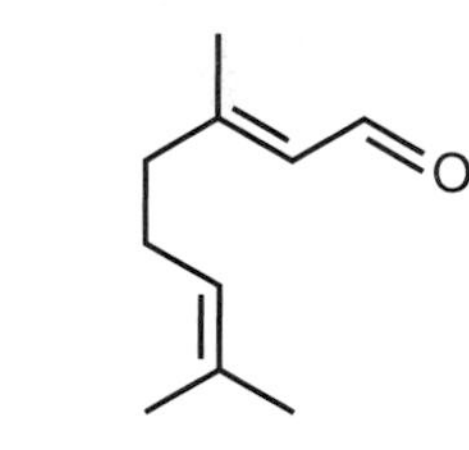

Figure 5-16 An aldehyde (A) contains a carbonyl group (B). an oxygen atom double bonded to a carbon) at the end of the carbon chain with a hydrogen atom attached to the carbon atom of the carbonyl group. The aldehyde Geranial (C).

Monoterpene Ketones

When the carbonyl group of a C-10 hydrocarbon is surrounded by carbon atoms on either side, it is called a monoterpene (C-10) ketone (Figure 5-17). Ketones are one of the most beneficial compounds for skin care, though they are also the one molecule that carries the most notorious contraindications as potential neurotoxins and abortifacients. Ketone compounds and the essential oils that contain them are useful as mucolytic agents. **Mucolytics** are able to liquefy and break down hardened mucous and other respiratory debris. Thujone and verbenone are ketones, which are identified with the *-one* ending.

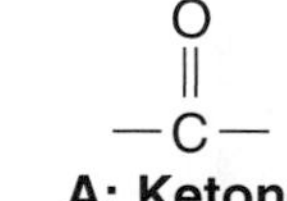

A: Ketone

B: 3-Octanone

O

Figure 5-17 A ketone contains a carbonyl group attached within the carbon chain with carbon atoms on either side of it (A). The ketone 3-Octanone (B).

Essential oils: *eucalyptus dives, Euc. polybractea*, hyssop, mugwort, rosemary verbenone type, thuja
Properties: promotes tissue and cell formation, mucolytic
Contraindications: neurotoxic, abortive

Sesquiterpene Ketones and Diketones

The action of the sesquiterpene (C-15) ketones and diterpene (C-20) ketones vary, depending on the specific molecule. Two examples of C-15 ketones are nootkatone, the molecule that gives grapefruit its fragrant identity, and atlantone in cedarwood. Italidione, a diketone, is a cell regenerative molecule that makes *Helichrysum italicum* the ideal regenerative skin conditioning essential oil used in aromatherapy.

32 Linalyl acetate

Figure 5-18 When an alcohol reacts with an acid it forms an ester compound. Pictured is the ester linalyl acetate.

Monoterpene Esters

Esters are fragrant compounds formed when a carboxylic acid reacts with an alcohol. Linalol, a monoterpene alcohol, reacts with a carboxylic acid to construct the ester linalyl acetate. Esters' fruity fragrance and sedative and antispasmodic properties make oils with ester compounds highly favored for use in aromatherapy. Esters are useful compounds for treating and preventing fungal infection; especially notable for this purpose is geranium. The ending *-ate* is a common suffix of ester compounds, such as bornyl acetate and geranyl tiglate (Figure 5-18).
Essential oils: lavender, bergamot, birch, clary sage, Roman chamomile, *Inula graveolens*, wintergreen
Properties: anti-inflammatory, anti-spasmodic, balancing to central nervous system, calming, fungicidal

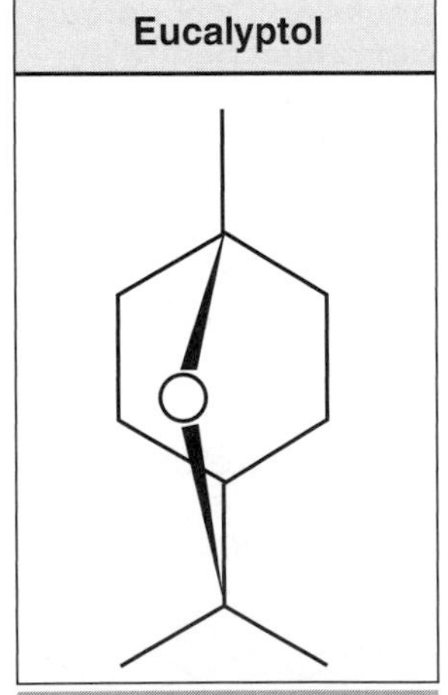

Figure 5-19 When an oxygen atom is integrated into a terpene ring system it is called an oxide. Pictured is the oxide 1,8 cineole or eucalyptol.

Monoterpene Oxides

The compound that emits the identifying scent of eucalyptus is an **oxide,** 1,8 cineole, also known as eucalyptol. The antiviral and expectorant activity of oxides, found in eucalyptus oils, tea tree, and ravensare are useful to treat colds and flu (Figure 5-19).
Essential oils: eucalyptus oils (especially globulus and radiata), tea tree, ravensare, MQV, green myrtle
Properties: anti-viral, expectorant

Phenols

The **phenol** group contains the most powerful antimicrobial compounds used in aromatherapy. Phenols are defined by an alcohol functional group (-OH) attached to an **aromatic compound**, a very stable class of compounds because of its equal distribution of the electrons. *Aromatic compound* is simply a chemical term and has nothing to do with aromatherapy or the aroma of the compound. The alcohol group in phenols is attached to the aromatic compound **benzene.** This is a 6 carbon, cyclic structure, an **aromatic ring,** containing three double bonds (Figure 5-20). Essential oils do not contain the synthetic, carcinogenic benzene that you may be familiar with as a solvent. The compounds in essential oils have a carbon side chain that brings the total carbon count to 10. Phenols end in *-ol* because of the attached alcohol functional group.

Because of their aggressive activity, essential oils containing phenols are potential irritants and not the best choice for skin care. The most common use of the phenolic essential oils is for infections and as disinfectants.

Essential oils: oregano, thyme (thymol type), savory
Properties: anti-fungal, anti-parasitic, strong bactericidal, heart tonic, immune stimulant, strengthening, warming
Contraindications: skin irritant, liver toxin (with prolonged use and high internal dosages)

PHENYLPROPANOIDS

Not all compounds found in essential oils are terpenoid hydrocarbons. Some occur as phenylpropanoids, a family of

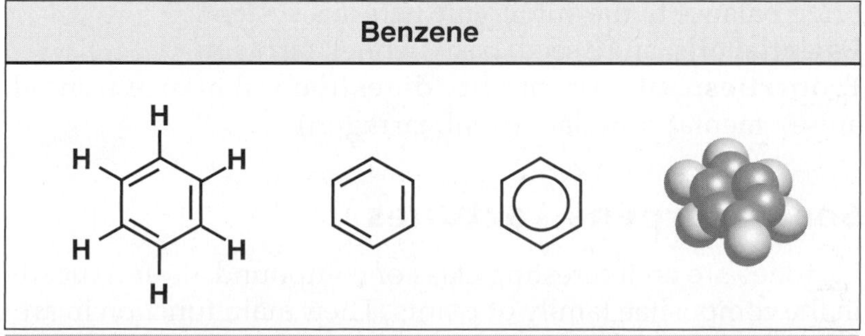

Figure 5-20 The benzene ring system, also called an aromatic ring, with its stable arrangement of 6 carbon atoms.

compounds resulting from the fatty acid or amino acid metabolism of the plant. Phenylpropanoid compounds contain two aromatic ring structures. The phenylpropanoids are classified in two categories for structure-effect identification. In one group are the "hot" compounds, which tend to have a strong antimicrobial effect, and the other group contains the "mild" compounds that can reduce stress. These in the second group are called the phenylpropane ethers.

Phenylpropanes

The "hot" group of phenylpropanoids includes two main components: cinnamic aldehyde and eugenol. These compounds are extremely beneficial for treating microbial infection and creating equilibrium during illness. Clove, with its high eugenol content, has been used in dentistry for infection and as an analgesic. As with phenols, avoid topical use or use them in very low dosages to avoid contact dermatitis and skin irritation.

Bay laurel is an interesting and beneficial oil, in that it derives some useful properties from its eugenol content without having topical irritant qualities.

Essential oils: cinnamon, clove, bay laurel
Properties: similar to those of phenols; analgesic (clove)
Contraindications: skin irritant, possible liver toxin at high dosages

Phenylpropane Ethers

Ethers are mild phenylpropanes and are well known for their soothing and antispasmodic properties. They are used to bring balance to the autonomic nervous system.

Essential oils: anise seed, basil, fennel, tarragon
Properties: anti-spasmodic, digestive imbalance (fennel, anise), mental stimulant (basil, tarragon)

Sesquiterpene Lactones

Lactones are an interesting class of compounds found mostly in the compositae family of plants. Their main function in aromatherapy is as a very powerful mucolytic.

Essential oils: Inula graveolens
Properties: strong mucolytic,[6] anti-inflammatory[7]
Contraindications: used with caution because information regarding lactones is scarce

IDENTIFYING A COMPOUND BY THE SUFFIX

The ability to identify a compound by its suffix is helpful when the compound of an essential oil is listed but not the group the compound belongs to. In this chapter, the common suffix, when applicable, has been included with the description of each chemical family. Because phenols, terpene alcohols, and some phenylpropane compounds all contain alcohol functional groups, the compounds in these families end with the suffix *-ol*. If you are reading through the literature and find a compound that is identified ending in an *-ol* but is not associated with a group (alcohol, phenylpropane, or phenol), you may identify it by making an educated guess according to the activity of the essential oil. If it lists irritating qualities, you may assume there are phenols or phenylpropanes present. Situations like this may be challenging if you don't have a chemical background. This deduction will get easier as you progress in your work with essential oils. This detective work is also one reason why it is helpful to understand the properties of all the chemical families and to learn how reference books like this one help you to be more thorough in your aromatherapy practice.

Aspects of the Structure-Effect Diagram

The Structure-Effect Diagram can be used to demonstrate several aspects of the chemical families. In Figure 5-21 the diagram is used to show some of the properties that each of the groupings, or more accurately the chemical compounds within the group, may have. Figure 5-22 contains essential oils that contain higher amounts of, or whose effects are strongly influenced by, the chemical group. Some of the molecular components found in essential oils are listed within their chemical group in Figure 5-23.

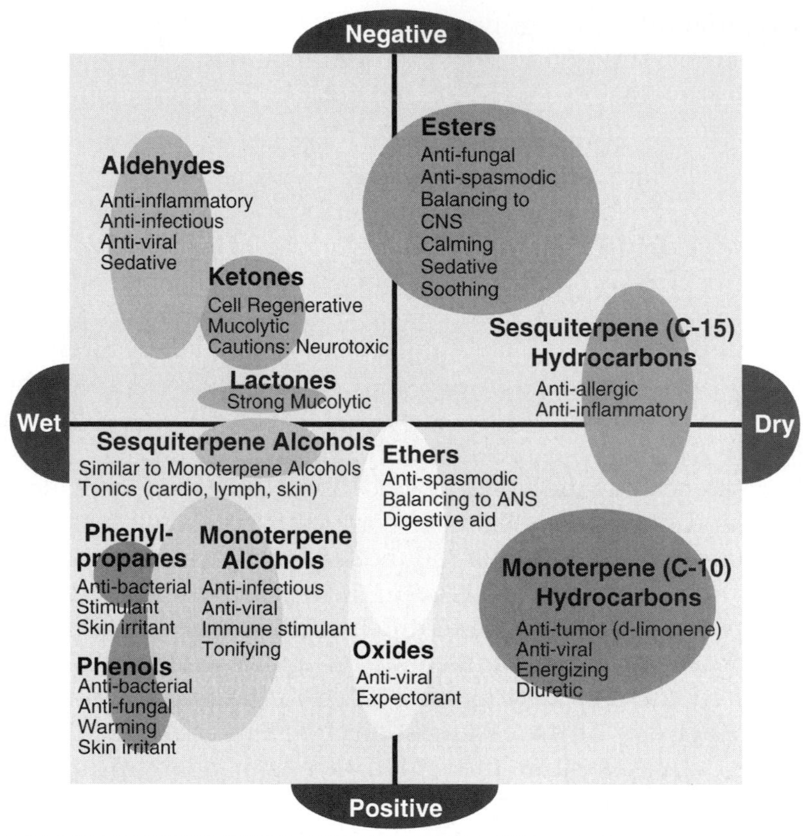

Figure 5-21 The therapeutic properties associated with each of the chemical groupings.

TRACE ELEMENTS

Essential oils contain many trace elements. Trace elements are those compounds that exist in very minute quantities but add an action or character that contributes in significant ways to the end result.

Coumarin

Coumarin is a trace element not included among the chemical families of the Structure-Effect Diagram. It is a compound produced within the same biosynthetic pathway as the phenylpropanes. Coumarins are found in many essential oils and considered one of the most pharmacologically active compounds. Coumarins provide a distinctive woodruff aroma and contribute spasmolytic properties to the oils that contain them.

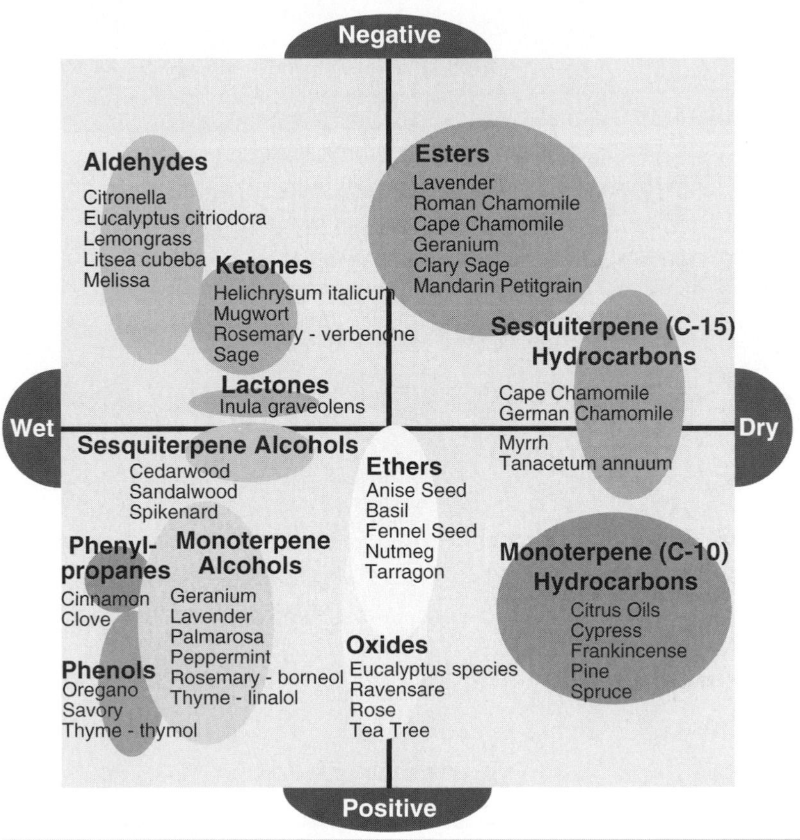

Figure 5-22 The essential oils associated with the chemical groupings. Essential oils contain many compounds and are listed here to show the compounds they may be most influenced by.

Essential oils: lavender, bergamot, angelica, khella
Properties: anti-spasmodic,[8] cooling, relaxing, sedative, nerve tonic

CHEMOTYPES

An interesting phenomenon takes place when a plant of one specified botanical origin produces oils of distinctly different chemical composition. The reason this variation happens is not entirely known, but the influences seem to be geographic location, altitude, photosynthesis, climate, and possibly genetic factors. Examples of this phenomenon are the *Thymus vulgaris* species and *Rosmarinus officinalis.* The main component found in the essential oil of these plants varies, depending on where the plant is grown.

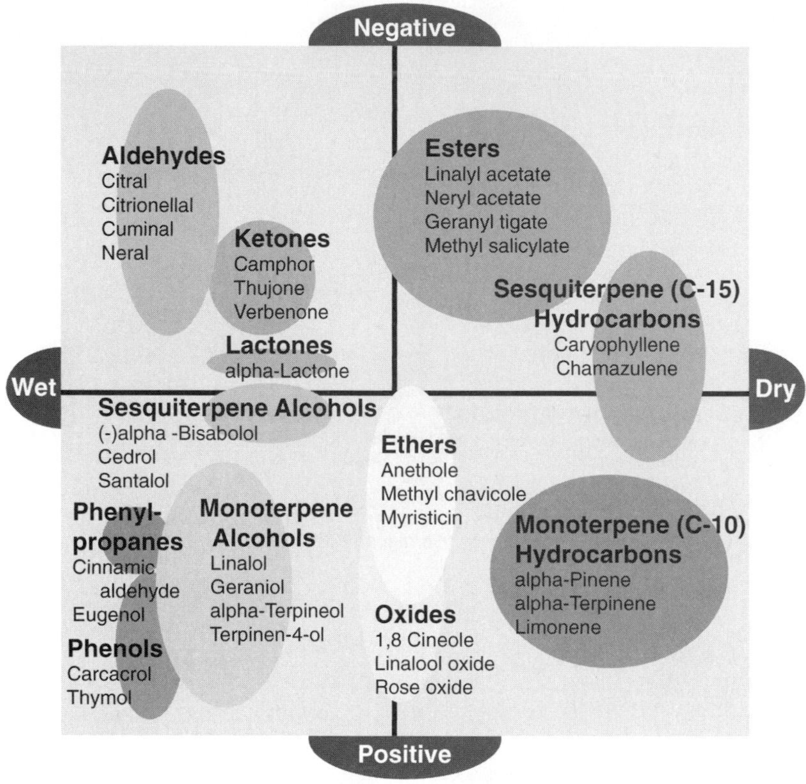

Figure 5-23 Some of the chemical compounds that are within the associated families of the Structure-Effect Diagram.

Different chemical composition produced by a plant from one specified botanical origin is called **chemical polymorphism.** In the case of rosemary (*Rosmarinus officinalis*) and thyme (*Thymus vulgaris*), the chemical composition can vary dramatically. These oils are identified not only by their botanical origin but are also identified by their main (active) components. These components are called **chemotypes.** In this instance, the molecule that best describes the main composition of an essential oil is tagged at the end of the oil's name. The oil extracted from *Rosmarinus officinalis* that contains a high amount of borneol is called borneol type. Cineol and verbenone types also exist. The most common *Thymus vulgaris* chemotypes used in aromatherapy are thymol, geraniol, linalool, and thujanol. The way these oils are used in aromatherapy depends on the chemotype of the essential oil and the properties that the main chemical component gives to the oil.

Chemotypes (CT) of *Thymus vulgaris*
Thymus vulgaris CT geraniol (Thyme geraniol type)
Thymus vulgaris CT linalol (Thyme linalol type)
Thymus vulgaris CT thujanol (Thyme thujanol type)
Thymus vulgaris CT thymol (Thyme thymol type)
Thymus vulgaris CT carvacrol (Thyme carvacrol type)
Chemotypes (CT) of *Rosmarinus officinalis*
Rosmarinus officinalis CT borneol (Rosemary borneol type)
Rosmarinus officinalis CT camphor (Rosemary camphor)
Rosmarinus officinalis CT 1,8 cineole (Rosemary cineole type)
Rosmarinus officinalis CT verbenone (Rosemary verbenone)
Chemotypes (CT) of *Eucalyptus polybractea*
Eucalyptus polybractea CT 1,8 cineole (*Eucalyptus polybractea* cineole type)
Eucalyptus polybractea CT crypton (*Eucalyptus polybractea* crypton type)

AUTHOR'S **NOTE**

HOW DO YOU USE THE STRUCTURE-EFFECT DIAGRAM?

You just made your way through some intense essential oil chemistry. Congratulations. I'd like to explain a few ways that I found the Structure-Effect Diagram useful. To begin with, if you aren't a chemist and have little interest in the chemistry of the oils, you can use this chart as a visual reference and guide to selecting essential oils. One technique is to use the color coding and symptom comparisons discussed in the section titled *The Color Connection.*

Skin provides a good example of how to use this information to select an essential oil. A rash or skin irritation is associated with, if not the actual color of, red. The lower left corner of the diagram is red. Follow the diagonal line from red to its opposite end. You are now in blue, at the upper right corner. The sesquiterpene hydrocarbons are the group that sits in this area. The compound chamazulene, a sesquiterpene hydrocarbon, is blue. This compound is found in the blue oils, German chamomile, *Tanacetum annuum*, and Cape chamomile. These are essential oils that would be selected to "cool" a red, irritated skin condition.

Continued

Be attentive to the composition of essential oils. They contain anywhere from a few to hundreds of different compounds. If you look at the properties of lavandin, which contains mostly linalool, linalyl acetate, and a few other compounds, you can assume that these two compounds will define the main properties of lavandin. The essential oil of wild lavender also contains mostly linalool and linalyl acetate. The difference is that wild lavender contains over 200 compounds, with almost every family in the diagram represented. This diversity accounts for lavender's exceptionally therapeutic properties. The diverse healing properties of lavender are well known. By looking at the Structure-Effect Diagram, you can see that lavender's diversity in healing is a result of the diversity in its structure (Figure 5-24).

Bay laurel contains compounds that, when placed on the chart, circle around the center. This pattern may be interpreted as suggesting that bay laurel is a balancing essential oil, which it is thought to be. Anise seed is quite the opposite but results in a similar suggestion. The essential oil contains around 90% anethole, a phenylpropane ether. This compound is positioned at the neutral mark of the chart. Anise seed, with a 90% concentration of a self-balanced compound, is considered balancing. From my own experience, I would have to say this is true of both anise seed and bay laurel. Anise is used to raise the activity of the parasympathetic nervous system and creates balance in times of stress when the flight or flight response is in overdrive. Bay laurel helps to balance the lymph system, bringing movement to congested lymph.

In my kindergarten days of aromatherapy, I owned a limited collection of essential oils. I referred to many books and used the recipes included. Time and again, a recipe called for an essential oil I didn't have. The solution came from looking up the essential oil composition and seeing where the compounds appeared on the Structure-Effect Diagram. If the recipe called for geranium, but I didn't have any, I could replace it with palmarosa, an oil composed primarily of geraniol, an important component in geranium. Geranium, because of its similarities to rose, would fill in for the more expensive rose essential oil. Roman chamomile could be replaced with clary sage or other oils that contain higher amounts of sedating ester compounds. This technique does not provide exact replacements and depends on the effects you're looking for. There is no exact replacement for any essential oil, because individual composition is the factor that gives an oil its unique qualities and personality.

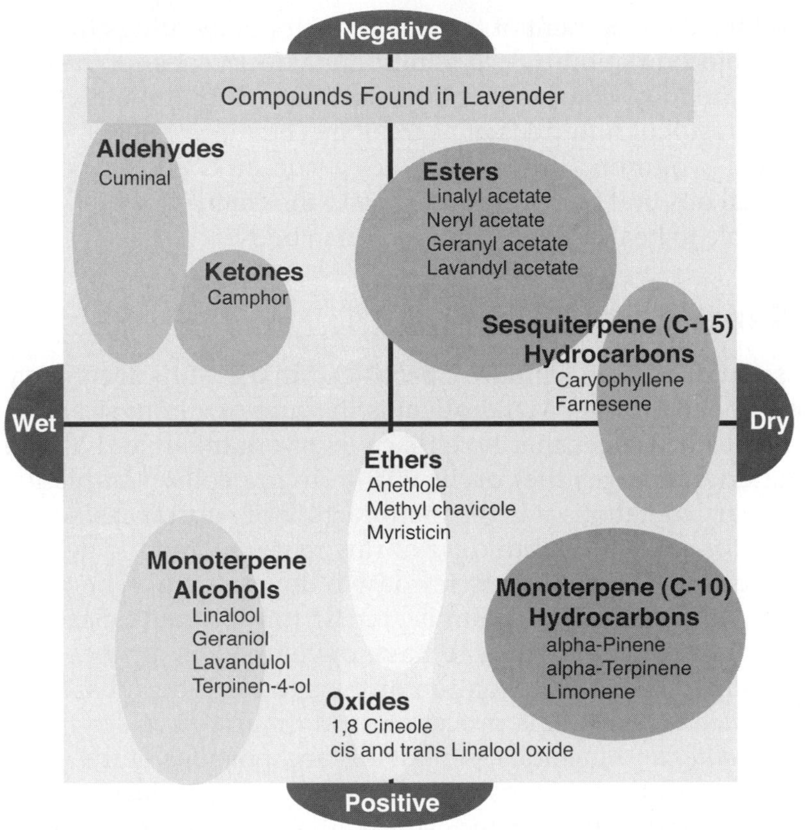

Figure 5-24 Lavender contains many compounds. This diagram gives a visual representation of the compounds contained in lavender. You can see that lavender contains compounds distributed throughout the diagram. This may help you to understand lavender's diverse activity. Keep in mind that this diagram does not show the ratios of the chemical compounds contained in lavender. To be visually accurate the circles representing the monoterpene alcohol group and the ester group would be the largest as lavender generally contains between 30–45% linalool, a C-10 alcohol and 30 – 45% linalyl acetate, an ester.

BIOLOGY OF ESSENTIAL OILS COMPOUNDS

Dr. Kurt Schnaubelt has written a valuable biological perspective of terpene molecules, essential oils, and the place they hold in human evolution.[9,10] This perspective has spawned a deeper understanding of essential oil use and its compatibility with the human body. Schnaubelt's analysis of plant biology and the development of terpenoid compounds brings to light the "biocompatibility, tolerability, and effectiveness of the natural chemical compounds that comprise essential oils [that] are a result of hundreds of years of biochemical trial and error called evolution."[11] It is the biology, not the chemistry, of essential oils that helps us comprehend the extent to which they are able to heal and protect the human body.

Plant Metabolism

Essential oils are primarily produced in a plant's secondary metabolic process. **Metabolism** is the sum of all physical and chemical changes that take place in an organism and all the material changes that occur within living cells.[12] In plants, primary metabolism is the manufacture of substances necessary for energy, the building of raw material and oxygen, or those materials necessary for day to day survival. The process of primary metabolism is similar for all plants. Secondary metabolism appears to have developed as a process to aid survival and propagation of the species. The substances produced during this process are summarized as *secondary metabolites* and include essential oils and portions of the plant that are useful as drugs and medicines.[13] Secondary metabolites found in many species of plants may have evolved as a response to protect the plant from pathogens, the environment, or herbivores. Essential oil components of secondary metabolic process also function as attractants for pollinating insects. The actions of secondary metabolites, or essential oils, within a plant are mimicked when used for human health, sexual attraction, and repelling insects.

BIOSYNTHESIS: SOME THINGS NEVER CHANGE

Throughout evolution, life has maintained its ongoing system of biosynthetic pathways. A **biosynthetic pathway** is the chain of events that occurs in the formation of chemical compounds in a living organism.[14] The chemicals used by mammals and all living organisms are produced, changed, restructured and eliminated using enzymes, water, and other compounds and atoms in a process called **biosynthesis**. All living organisms, from one-celled bacteria to human beings, use identical pathways to generate important molecular structures. The biosynthetic pathway that forms essential oil compounds, the terpenes, has been in place since very early on in life's history. The very earliest one-celled life forms had a triterpene structure that is generated through the same biosynthetic pathway used by mammals to form cholesterols and hormones.[15]

Terpenoid compounds, which represent the bulk of essential oil components, are within the biosynthetic pathway that builds many vital structures including hormones, carotenoids, and cholesterol.[16] This fact supports the logic for use of natural substances, such as genuine and authentic essential oils, over synthetics and is summed up by Dr. Kurt Schnaubelt: "Essential oils possess emergent properties of whole organisms and interact with humans in ways not available to agents (aka synthetic drugs) which do not share with us common evolutionary development."The biosynthetic pathway of terpenoid compounds was especially useful in the study of terpene compounds and tumor apoptosis, or cell death.[17] The results showed that the compounds, including limonene, would shut off the mechanism necessary for cell strength, causing only the tumor cells to die, leaving the healthy cells unaffected.[18]

ESSENTIAL OILS AND HUMANS: THE EVOLUTIONARY CONNECTION

An overview of evolution may seem far removed from the practical use of essential oils and aromatherapy. Understanding evolutionary concepts is valuable for comprehending the harmony natural substances have in the human body, the genetic relationship we share with plants, and the biological similarities between plants and humans that may be influential in the therapeutic properties of essential oil use. In general, these areas of study lend depth to the concepts of holistic health.

Humans' Botanically Rich Evolutionary Environment

The evolutionary link humans have with the plant kingdom is expressed within the body's structure, chemistry, and genetics. The human race's intimate association with the plant

For Your Information

Actions of Terpenoid Compounds

Schnaubelt expresses the importance seen in the relationship between terpenoid compounds and human physiology by stating "how intricately the synthesis of terpenoids in animal or plant cells is connected to the chemistry of life."[19] Terpenoid compounds may influence human physiology or psyche by:

- Inducing the attachment of lipophilic anchors, which bind proteins to cell membranes.
- Precipitating changes in calcium ion transport through the cell membrane.
- Acting as precursors to sex hormones and steroids.
- Interacting with cholinergic receptors of the autonomic nervous system.

Cholinergic receptors release acetylcholine, a neurotransmitter at the neuromuscular junctions responsible for nerve to muscle response.

kingdom has progressed to become an interdependent relationship. The exchange of carbon dioxide (CO_2), used by plants and emitted by animals, is an example of this interdependence. The oxygen (O_2) emitted by plants is essential to maintaining animal life. Humans cannot survive without the carbohydrates and nutrients plants provide, and we benefit as well from other materials derived from plants, which provide shelter, medicines, tools, and clothing.

By the time humans appeared on the planet, the plant kingdom was fully established, though like all life forms, it continues to adjust and evolve with the environment and in reaction to other life forms. Plants, in their development of the secondary metabolites, have been using essential oils as communicators long before humans existed. As humans evolved, the planet's atmosphere was rich in the terpenoid compounds emitted by plants. This history reveals a very intimate relationship between humans and the fragrant essential oils of the plant kingdom. Response and attraction to the aromas of flowers in bloom, a mountain forest, and a field of sweet grasses are a consequence of the evolutionary familiarity with plant odorants.

EMERGING PROPERTIES

Life is highly organized into a hierarchy of structural levels. **Emerging properties** are the special quality that arises from the hierarchical order at each stage of development. A cat is composed of many of the same elements, molecules, and organs as a dog. So, what gives a cat its distinctive qualities? The elusive personality and other cat traits result from properties that emerge from the union of atoms, molecules, and organs. The parts themselves cannot explain the uniqueness of a cat. And this situation does not end with cats as a group. Each cat also has its own emergent design that results in the individuality of the single cat. Emergent properties are a biological interpretation of this phenomenon.

Everything evolves with emerging properties. Atoms, which become specific atoms because of the emerging properties of the subatomic particles that build them, bond to form molecules, each with its own, very specific, set of properties that include and expand on the properties of its atomic parts. This process continues with the development of cells, and cells into organisms. Life on this planet is a composition of emergent properties that developed from the structure of hierarchical levels. From the "Big Bang" to atomic chemistry to molecular structure to the formation of planet earth to the emergence of cells to organism to human beings, hierarchical emergent properties are evident. Where in the process of emerging properties, from atom to cell, does life begin?

Emerging Properties and Holism

Emergent properties are illustrated in order to better comprehend the actions of essential oils, the unique physiology of the human being, and the resulting interaction between the two. The myriad healing possibilities and results that may occur with aromatherapy serve as a constant self-reminder that both essential oils and humans are a consequence of emergent properties.

The description that is often used to explain these emergent properties is "the sum of the whole is greater than the individual parts." Collaboration exists among all of the individual structures in an organization, which the individual parts could not achieve on their own or without the complicity of the other parts. Neil Campbell, editor of *Biology,* explains it this way: "The organism we recognize as an animal or plant is not a random collection of individual cells, but a multi-cellular cooperative."[20] The concept of holism used in this text is inspired by the knowledge that humans are not a series of parts but are a multi-cellular cooperative.

THE INDIVIDUAL VS. THE BIOLOGICAL WHOLE

We began this chapter with a review of the individual compounds and chemical families contained in essential oils. Though much of the effectiveness of essential oils may be understood from its chemical properties, the pharmacological approach of focusing on one active component has limitations in truly uncovering the potential for therapeutic possibilities derived from essential oils. This disconnect is evident when one acknowledges emerging properties and the co-evolution of plants and mammals. Essential oils are complex in their action and do not easily fit into **reductionist** pharmacology.

Reductionist science believes that the "properties of the whole can be reduced to the effects of single components."[21] Reductionism ignores the relationships that exist between the parts. Reductionist pharmacology looks at an individual component of the essential oil, such as cineole in tea tree oil, and identifies the activity of the whole oil with the properties of this one molecule. This approach ignores the overall activity of the emerging properties of the cineole with the other compounds that compose tea tree oil. Isolated cineole is not the same as the cineole in the composition of the whole oil.

The interaction of the essential oils and human physiology also cannot be reduced to the oil, or individual compound, interacting with one single cell or one system. The holistic biological responses to essential oils on the physiology and psyche of the human being, including the sensory impact, must be considered in the therapeutic use of essential oils. Precise evaluation and prediction of results with essential oils are not always possible, because of the complexity and multitude of interactions with mucous membranes, the endocrine, limbic, and nervous systems, the digestive and respiratory tracts, and other systems of the body.

CHAPTER SUMMARY

The sciences of chemistry and biology are used to support and understand the therapeutic activity of essential oils. In this chapter, a review of basic chemistry, including atoms, chemical bonding and polarity, is provided as a foundation to understand the structure and function of essential oil compounds. The Structure-Effect Diagram, a system that depicts chemical families, terpene hydrocarbons, and functional groups, is introduced to illustrate the molecular structures of essential oils. The Structure-Effect Diagram is a tool and guide to selecting essential oils for their therapeutic properties and functions expressed by their chemical activity. Selection and use are further developed through the introduction of biological concepts such as that of emerging properties and the co-evolution of plants and animals. These newly developed ideas strengthen comprehension and holistic use of aromatherapy.

REVIEW QUESTIONS

1. How do the sciences of chemistry and biology support the use of essential oils?
2. What is organic chemistry?
3. Describe two features of a terpene hydrocarbon.
4. What features of the chemical family does the Structure-Effect Diagram represent?
5. How can the Structure-Effect Diagram be used to select a symptom specific formula of essential oils?
6. What are emerging properties and how do they relate to holistic aromatherapy?

CHAPTER REFERENCES

1. Clancy, C. (2001). Acting Director, Agency for Healthcare Research and Quality. Presentation before the House Subcommittee on Oversight and Investigation. May 23, 2001.
2. Campbell, N., Reece, J. & Mitchell, L. (1999). *Biology* (5th edition). Menlo Park, CA: Benjamin Cummings.
3. Franchomme, P. & Pénoël D. (1990). *L'aromathérapie exactement.* Limoges, France: Roger Jollois Editeur.
4. Schnaubelt, K. (1995). *Advanced Aromatherapy: The Science of Essential Oils.* Rochester, VT: Healing Arts Press.
5. Wagner, H. & Sprinkmeyer, L. (1973). "Über die pharmakologische Wirkung von Melissengeist." *Deutsche Apootheker Zeitung 113* (30): 1159–1166.
6. Schnaubelt, K. (1985). *The Aromatherapy Course.* San Rafael, CA: Pacific Institute of Aromatherapy.
7. Lyb, G., Knorre, A., Schmidt, T. J., Pahl, H. L. & Merfort, I. (1998). "The anti-inflammatory sesquiterpene lactone henenalin inhibits the transcription factor NF-KB by directly targeting p65." *The Journal of Biological Chemistry 273* (50): 33508–33516.
8. Veterinary Institute of Integrative Medicine. (n.d.). *Dong quai.* Accessed on July 25, 2007 at http://www.viim.org.
9. Schnaubelt, K. (2002). *Biology of Essential Oils: Pacific Institute of Aromatherapy Masters Series.* San Rafael, CA: Terra Linda Scent and Image.
10. Schnaubelt, K. (2002). *Chemistry of Essential Oils: Pacific Institute of Aromatherapy Masters Series.* San Rafael, CA: Terra Linda Scent and Image.

11. Schnaubelt, K. (1999). *Medical Aromatherapy: Healing With Essential Oils.* Berkeley, CA: Frog, LTD.
12. Venes, D. (ed.) (1997). *Tabor's Cyclopedic Medical Dictionary* (18th edition). Philadelphia, PA: F. A. Davis Company.
13. Schnaubelt, K. (2002). *Biology of Essential Oils: Pacific Institute of Aromatherapy Masters Series.* San Rafael, CA: Terra Linda Scent and Image.
14. Venes, D. (ed.) (1997). *Tabor's Cyclopedic Medical Dictionary* (18th edition). Philadelphia, PA: F. A. Davis Company.
15. Schnaubelt, K. (2001). *Chemistry of Essential Oils; Pacific Institute of Aromatherapy Masters Series.* San Rafael, CA: Terra Linda Scent and Image.
16. Herbert, R. (1989). *The Biosynthesis of Secondary Metabolites* (2nd edition). New York, NY: Chapman and Hall.
17. Schnaubelt, K. (ed.) Franchomme, P. (2000, November). "Pharmacology of R (+)-limonene and some citrus peel essences." In: *Essential Oils and Cancer. Proceedings of the 4th Scientific Wholistic Aromatherapy Conference.* San Rafael, CA: Terra Linda Scent and Image.
18. Schnaubelt, K. (ed.) Elson, C. E., Peffley, D., Hentosh, P. & Mo, H. (2000). "Functional consequences of isoprenoid-mediated inhibition of mevalonate synthesis: Application to cancer and cardiovascular disease." In: *Essential Oils and Cancer. Proceedings of the 4th Scientific Wholistic Aromatherapy Conference.* San Rafael, CA: Terra Linda Scent and Image.
19. Schnaubelt, K. (2001). *Chemistry of Essential Oils: Pacific Institute of Aromatherapy Masters Series.* San Rafael, CA: Terra Linda Scent and Image.
20. Campbell, N., Reece, J. & Mitchell, L. (1999). *Biology* (5th edition). Menlo Park, CA: Benjamin Cummings.
21. Weil, A. (1995). *Spontaneous Healing.* New York, NY: Alfred A. Knopf.

Therapeutic Effects of Essential Oils

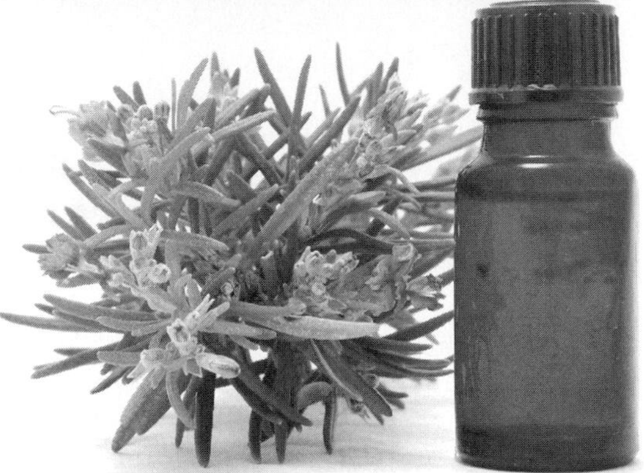

CHAPTER 6

My medical training made me want to flee from the world of invasive, technological treatment toward a romantic ideal of natural healing.[1]

–*Andrew Weil*

LEARNING OBJECTIVES

1. Increase your knowledge of the therapeutic uses for essential oils.
2. Recognize the activity of an essential oil in relation to its molecular components.
3. Review useful and valuable essential oil research and clinical results.
4. Discover why essential oils pose little risk when used appropriately.
5. Examine the contraindications for safe and correct use of essential oils.

THERAPEUTIC PROPERTIES OF ESSENTIAL OILS

The value of essential oils comes from their ability to act as healing agents. Their therapeutic properties are found in individual components as well as the combination of components within specific oils. The Structure-Effect Diagram and the chemical groupings in Chapter 5 are basic information needed to understand the activity and properties of the individual components that make up essential oils. A deeper evaluation of these therapeutic properties will help you to become more proficient in their use and function in aromatherapy.

Antiseptic and Antimicrobial Properties

The antimicrobial (antibacterial, antifungal, antiviral) action of essential oils is one of the most successful applications in aromatherapy. Antimicrobial properties are well documented by extensive research and evaluation. Essential oils are used to treat bacterial and viral infections of the throat or as disinfectants to protect wounds. Aromatherapy is an accepted remedy for the common cold and other viral infections. The broad antimicrobial properties of tea tree oil have made it one of the most popular medicinal oils used in many applications including treatment for warts or athlete's foot. The antimicrobial use of essential oils is strongly supported by valid scientific research.

Gattefossé provides several studies of antimicrobial activity including a 1918 experiment that successfully prevented and cured influenza.[2] The current use of essential oils as a room disinfectant is supported by the 1954 study by Kober and Keller demonstrating the airborne antimicrobial activity of essential oils.[3] French hospitals make use of the antimicrobial properties of essential oils by disinfecting against airborne fungus and bacteria.[4] In 1995, Dr. Rolf Deininger reviewed the activity of essential oils and concluded that they were especially effective against infections of the respiratory system, skin infections, and diseases of the gastrointestinal and urinary tracts.[5]

To explain the antimicrobial properties of essential oils, most studies focus on individual compounds, such as the phenol compound, thymol, found in thyme oil. This approach may limit the true knowledge of how essential oils actually work. One study demonstrated the antibacterial effectiveness of low phenol containing thyme oils to be equal to high phenol containing oils.[6] This result supports the position that there is more to understanding how essential oils work than merely knowing about the isolated activity of individual components.

Antibacterial Essential Oils: An Alternative to Antibiotics

The use of essential oils may prove to be a more effective and safer alternative than pharmaceutical antibiotics. Bacteria do not become resistant to the effectiveness of essential oils, as they do with antibiotics. Dr. Daniel Pénoël at the *Aroma '93* conference emphasized the harmony essential oils have with the body over antibiotics by saying, "where antibiotics inflict extensive damage on human bacterial flora, essential oils respect the integrity of the necessary 'friendly' bacteria of the organism, a condition for true and lasting healing."[7] Michael Schmidt, et al., in the book *Beyond Antibiotics,*[8] describe the negative aspects of overuse of antibiotics and the proven detriment to health:

- They kill bacteria but foster the development of bacteria resistant to antibiotics.
- They may undermine immune response.

Antibiotics have saved many lives and have a purpose in health and healing. Only abuse and overuse of these substances have made them a danger to health. Essential oils may one day prove to be an effective replacement for antibiotics. Their antibacterial applications could help decrease the overuse of antibiotics and allow those powerful pharmaceuticals to be used for more serious cases of infection.

If you are a non-medical licensed practitioner you should ensure safety and account for the restrictions of law by presenting the use of essential oils for preventive measures, rather than for treating bacterial infections.

Effectiveness of Essential Oils against Viral Infection

Antiviral properties of essential oils fill a void in health care and medicine that has not been resolved by pharmaceutical chemistry. Essential oils are extraordinarily effective at halting viral activity. The use of essential oils against viral infections extends well beyond the common cold or flu. Recent research has shown essential oil of lemongrass to be effective against the herpes type-1 virus.[9] The virus, varicella-zoster, that produces shingles, has been successfully treated with a combination of 50 percent *Calophyllum inophyllum* and 50 percent *Ravensare aromatica*.[10]

Here again is a situation in which essential oils provide the benefit of prevention as well as treatment.

Essential Oils for Fungal and Yeast Infection

The use of essential oils, especially tea tree, in the treatment of **candidiasis,** an infection with the yeast *Candida albicans*, is well documented.[11,12] Essential oils are used for several types of fungal infection including ringworm, toe fungus, and vaginal yeast infection. Geranium, lavender, oregano, and tea tree are oils that have antifungal properties.

Topical application of essential oils provides relief from a variety of fungal and yeast related infections. The benefits of tea tree oil in treating seborrheic dermatitis, thought to be associated with the Malassezia yeast, was demonstrated in a study published by the *American Journal of Clinical Dermatology*, validating the use of this oil in treatment shampoos.[13] Tea tree oil has been used successfully to treat tinea pedis, or athlete's foot. Several oils are mentioned in the aromatherapy literature for clearing ringworm, tinea corporis, from the skin, including *Eucalyptus pauciflora*, an oil that contains high amounts of citronellal and is similar to the more common *Eucalyptus citriodora*.[14]

ANTI-INFLAMMATORY PROPERTIES

The ability of essential oils to reduce inflammation makes them a valuable treatment for skin care. German chamomile (*Matricaria recutita*) and *Helichrysum italicum* are best known for reducing inflammation. German chamomile tested as effective as steroidal and non-steroidal.[15] Both oils are high in anti-inflammatory sesquiterpene hydrocarbons. Helichrysum is renowned for its effectiveness in reducing hematoma (bruising) and swelling when applied immediately after an injury, especially a sports injury. *Tannacetum annuum* (sometimes called Moroccan chamomile) is unrivaled in its application for allergic responses and inflammation.[16]

Essential Oils for Anti-Inflammatory Skin Care

Considering the fact that all imbalances of the skin result from or include symptoms of inflammation,[17] the protection to the skin provided by the anti-inflammatory properties of essential oils warrants their use in all skin care formulas. Essential oils offer everyday protection from inflammation when included in a skin care maintenance program. Essential oils are also valued as an effective treatment and anti-inflammatory relief of burns, sun damage, rashes, hives, and insect bites. See Table 6-1 for a list of beneficial essential oils that are highly effective for use on inflammatory skin conditions.

Counter-Irritation

Some irritant essential oils also have an anti-inflammatory action. These oils, clove, thyme (thymol type), and oregano, may trigger secondary biochemical reactions called counter-irritation. In this situation, the irritation caused by the oil triggers an anti-inflammatory action within the body. This response is accomplished with very small amounts of the irritant oil because larger amounts ultimately cause inflammation.

Table 6-1 Essential Oils for Inflammatory Skin Conditions
Black pepper (*Piper nigrum*)
Cape chamomile (*Eriocephalus punctulatus*)
Eucalyptus globulus
Frankincense (*Boswellia carterii*)
German chamomile (*Matricaria Recutita*)
Helichrysum italicum
Kunzea ambigua
Lavender (*Lavandula angustifolia*)
Myrrh (*Commiphora molmol*)
Tanacetum annuum
Yarrow (*Achillea millefolium*)

SEDATIVE PROPERTIES

Probably the most popularized effects in aromatherapy are the sedative properties of essential oils. Lavender is generally marketed for its ability to calm stressed nerves and for providing relief from insomnia.[18] Many oils are listed as being sedative, calming, and relaxing, especially those oils that contain large amounts of ester and aldehyde compounds. Some of the most effective sedative compounds are citral and citronellal,[19] found in melissa and lemon verbena, and the linalool[20] and linalyl acetate compounds common in lavender and ylang-ylang. Research demonstrates that these essential oil compounds produce a strong sedative action.

Stress and Skin Care

Stress and anxiety are factors that potentially cause many disruptive skin conditions. Considering the holistic effects of an oil such as lavender, you can see how this oil can be used as a beneficial treatment that would address both the physical skin condition, such as acne or inflammation, and the stress related issues that may be aggravating the condition. Many beneficial skin treatments using essential oils are formulated with this dual action in mind. Use of essential oils from the list in Table 6-2 may help relieve the tension and stress that create symptoms of imbalance in the skin.

Table 6-2 Stress Reducing and Calming Essential Oils
Anise seed (*Pimpinella anisum*)
Bergamot (*Citrus aurantium ssp. bergamia*)
Cape chamomile (*Eriocephalus punctulatus*)
Cardamom (*Elettaria cardamomum*)
Clary sage (*Salvia sclarea*)
Lavender (*Lavandula angustifolia*)
Mandarin petitgrain (*Citrus reticula*)
Melissa (*Melissa officinalis*)
Neroli (*Citrus aurantium*)
Roman chamomile (*Anthemis nobilis*)
Rose (*Rosa damascena*)
Tarragon (*Artemisia dracunculus*)

Appropriate Use of Sedative Oils

More is not better for sedative effects. Testing the sedative results of essential oils demonstrated that the lowest concentrations were most effective for sedation, 1 milligram per kilogram of body weight. This amount equals approximately 2 to 5 drops of essential oil per 70 kilograms (154.3 pounds) body weight.[21] Higher concentrations actually *reduced* the sedating effects.

In practice, 2 to 5 drops is more essential oil than you are likely to absorb at one time, because you will be learning to dilute them. If you are using essential oils to scent a room, the desirable amount is at the level of detection. Avoid over diffusing the oil so much that it is considered overpowering. Chapter 8 includes application methods and is a guide to determine the effectiveness of lower concentrations.

ANTISPASMODIC PROPERTIES

The essential oils with higher ester content, such as lavender, neroli, and Roman chamomile,[22] are well suited to relieve spasms caused by tension and nervousness. The soothing effects on the nervous system make ester containing oils the choice for spasms related to nervous tension and stress. Digestive spasms, often related to anxiety and stress, are alleviated with anise seed, cardamom seed[23] and coriander seed.[24] Their main components are phenylpropane ethers. These ether-containing oils tend to be ideal for digestive spasm or nervous stomach.

The ester content of clary sage often soothes premenstrual discomfort[25] and cramping.[26] It also has estrogen like qualities and is used to balance female reproductive issues. Clary sage is then a holistic treatment, with esters to subdue the symptoms and a sesquiterpene compound that balances the hormones that may be the cause of these symptoms.

EXPECTORANT AND MUCOLYTIC PROPERTIES

Eucalyptus oils are known for their ability to clear the lungs and sinuses. This action comes from the expectorant and mucolytic properties of the eucalyptus oils, primarily *Eucalyptus globulus*, *Eucalyptus radiata*, and *Eucalyptus polybractea*. The oxide compound, eucalyptol (1,8 cineole), is largely responsible for their expectorant activity. 1,8 cineole is also found in other essential oils, such as tea tree, MQV, and ravensare.[27,28] These oils tend to have a synergistic composition that includes strong antiviral properties. The expectorant activity of the essential oils is most effective at low dosages and through inhalation. The dosage should be at a level where the aroma is faint or not detectable.

Oils that contain ketone components and sesquiterpene lactones are able to soften or liquefy mucus and clear the bronchial capillaries. *Eucalyptus dives* is a safe ketone containing oil with beneficial mucolytic action.

CELL REGENERATIVE AND WOUND HEALING PROPERTIES

Essential oils are particularly useful to condition and heal the skin. Gattefossé's interest in aromatherapy was enhanced by his experience with the wound healing properties of lavender. Many essential oils, such as frankincense, *Helichrysum italicum,* and rose, have an established use in skin care because of their cell regenerative properties. Essential oils that contain large amounts of ketone compounds are generally best for cellular regeneration and wound healing.[29] Oils of *Eucalyptus dives* and rosemary verbenone, with the ketone compounds piperitone and verbenone, respectively, are used in skin care extensively with satisfying results. Helichrysum contains a diketone that offers extraordinary wound healing properties. Helichrysum provides enhanced benefits to any skin care treatment including acne, eczema, psoriasis and wrinkle reduction.[30,31] The use of essential oils for healthy cell regeneration supports all skin conditions including a healthy aging benefit.

Many essential oils assist in proper and healthy regeneration of the skin. This quality is assumed to be, in part, a result of their antioxidant properties. Quite a number of essential oil components have antioxidant activity.

Seeing Is Believing

The wound healing activity of essential oils is often profound and one of the more intriguing properties of the oils. Seeing how quickly healing takes place when applying essential oils to a burn, a cut, or a surgical wound offers visible proof that essential

AUTHOR'S **NOTE**

PERSONAL EXPERIENCES WITH ESSENTIAL OILS

The opportunity to personally test essential oils will present itself to you. Once you've had this experience, it will provide the proof you need to inspire your continued use. This event happened to me, and to all my aromatic associates. We all have personal stories that are the inspiration that keeps us involved in aromatherapy. Many of the formulas I include in this text are a result of a personal experience. My experiences have been many including the use of antimicrobial oils to successfully put an end to my son's chronic childhood ear infections. I treated my own third degree burn using lavender and German chamomile followed by antimicrobial and cell regenerative oils. My healing was clean and left no scarring. These are both relatively serious conditions that you do not want to attempt without full awareness of what you are doing. Even with less serious conditions you'll soon be able to tell tales of aromatic success and share these with other people, your friends, family and clients.

oils assist biological functions of the body. Lavender and German chamomile's wound healing properties have been successfully used on aging patients with slow-to-heal wounds.[32] Ron Guba, an Australian aromatherapist, used his formulation skin cream on elderly patients and demonstrated healing in 12 weeks, rather than the 26 weeks required for healing in the control group.[33]

MODERN AROMATHERAPY: RESEARCH AND CLINICAL STUDIES

To define modern use of essential oils in aromatherapy we begin with Gattefossé, who was the first to conduct scientific studies that focused on therapeutic essential oil activity according to their principal constituents. He believed that the action of the oil was attributable to individual components, though he did support the use of the whole oil. An emphasis on individual components allows for adulteration to achieve a correct balance of therapeutic compounds. The focus on active compounds alone should be limited and not seen as the complete understanding of the therapeutic results of the essential oil. This view has already been expressed in this text and is also the standard mantra of many clinicians and researchers who view the combination of individual compounds as necessary to provide a therapeutic result. This point was made earlier in reference to the non-phenolic containing thyme oils being equally antimicrobial to those containing the phenolic compounds. Some experimental results cannot be explained by the chemistry of individual compounds; therefore, the results may be ignored by reductionist science. At this time, essential oils, though well studied, still remain a somewhat mysterious treatment modality. The therapeutic validity of essential oils will develop as more holistic procedures are put into place or methods are developed for analysis that incorporate non-specific and holistic activity of the oils within the body plus the synergistic activity of the complete, not just the known active compounds of, essential oil.

Many published studies that relate to the use of essential oils are available. These can be accessed through the Internet, on sites such as http://www.pubmed.com, or other research related search engines. Published research results may vary dependent upon the study design and variables studied. As a general rule, studies conducted on animals may not parallel results found in studies using humans under true clinical conditions.

PAUL BELAICHE'S AROMATOGRAM: STUDIES OF ANTI-MICROBIAL EFFECTIVENESS

In 1979 Paul Belaiche published *Traité de Phytothéapie et d' Aromathérapie*, a three volume work demonstrating the antimicrobial effectiveness of essential oils. This study has become an important work that has advanced the practical use of essential oils. In this work, Belaiche uses the aromatogram to test the ability of the whole oil, or individual compounds, to inhibit or kill specific microorganisms. His tests were carried out in labs using 40 different essential oils as well as in clinical studies treating illnesses such as angina, bronchitis, malaria, sinus infection, and tuberculosis. Belaiche's work is documented with charts that compare each oil's effectiveness against specific microorganisms. The ability of the essential oil against the

AUTHOR'S **NOTE**

LIVING IN A "PROVE IT" SOCIETY

When I began my aromatherapy studies I did not fully question the information I was hearing. I liked what I was hearing. I knew enough about herbs and nutrients from my previous studies that I was not a novice in natural healing. I approached essential oils with open curiosity. I wanted essential oils to do the magic they were proposed to do. I didn't want written proof. I wanted essential oils to perform. I wholeheartedly, and without hesitation, began using them. They did all the things I was expecting of them. Wait, sorry: I'm still bald. Then again, that was my own wishful thinking, not anything I was told the oils would change.

Valid studies are available that provide proof that essential oils heal. My interest in the oils extends to wanting to know the mechanisms, or how they work in the body. I find studies to be useful and sometimes fascinating. There's no doubt of the value of having "proof" and validation that essential oils have identifiable healing capabilities, but I will always prefer the experience of essential oil efficacy over laboratory or clinical research.

organism is rated 0 to 1, with 1 being the most effective. As an example, oregano is rated 0.83 in effectiveness against the streptococcus bacteria, whereas clove is rated 0.44 against the same pathogen. Belaiche's aromatogram is very useful in medical settings where testing for specific infectious agents is possible.

L'AROMATHÉRAPIE ÉXACTEMENT: CLINICAL APPLICATION BY PIERRE FRANCHOMME AND DR. DANIEL PÉNOËL

L'aromathérapie éxactement by Pierre Francomme and Dr. Daniel Pénoël (1990) is considered to be *the* medical text in aromatherapy. This text is a combination of research and clinical study that provides scientific data with a holistic orientation. Several practical uses of essential oils found in this text are constantly referenced in aromatherapy practice and literature.

Although the text has not been translated into English, it is useful to non-French speaking clinicians as a resource guide because of the familiarity of the botanical names and the Latin terms used for medical descriptions.

CONTRAINDICATIONS, SENSITIVITIES, AND TOXICITY

The most confusing concerns regarding aromatherapy are the potential sensitivities and contraindications of the essential oils. Aromatherapy literature is riddled with contradictory information regarding the safe use of essential oils. The issue of toxicology is directly addressed by Ron Guba in his presentation, *Toxicity Myths – The Actual Risk of Using Essential Oils*.[34] He begins by pointing out how most of the contraindications are rarely supported by research or clinical experience. This observation initiates curiosity about the origin of the "toxicity myths." Guba attributes the diversity of opinion regarding essential oil toxicity to three sources: philosophical differences, lack of knowledge among practitioners, and the fear of public misuse. Authors and practitioners commonly express cautions and contraindications as "never" and "don't" to avoid problems with readers and clients, or to avoid law suits. These cautions and contraindications may be passed on as statements of fact and continually repeated to become, as Guba says, "common perception that the therapeutic use of essential oils is a risky business."

In response to Guba's Toxicity Myth, another well known author of aromatherapy has written *10 Sensible Aromatherapy Practices, Phenolic Oils and Ron Guba*.[35] In this article Tony Burfield lists conditions that, if followed according to Guba's suggestions, could lead to legitimate sensitivities. Determining which author to believe is a frustrating situation for the practicing aromatherapist.

Many conditions contribute to the "facts" and opinions stated regarding essential oil dangers and safety. These conditions include the testing methods used in the scientific study of essential oils as well as the translation of these studies. It is important in any study that the essential oil used is genuine and authentic. As you've read in this text, adulterated or synthetic oils do have risks, the most serious of which is possible irritation. Tested oils must clearly state the botanical origin and their quality.

Business Related Claims of Hazards and Efficacy

Economic issues may contribute to the warnings found regarding essential oil use and their possible toxicity. Lobby groups of industries that could suffer from extended use of essential oils may be interested in keeping this un-patentable product from receiving favorable attention. Economics, or more accurately business practice, also colors the claims of essential oil efficacy. Those groups that benefit financially from essential oils would strive to use whatever means to support their safety and use. This confusing arena of essential oil contraindications, toxicity, and safety requires clarity based on sound research rather than hearsay.

Common Sense and Safety

Common sense makes safe scents. Common sense suggests that essential oil toxicity is over-exaggerated based on the fact there have been few injuries, fatalities, or other problems in the hundreds of years of their use. Appropriate use of essential oils appears safe and generally free of complications. If complications do occur, simply discontinuing the use of the problematic essential oil can alleviate the situation. There are, however, valid contraindications and potential toxicity issues that aromatherapists must understand.

Risk and Responsibility

Essential oils, used responsibly, have minimal risks. The conclusion that one would expect to derive from any presentation on aromatherapy is to use essential oils responsibly. This entire manuscript is dedicated to knowledgeable and responsible use of essential oils. We will proceed on the assumption that caution is advisable and fear is unnecessary. The path to safe use of essential oils is to become aware of all the precautions, based on legitimate and relevant studies that are available regarding the oils that you use.

"FRENCH" AND "BRITISH" AROMATHERAPY REVISITED

The evolution of aromatherapy spawned the two "schools," or philosophies, of aromatherapy first mentioned in Chapter 2. The French method developed from the medicinal practice of using essential oils based on their chemistry and pharmacology.

The development of medical scientific aromatherapy began in France and spread into Germany and Switzerland, carrying with it this medical style that incorporated large dosages and internal use of essential oils.

The "British" style of aromatherapy is attributed to Maugerite Maury, a French woman who pursued a more "energetic" practice of essential oil use. Her idea was to leave large dose applications to the medical practitioner and expand the use of essential oils by incorporating them into massage and beauty practices, using a common dilution of 2 to 5 percent essential oil. This style was popularized in England and has become the dominant method practiced in English speaking countries. It commonly teaches employing low dosage "energetic" formulation and avoiding internal use or high dosage amounts. Guba suggests that this "bias has served as the 'philosophical base' on which many of the common statements regarding essential oil toxicity are based." The "aggressive" and "radical" French methodology, using high dosages, undiluted oils applied topically, and the internal applications of essential oils, is seen as irresponsible according to the more "gentle" style of the "British" practitioner.

The intent of this book is to present sensible methods and safety issues without a labeled identity of "French" or "British" or the promotion of any unnecessary fears. Essential oils can then be used responsibly according to the individual's knowledge and professional status and licensing.

IRRITATION, CONTACT DERMATITIS, AND ALLERGIES

This text is primarily focused on topical application of essential oils for skin health and beauty. It would be sensible, then, to offer some insight into the potential negative effects of essential oils when applied to the skin. Irritation and sensitivity is possible with the use of almost any essential oil. Some oils have known sensitizing properties, but irritation may also be caused by an individual's sensitivity and not an irritant quality of the oil. This is not a situation that can be anticipated according to the composition or normal activity of essential oils. It is an immune response that is specific to the individual, whether it is an allergic response or some other random anomaly. To determine sensitivity of an individual to specific oils, perform a patch test. To do this, simply apply a small amount of the formulation to be used to the inner elbow. Wait 24 hours and check for reactions. A consultation may also reveal a potential allergy, though an allergy to a flower does not necessarily translate to an allergy or reaction to the essential oil. Other reasons for essential oil irritation are cross reactions from medications and sensitivities accumulated from persistent use of fragrance compounds (perfumes) or environmental toxins.

Using Undiluted Essential Oils

The use of essential oils applied undiluted on the skin is spurned by most aromatherapy experts. This is a reasonable precaution when presented as "erring on the side of safety" and recommended to the beginner who does not yet have the experience to know which oils are skin irritants and which are not. The emphasis should be placed on caution, not fear. The contradictory back and forth of whether essential oils should or should not be used undiluted is alleviated by the knowledge that the oils work quite effectively in dilution; therefore, using them undiluted is not necessary. From another perspective, a personal discovery of which oils are irritant and which are not is a harsh, not a dangerous, lesson. An undiluted essential oil is not likely to cause serious injury or a lasting injury.[36]

SENSITIZATION

Sensitivity to an essential oil can develop over time. If an oil is used on an ongoing daily basis the body may begin to recognize it as an allergen and respond accordingly. The development of an allergic reaction that occurs over a period of time is called **sensitization**. Signs of sensitization include rash, itch, sneezing or shortness of breath. This may occur at any interval from weeks to many years of using the same essential oil.

Sensitizing Oils

The essential oils that are considered sensitizing are those containing high amounts of phenols and aromatic aldehydes (cinnamic aldehyde). These oils are most likely to irritate. Thyme thymol type, oregano, cinnamon, and clove are well known irritant oils. When used alone and undiluted on the skin, these oils predictably cause irritation and possible burning. Caution should be exercised at any dilution containing more than 2.5 percent of these oils, and they are said to be safest under a 10 percent dilution. If irritation occurs when an oil is applied, or spills, on the skin, remove it by applying a fair amount of vegetable oil, such as olive or safflower, and wipe it from the skin. Water should not be used alone to wipe off an irritant oil. Water will push the essential oils deeper, and more aggressively, into the skin.

Other oils that may cause irritation contain the lemon fragranced aldehydes, like lemongrass or melissa, especially when used in higher dosages of over 5 to 10 percent. This is generally only an issue when using adulterated oil or the isolated aldehyde compound alone.[37] Should a citrus oil, or needle tree oil (juniper, cypress or pine) **peroxidize,** a chemical change in the oil caused by an oxygen reaction, it becomes an irritant. If bought from a reputable source and stored properly, a good citrus or needle oil should remain stable for quite some time before peroxidizing.

The oils that contain the 1,8 cineole molecule, like *Eucalyptus radiata*, tea tree and rosemary cineole may be irritating and cause inflammation on some skin types. This is especially likely for skin that is already irritated but is not generally a problem when used in dilutions even as great as 50 percent.

The aforementioned oils are the most likely candidates for irritation, but even soothing and calming lavender can become an irritant under the right conditions, especially when used undiluted. Using any essential oil in the bath or applying it to wet skin increases the chances of irritation. The emphasis again is on caution. Your experience will be your guide to avoiding sensitivity.

Photosensitizing Oils

Photosensitivity refers to sensitivity to light caused by ingredients or drugs that may cause a chemically induced change in the skin that makes an individual unusually sensitive to light.[38] This unusual sensitivity translates into avoiding sun light or any ultraviolet light source when photosensitizing essential oils are being used. Oils containing furanocoumarin are the most common photosensitizing agents and include bergamot and lemon. Lime, bitter orange, and angelica have a milder potential for photosensitivity activity. Reactions can vary from discoloration to blistering.

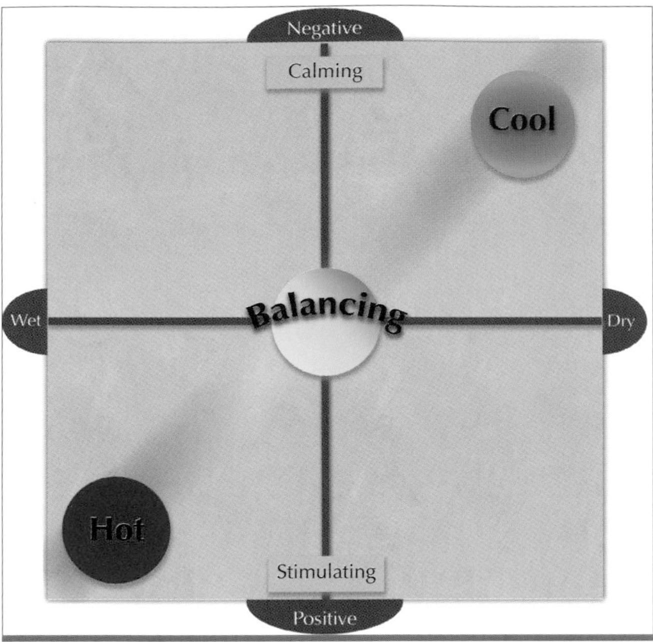

Plate 1 Color provides a visual support to understanding the activity of essential oil compounds in relation to their position on the Structure-Effect Diagram.

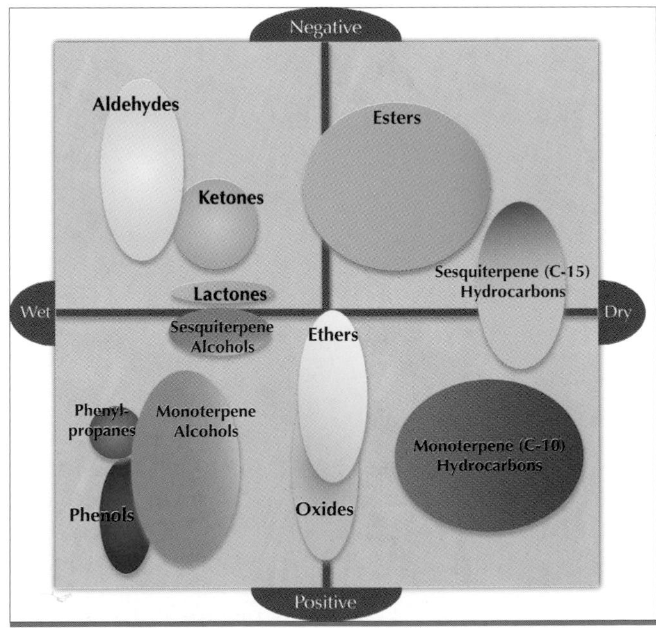

Plate 2 The chemical family groupings and their position on the Structure-Effect Diagram. Be aware that the exact polarity and electropositive or negative position is determined by the individual molecules found in each family. The positions of the family groupings in this chart are only an approximation.

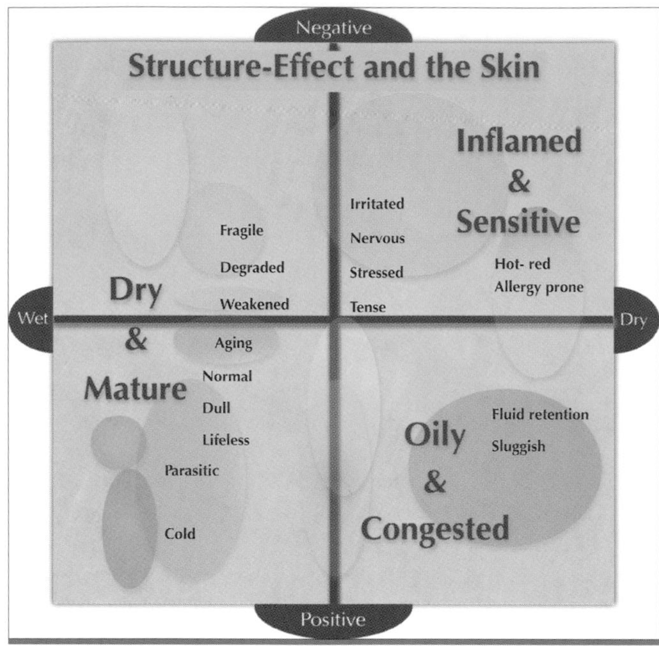

Plate 3 The Structure-Effect Diagram and the skin. Each skin type or condition is positioned in the area relating to the chemical grouping that would be most efficient in creating balance or treatment.

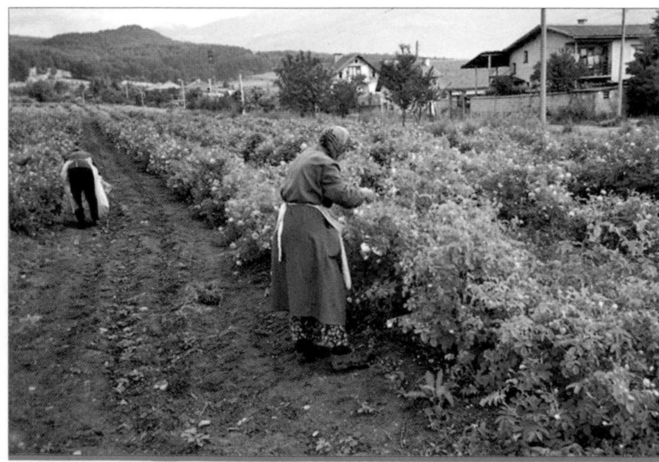

Plate 4 The famous Bulgarian Valley of Roses. It takes a very skilled hand to pick the extremely delicate rose petals (*Rosa damascena*).

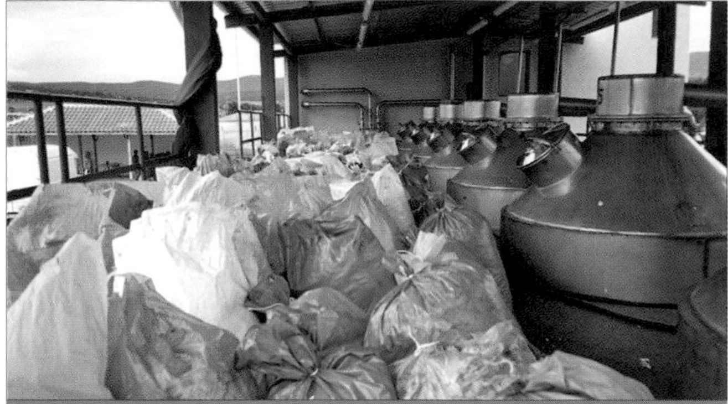

Plate 5 Rose petals are brought to the distillation units. Experienced Bulgarian distillers produce the finest Rose Otto (steam distilled rose) in the world.

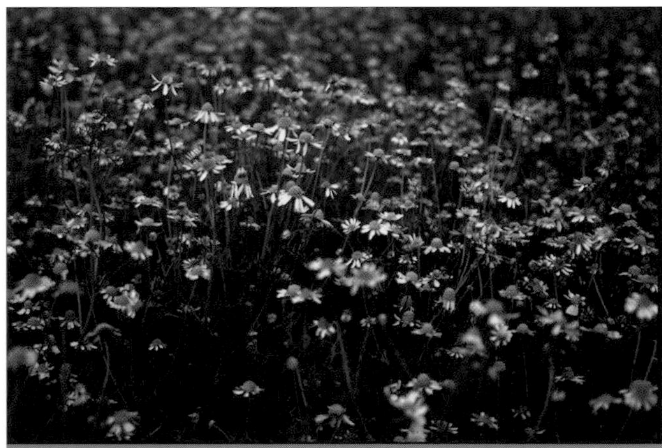

Plate 6 German Chamomile (*Matricaria recutita*)

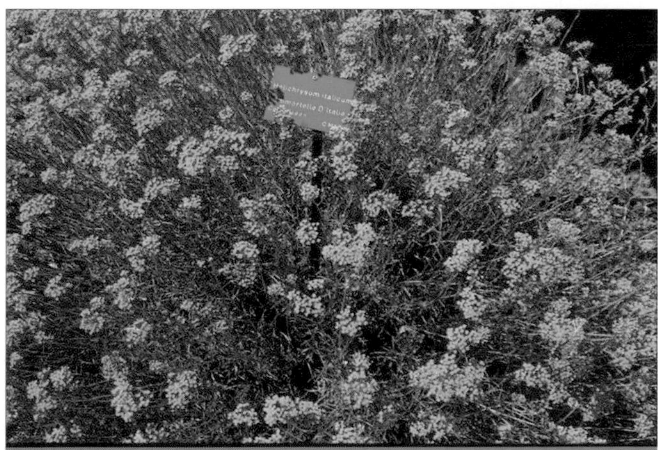

Plate 7 *Helichrysum italicum*

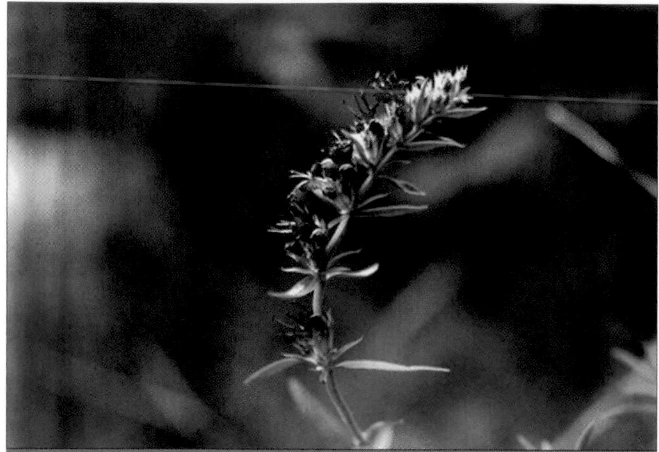

Plate 8 Hyssop (*Hyssopsus officinalis*)

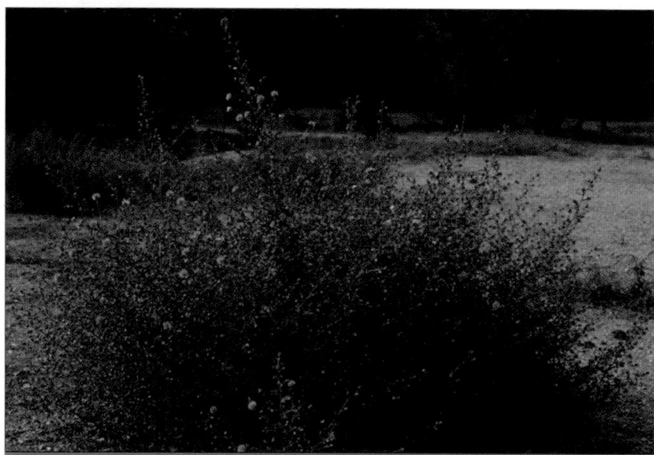

Plate 9 *Inula graveolens*

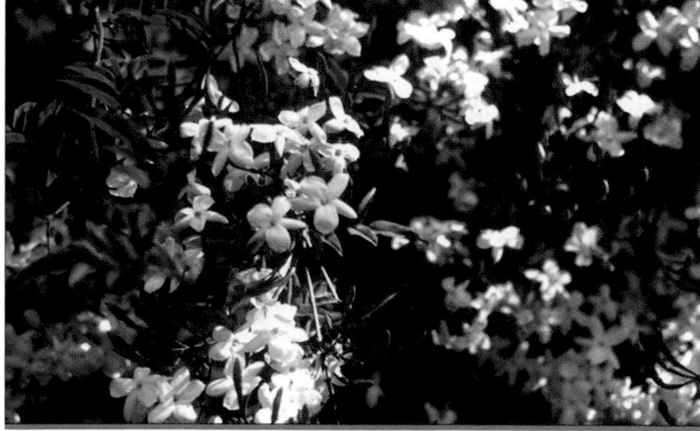

Plate 10 Jasmine (*Jasminum grandiflorum*)

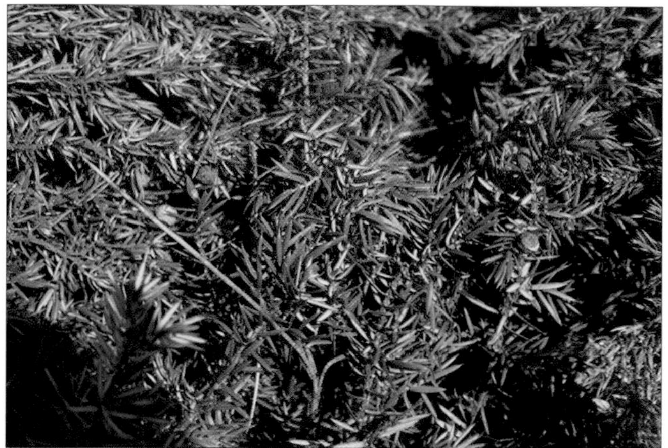

Plate 11 Juniper (*Juniperus communis*)

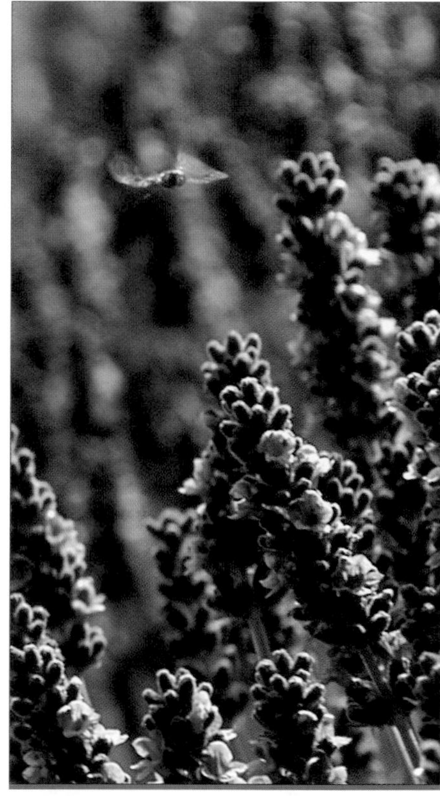

Plate 12 Lavender (*Lavandula angustifolia*)

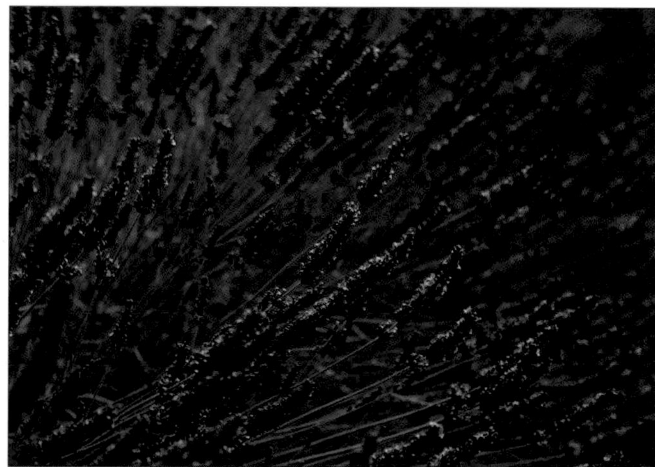

Plate 13 Lavandin (*Lavandula hybrida*)

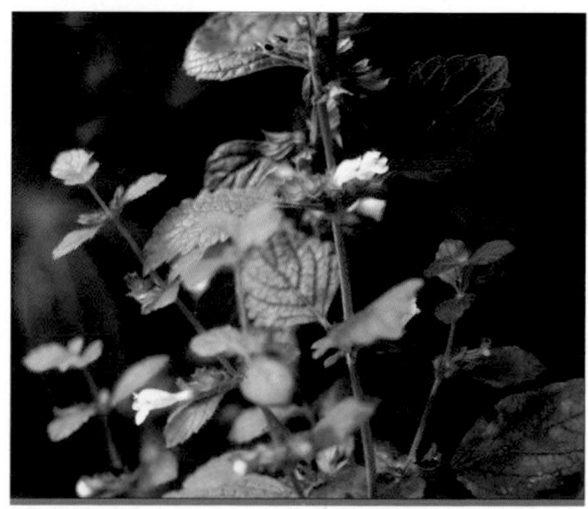

Plate 14 Melissa (*Melissa officinalis*)

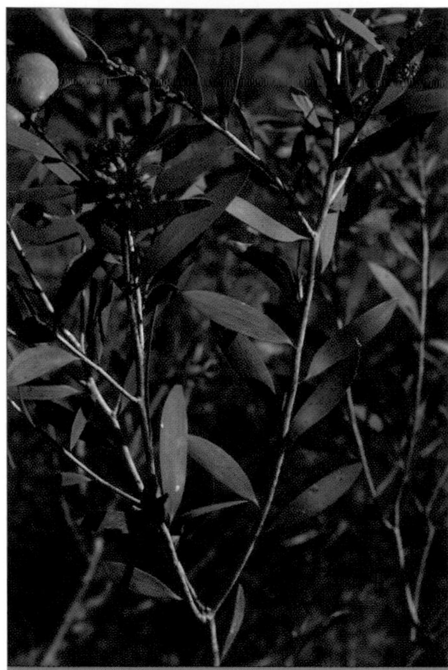

Plate 15 MQV (*Melaleuca quinquenervia viridiflora*)

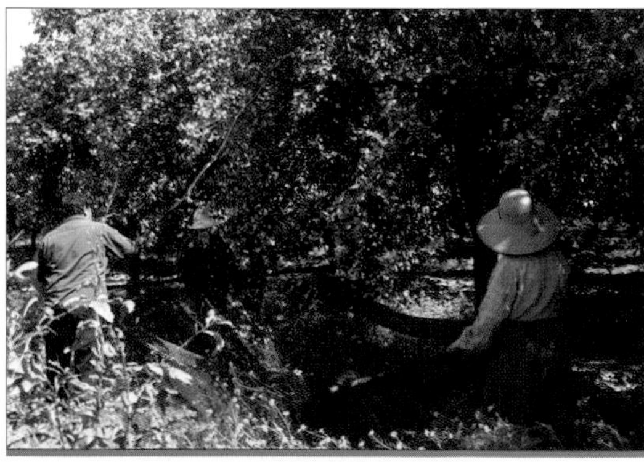

Plate 16 Harvesting orange blossoms for the production of neroli essential oil in Seville, Spain.

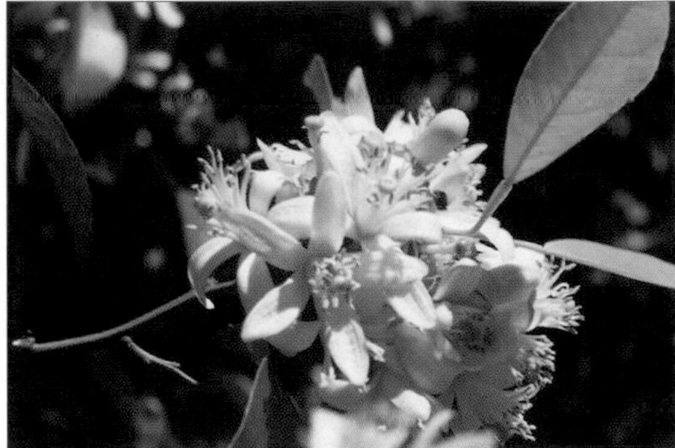

Plate 17 Orange blossom/neroli (*Citrus aurantium*)

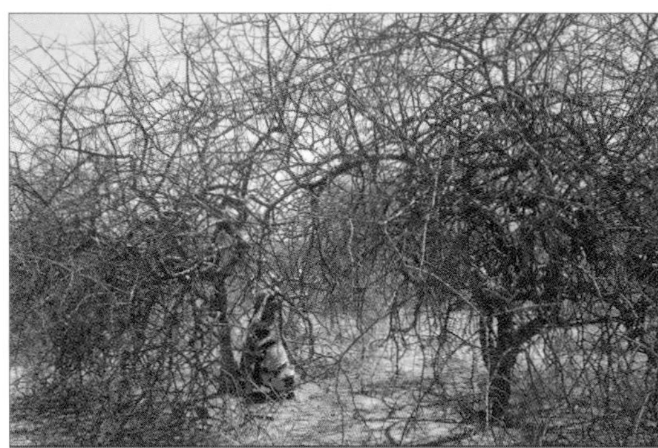

Plate 18 The Somalian women work their way to the center of the thorny *Boswellia carteri* (frankincense) bush to gather the gum for distillation.

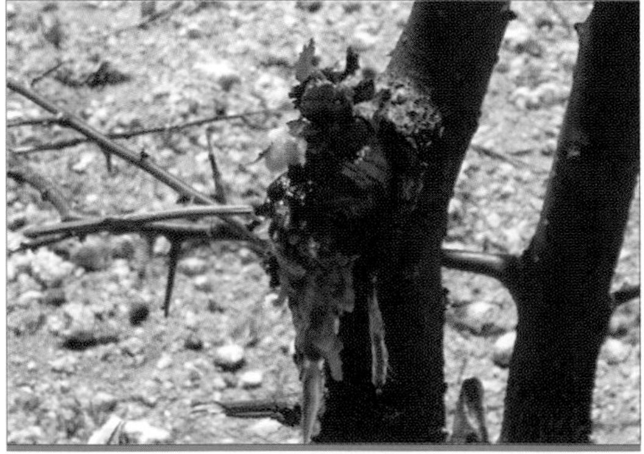

Plate 19 The sap of the Boswellia bush naturally seeps from the bark forming the hardened frankincense gum.

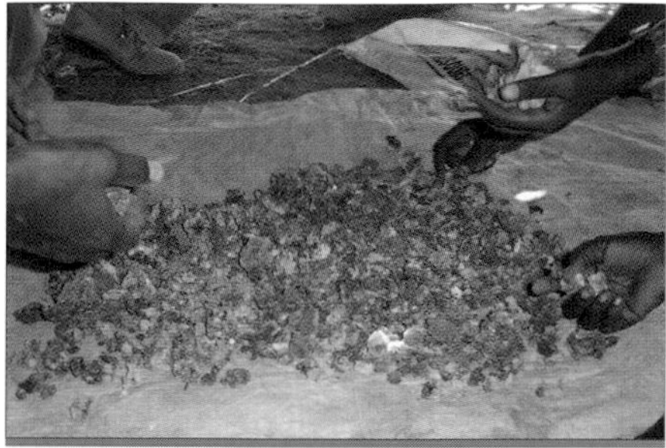

Plate 20 Sorting through the Somalian frankincense gum prior to distillation.

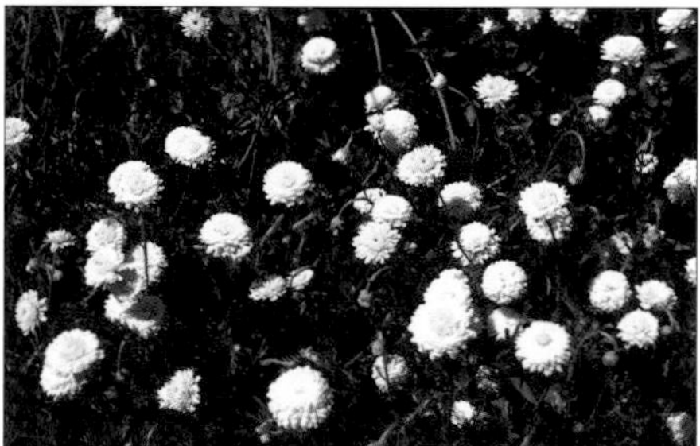

Plate 21 Roman chamomile (*Anthemis nobilis*)

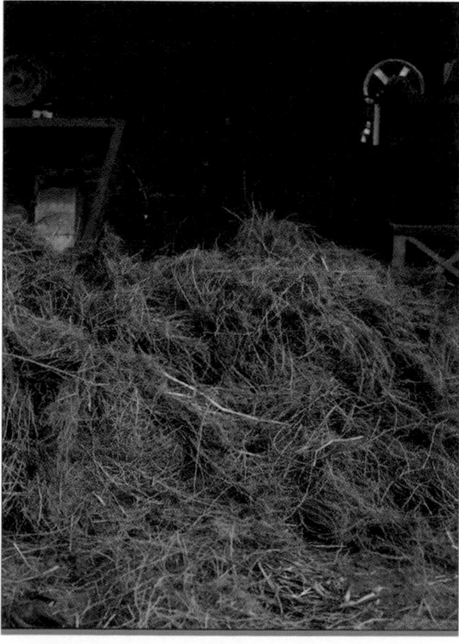

Plate 22 Vetiver root (*Andropogon muricatus*)

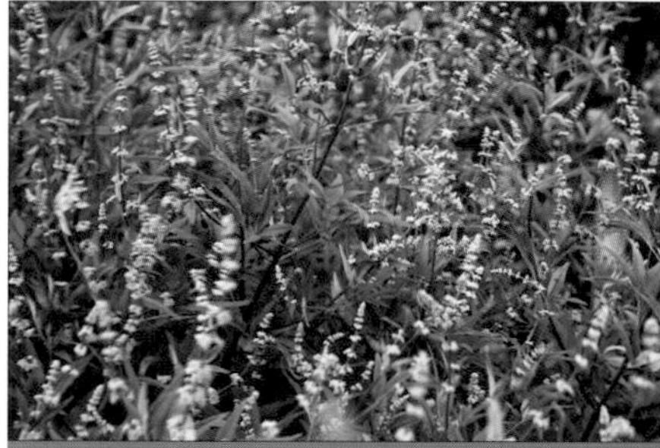

Plate 23 Vitex (*Vitex agnus costus*)

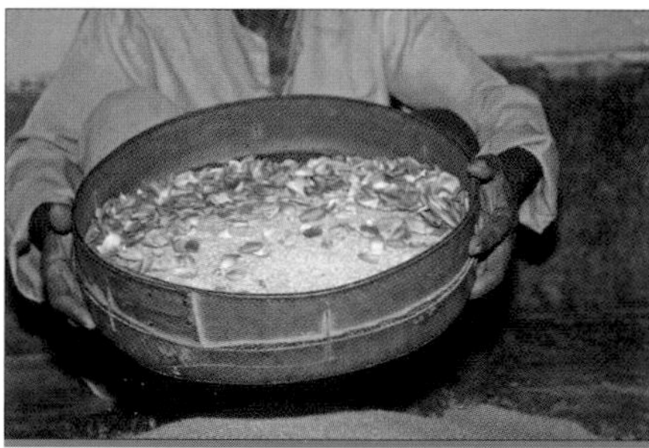

Plate 24 The sesame seeds are sifted, after absorbing the essence from the rose petals, in the traditional Indian process of making enfleurage.

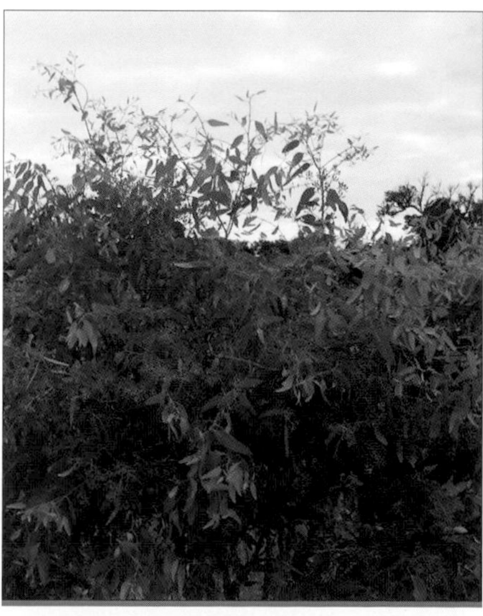

Plate 25 *Eucalyptus staigerianna.*

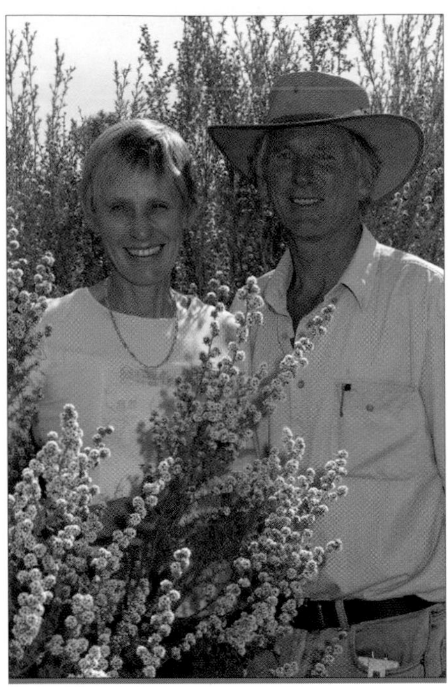

Plate 26 John and Peta Day with Fragonia™ (see Appendix D)

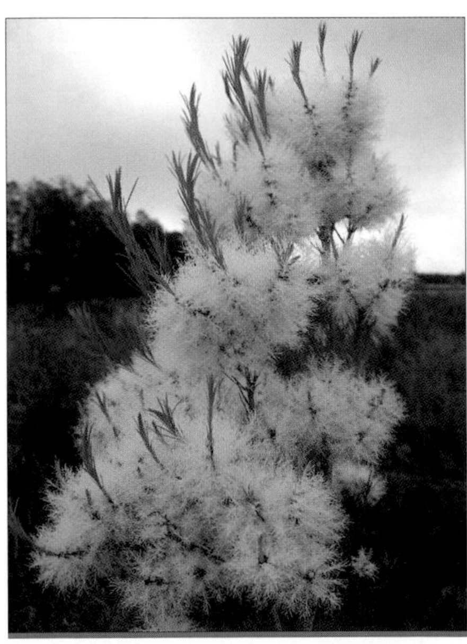

Plate 27 Flowering tea tree (*Melaleuca alternifolia*)

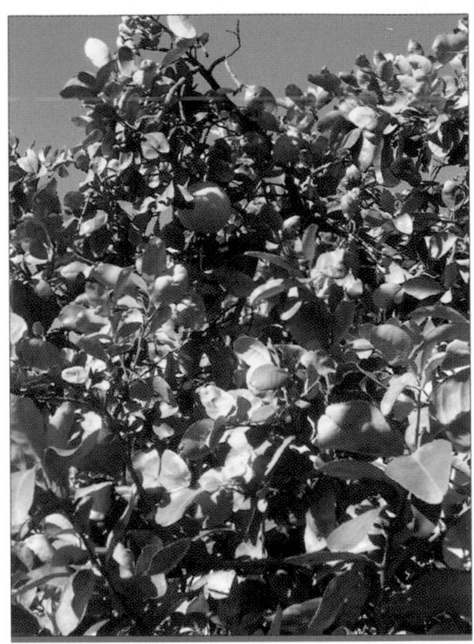

Plate 28 Grapefruit (*Citrus paradisi*)

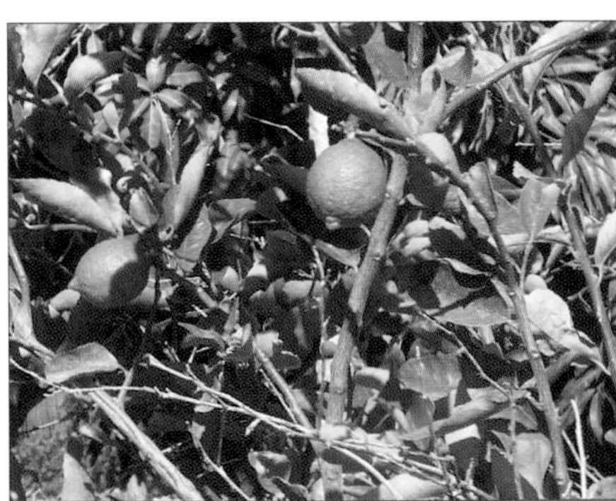

Plate 29 Lime (*Citrus limetta*)

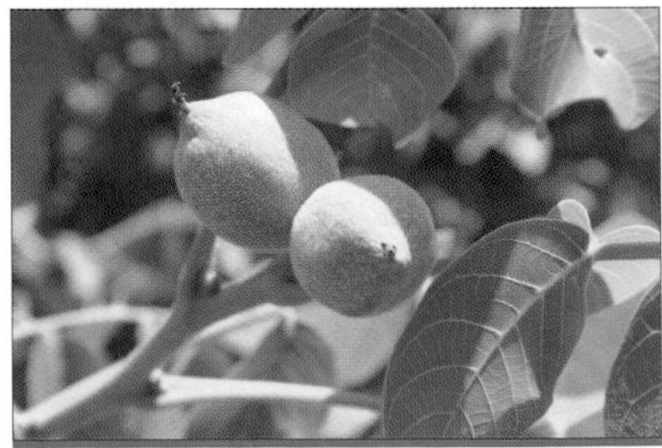

Plate 30 Sweet almond (*Prunus dulcis*)

NEUROTOXICITY AND HEPATOTOXICITY OF KETONES

Ketones are the compounds that carry the most notorious toxicity issues. In studying the chemistry in Chapter 5 it was noted that ketone compounds are potentially toxic to the nervous system (neuro-toxin) and a liver toxin (hepato-toxin). Ketone molecules can build up in the liver and cause irreversible liver damage. Toxic effects are usually produced using larger, oral dosages. Ketones penetrate the blood-brain barrier and can produce convulsive effects. Extra caution is made for using ketones with those who are prone to seizures. Precautions are also stated for use during pregnancy because of the potential abortive effects of ketones. These claims are unsubstantiated, though it is advisable to use precautions with essential oils during pregnancy.[39]

Essential oils with ketone content are valuable cosmetic ingredients for skin conditioning and treatment. Rather than discount their use, you should learn the potential risks and use these oils sensibly and with caution.

Safe dosage amounts for percutaneous application applied a maximum of five times per day, according to Francomme and Pénoël, are as follows:

Adults	0.5 mL	(approximately 15 drops)
Older Children	0.25 mL	(approximately 7 drops)
Small Children	0.1 mL	(approximately 3 drops)

As you will see in Chapter 8, these are much higher dosages than occur in most applications used in massage and therapeutic skin care.

HEPATOTOXICITY OF PHENOLIC COMPOUNDS

A review of safety issues indicates repeated warnings of potential liver toxicity with all essential oils. This caution is entirely relevant if large amounts of essential oils are consumed orally. As with anything, including water, using an excess of a substance has consequences. The oils of most concern for liver toxicity are the ketones, as already mentioned, and the phenolic oils. Oils rich in phenols, such as oregano, savory, and thyme thymol type, are prescribed for internal use owing to their powerful antiseptic activity and tolerance to internal use.

At low dosages over short periods (2 to 4 days), this practice is not problematic. Higher dosages and long term use are likely to cause liver damage.

POTENTIAL KIDNEY IRRITATION WITH MONOTERPENES

The irritating quality of juniper to the kidneys is well known. This quality is attributed to the monoterpene, pinene. Though it is juniper that carries the caution related to kidney-tissue damage, it is a suitable warning for all oils high in monoterpene hydrocarbons. Guba explains the experiments regarding kidney damage to be unfounded and use of oils such as pine, also high in pinene, showed no kidney damage.[40] It is wise to be aware of concentrations of monoterpene hydrocarbons that are in the oils used in higher amounts or over long periods of time. The needle tree oils, pine, spruce, and fir included, and the citrus oils are the most suspect in kidney irritation.

OTHER PRECAUTIONARY CONSIDERATIONS

When used responsibly, essential oils are very safe. The precautions listed in this chapter, descriptions of the molecular compounds (Chapter 5), and the essential oil profiles (Chapter 7) will guide you for safe practice with essential oils. Other considerations that may present themselves when exploring therapeutic aromatherapy are pregnancy, drug combining, medical conditions, and the use of essential oils with children.

Pregnancy

Fears and cautions are often expounded for essential oil use during pregnancy. Midwives have been using essential oils during pregnancy and at the time of birth for quite some time. It is not necessary to avoid essential oils in the average dosage of 2 to 5 percent concentrations or through periodic inhalation, though it goes without saying that there are special, mostly individual, considerations for use during pregnancy. For instance, you may wish to avoid peppermint and replace this effective oil for nausea with spearmint. An additional cautious approach is to begin with the lower dosages of 1 to 2 percent essential oil, because the sense of smell is altered and at times more sensitive during pregnancy.

Medical Conditions

Topical use of essential oils will, in general, not affect most medical conditions. There is always reason for caution, depending on the condition of the individual. Using common sense may be your most reasonable ally. For example, don't use essential oils with compounds known to be potential liver irritants on an individual with any type of liver ailment. A good rule to follow is, when in doubt, don't do it.

Drugs and Essential Oils

Jane Buckle suggests theoretical cautions when combining essential oils with medications, because the oils may interact by combining with similar cellular receptors and somehow alter the chemistry of the drug.[41] Potential interactions between essential oils and prescription drugs are beyond the scope of this text.

Children

Precautions apply when essential oils are used for children. Children tend to be more sensitive and responsive than adults to essential oils. Start with much lower concentrations of essential oils. Many formulas found in aromatherapy literature give specific amounts. For our purposes, we will consider a lower dosage to be between 1 drop per ounce of carrier or up to 1 percent of essential oil in dilution to be appropriate. Children also respond well when the oil blend is applied to the soles of the feet.

A specific precaution is noted for peppermint, which is generally a safe oil but should not be used on children younger than 30 months of age.

CHAPTER SUMMARY

The many properties of essential oils offer a wide range of therapeutic effects. These properties have been well researched and include antimicrobial, anti-inflammatory, sedative, cell regenerative, expectorant, and wound healing effects. When working with the skin, select essential oils for properties that holistically and directly assist in maintenance, repair, and balance in all skin conditions.

Some contraindications and cautions are associated with essential oils. The aromatherapy literature and common knowledge include contradictory and legitimate warnings of irritation and other possible contraindications. It is up to you, the aromatherapy practitioner, to research, experience, and fully understand precautions associated with essential oil use. When used responsibly and respectfully, essential oils are a safe and effective therapeutic treatment modality.

REVIEW QUESTIONS

1. Name six therapeutic properties of essential oils.
2. What are the benefits of the anti-inflammatory properties for skin care?
3. What are some of the skin conditions that benefit from cell regenerative properties of essential oils?
4. What are the contraindications of using essential oils that contain ketone?
5. Name three reasons for irritation and sensitivity other than that expected of irritant oils or compounds.
6. What precautions should be taken when using essential oils on clients with a known medical condition?

CHAPTER REFERENCES

1. Weil, A. (1995). *Spontaneous Healing*. New York, NY: Alfred A Knopf.
2. Gattefossé, R-M. (1937). *Aromathérapie: Les Huiles essentielles hormones végétales*. Paris, France: Librairie des Sciences Girardot.
3. Keller, W. & Kober, W. (1954). "Possibilities of using essential oils for disinfection." *Arzneimittelforschung 5* (4); 224–229.

4. Buckle, J. (2002). "Clinical aromatherapy and AIDS." *The Journal of the Association of Nurses in AIDS Care 13* (3); 81–99.
5. Schnaubelt, K. (ed.). & Deininger, R. (1995, November). *The spectrum of activity of plant drugs containing essential oils (especially their antibacterial, antifungal and antiviral activity)*. Proceedings of Wholistic Aromatherapy: A Conference on the Therapeutic Uses of Essential Oils, San Francisco, California.
6. Jansen, A. M., Sceffer, J. J. C. & Baerheim-Svedsen, A. (1987). "Antimicrobial activity of essential oils: Aspects of the test method." *Planta Medica 53*; 395–398.
7. Pénoël, D. (1994). *The immune system of mankind*. Aroma '93, Conference Proceedings, Hove.
8. Schmidt, M., Smith, L. & Sehnert, K. (1993). *Beyond Antibiotics: 50 (or so) Ways to Boost the Immunity and Avoid Antibiotics*. Berkeley, CA: North Atlantic Books.
9. Minami, M., Kita, M., Nakaya, T., Yamamoto, T., Kuriyama, H. & Imanishi, J. (2003). "The inhibitory effect of essential oils on herpes simplex virus type-1 replication in vitro." *Microbiology and Immunology 47* (9); 681–684.
10. Francomme, P. & Pénoël, D. (1990). *L'Aromathérapie Exactement*. Limoges, France: Jollois.
11. Hammer, K. A., Carson, C. F. & Riley, T. V. (2004). "Antifungal effects of *Melaleuca alternifolia* (tea tree) oil and its components on *Candida albicans, Candida glabrata* and *Saccharomyces cerevisiae*." *Journal of Antimicrobial Chemotherapy 53* (6); 1081–1085.
12. D'Auria, F. D., Laino, L., Strippoli, V., Tecca, M., Salvatore, G., Battinelli, L. & Mazzanti G. (2001). "In vitro activity of tea tree oil against *Candida albicans* mycelial conversion and other pathogenic fungi." *Journal of Chemotherapy (Florence, Italy) 13* (4); 377–383.
13. Gupta, A. K., Nicol, K. & Batra, R. (2004). "Role of antifungal agents in the treatment of seborrheic dermatitis." *American Journal of Dermatology 5* (6); 417–422.
14. Shahi, S. K., Shukla, A. C., Bajaj, A. K., Banerjee, U., Rimek, D., Midgely, G. & Dikshit, A. (2000). "Broad spectrum herbal therapy against superficial fungal infections." *Skin Pharmacology and Applied Skin Physiology 13* (1); 60–64.

15. Aertgeerts, P., Albring, M., Klaschka, F., Nasemann, T., Patzelt-Wenczler, R., Rauhut, K. & Weigl, B. (1985). "Comparative testing of Kamillosan cream and steroidal (0.25% hydrocortisone, 0.75% fluocortin butyl ester) and non-steroidal (5% bufexamac) dermatologic agents in maintenance therapy of eczematous diseases." *Zeitschrift Für Hautkrankheiten 60* (3); 270–277.
16. Francomme, P. & Pénoël, D. (1990). *L'Aromathérapie Exactement*. Limoges, France: Jollois.
17. Perricone, N. (2002). *The Perricone Prescription*. New York, NY: HarperCollins Publishers.
18. Lee, I. S. & Lee, G. J. (2006). "Effects of lavender aromatherapy on insomnia and depression in women college students." *Taehan Kanho Hakhoe Chi 36* (1); 136–143.
19. Wagner, H. & Sprinkmeyer, L. (1973). "Über die pharmakologische wirkung von mellisengeist." *Deutsche Apotheker Zeitung 113* (30). 1159–1166.
20. Elisabetsky, E., De Souza, G., Dos Santos, M., Siquieira, I., Amador, T. & Nunes, D. Sedative properties of linalool. *Fitoterapia 66* (5); 407–415.
21. Newmark, T. & Schulick, P. (2000). *Beyond Aspirin: Nature's Answer to Arthritis, Cancer and Alzheimer's Disease*. Prescott, AZ: Holm Press.
22. Schnaubelt, K. (1998). *Advanced Aromatherapy*. Rochester, VT: Healing Arts Press.
23. El Tahir, K. E. H., Shoeb, H. & Al-Shora, H. (1997). "Exploration of some pharmacological activities of cardamom seed *(Elettaria cardamomum)* volatile oil." *Saudi Pharmaceutical Journal 5* (2–3); 96–102.
24. Emamghoreishi M, Khasaki M, Aazam MF. (2005). "*Coriandrum sativum*: evaluation of its anxiolytic effect in the elevated plus-maze." *Journal of Ethnopharmacology Jan 15; 96 (3)*;365–370.
25. Haas, M. (2004). *Quick Reference Guide for 114 Important Essential Oils*. San Rafael, CA: Terra Linda Scent and Image.
26. Holmes, P. (1993). "Clary sage." *International Journal of Aromatherapy 5* (1); 15.
27. Boyd, E. (1954). "Expectorants and respiratory tract fluid." *Pharmacological Review 6*; 521–542.
28. Dorow, P. Weiss, T., Felix, R. & Schumutzler, H. (1987). "Effect of secretolytic and a combination of pinene, limonene and cineole on mucociliary clearance in patients with chronic pulmonary disease." *Arzneimittelforschung 37* (12); 1378–1381.

29. Buckle, J. (2003). *Clinical Aromatherapy Essential Oils in Practice*. Philadelphia, PA: Churchill Livingstone.
30. Schnaubelt, K. (1998). *Medical Aromatherapy.* Berkeley, CA: Frog, LTD.
31. Schnaubelt, K (ed.) Harrison, J. (2005). "Difficult skin disorders," *Proceedings for the 6th Scientific Wholistic Aromatherapy Conference*, 92–105; Terra Linda Scent and Image, San Rafael, CA.
32. Leach, M. J. (2004). "A critical review of natural therapies in wound management." *Ostomy/Wound Management 50 (5)*; 36–51.
33. Guba, R. (1998). "Wound Healing." *International Journal of Aromatherapy 9* (2) 67–74.
34. Guba, R. (1998). *Toxicity Myths.* Victoria, Australia: The Centre for Aromatic Medicine, Balwyn North.
35. Burfield, T. (2004). *10 Sensible Aromatherapy Practices, Phenolic Oils and Ron Guba*. Accessed on July 29, 2007 at http://www.users.globalnet.co.uk.
36. Schnaubelt, K. (2004). *Aromatherapy Lifestyle*. San Rafael, CA: Terra Linda Scent and Image.
37. Buckle, J. (2003). *Clinical Aromatherapy Essential Oils in Practice.* Philadelphia, PA: Churchill Livingstone.
38. Venes, D. (ed.) (1997). *Tabor's Cyclopedic Medical Dictionary* (18th edition). Philadelphia, PA: F. A. Davis Company.
39. Tisserand, R. (1990). *The Essential Oil Safety Data Manual*. Tisserand Aromatherapy Institute. E. Sussex, England: Hove.
40. Guba, R. (1998). *Toxicity Myths.* Victoria, Australia: The Centre for Aromatic Medicine, Balwyn North.
41. Buckle, J. (2003). *Clinical Aromatherapy Essential Oils in Practice.* Philadelphia, PA: Churchill Livingstone.

The Essential Oils for Therapeutic Use

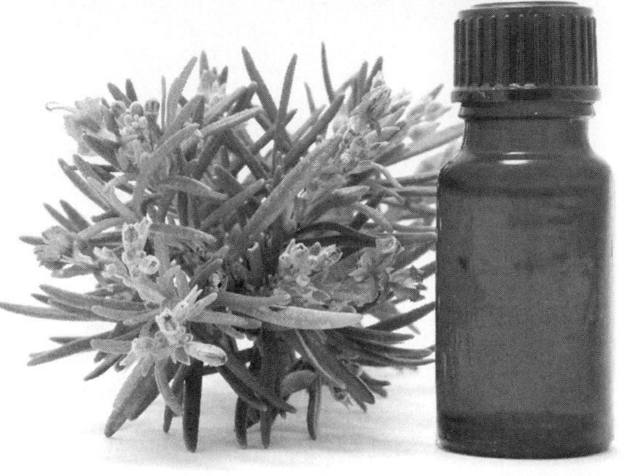

CHAPTER 7

Incidentally, all plants have a smell, and consequently contain a volatile oil: essential oils not yet extracted will be put to good use in the fullness of time.

–René-Maurice Gattefossé

LEARNING OBJECTIVES

1. Describe a basic collection of thirteen essential oils for therapeutic practice.
2. Review twenty additional essential oils used to expand therapeutic potential.
3. Acquire skills in selecting essential oils for the treatment of conditions based on a therapeutic focus.

THE ESSENTIAL OILS

Aromatherapy defines a skill based on knowledge of essential oils. Hundreds of essential oils are available for use in aromatherapy, with new ones consistently being introduced to the marketplace. To the novice, becoming familiar with so many oils may seem like an overwhelming undertaking. The goal is not to become familiar with every essential oil available for use. A generous assumption is that most aromatherapists are familiar with fewer than half of the oils distilled for aromatherapy purposes. A sensible beginning for the novice aromatherapist is to work with a few oils at a time and build knowledge. This gradual approach is the way every seasoned aromatherapist became familiar with the oils they use in practice. Most aromatherapists have a chosen arsenal of essential oils that includes their standard, specialty, and rare selections. This collection could encompass as few as 15 to several hundred oils.

Working with formulas from this text and other sources is a good way to become familiar with a variety of essential oils. The process of learning aromatherapy cannot be rushed and is not something that comes from memorizing what is presented in a class or book. Your experience with the essential oils is really the only way to develop the skills necessary to become expert in this field. The beauty of this method is that you can start to practice and create effective blends right away. In fact, this practice, as with any skill, is the way to become an experienced aromatherapist.

THIRTEEN ESSENTIAL OILS

The following list is an adequate starting point to become familiar with a group of essential oils that are therapeutically complete and fulfill most needs. The oils on this list are completely compatible for any holistic health practice, esthetics, spa, and massage therapy. The list includes information pertinent to efficient use and knowledge of the oils: common and botanical name, botanical family, main chemical composition of the essential oil, characteristic and the therapeutic properties, and the fragrance character.

Cedarwood (Atlas Cedar)

Botanical Name: *Cedrus atlantica*
Botanical Family: Cupressaceae
Derived From: The wood (sawdust) of the tree
Origin: Most cedarwood is produced in Morocco
Cost: Low to moderate
Fragrance Character: Base note, woody, moderate to low odor intensity
Blends Well With: Citruses, florals, other conifer oils such as cypress, juniper, spruce and cineole type oils like MQV, Tea tree and eucalyptus oils
Application: Topical, inhalation, bath
Main Components: Cedrol (sesquiterpene alcohol); atlantone-7 (sesquiterpene ketone); monoterpenes

Therapeutic Uses

Properties: Antiseptic, autonomic balance, circulatory and metabolic stimulant, fungicidal, grounding, relaxing, glandular and respiratory tonic
Medicinal Use: Cellulite, poor circulation, sluggish metabolism, energizing, urinary infection, varicose veins, autonomic nervous system balance (activates parasympathetic nervous system)
Skin, Hair & Body: Strengthen skin tone, aging skin, general skin and body care, dermatitis, detoxifies scalp, dandruff
Mind/Emotions: Reduce anxiety, aggression, fear and nervousness
Spiritual: Meditation
Contraindications: None known. Contains ketones.

Cape Chamomile

Botanical Name: *Eriocephalus punctulatus*
Botanical Family: Asteraceae
Derived From: Leaves
Origin: South Africa
Cost: Moderate to high
Fragrance Character: Middle note, fruity, moderate to high odor intensity
Blends Well With: Citruses, some florals, lavender, *Helichrysum italicum,* vetiver
Application: Topical, inhalation, bath
Main Components: Chamazulene (sequiterpene hydrocarbons); esters; terpinen-4-ol (monoterpene alcohol)

For Your Information

Fragrance Notes

The listed essential oils include a reference to base, middle, or top note. These terms refer to the fragrance quality of the essential oil and are useful in developing a pleasing aromatic scent. The note of the essential oil is determined by its evaporation rate. The more viscous oils that do not evaporate quickly have a deep fragrance, or base note. Oils such as orange and other citruses evaporate easily and have a lighter top note fragrance. A middle note comes from oils with a moderate evaporation rate. The fragrance character is used in blending and is addressed more fully in Chapter 8.

Therapeutic Uses

Properties: Anti-inflammatory, nervous system relaxant, sedative, antispasmodic, analgesic, euphoric
Medicinal Use: Cramps, inflammation, muscle spasm
Skin, Hair & Body: Acne, atopic dermatitis, psoriasis, rosacea, general skin care
Mind/Emotions: Stress, tension, anxiety, nervousness, depression
Spiritual: Chakra balance, meditation, spiritually uplifting
Contraindications: None known

Eucalyptus

Several eucalyptus species are used in aromatherapy. The two that are commonly called "eucalyptus" are the radiata and globulus species. Both have similar composition with some slight differences noted in this section.

Botanical Names: *Eucalyptus radiata* and *Eucalyptus globulus*
Botanical Family: Myrtaceae
Derived From: Branches and leaves
Origin: Radiata: Australia; *Globulus:* Australia, Corsica (preferred), Spain, Portugal
Cost: Low to moderate
Fragrance Character: Top/middle note, fruity, "eucalyptus" like, airy, moderate odor intensity
Blends Well With: Citruses, medicinal oils (tea tree, ravensare, thyme), lavender, *Helichrysum italicum*
Application: Topical, inhalation, bath, shower
Main Components: Terpene alcohols including terpinen-4-ol; 50 – 70 percent of the oxide 1,8 cineole; aldehydes (higher in radiata); sesquiterpenes (globulus)

Therapeutic Uses

Properties: Medicinal, expectorant, antiviral, antibacterial
Medicinal Use: Decongestant, colds, flu
Skin, Hair & Body: Acne, general skin care, scalp cleanser, cellulite
Mind/Emotions: Radiata may relax because of its higher aldehyde content
Spiritual: None specified
Contraindications: None known

Geranium (Figure 7-1)

Botanical Name: Pelargonium asperum
Botanical Family: Geraniaceae
Derived From: Whole of upper plant parts
Origin: Egypt, Reunion, Madagascar
Cost: Moderate
Fragrance Character: Middle note, floral, rose-like, round, moderate odor intensity
Blends Well With: Good blending oil, works with other alcohol/ester oils and florals
Application: Topical, inhalation, bath
Main Components: Terpene alcohols (55 percent) and esters (20 percent)

Therapeutic Uses

Properties: Adaptogenic (the ability to adjust to the body's needs), antiseptic, fungicidal
Medicinal Use: Viral infection, *Candida albicans* infection, PMS, systemic balance
Skin, Hair & Body: General skin care, herpes simplex
Mind/Emotions: Balancing
Spiritual: Balancing
Contraindications: None known

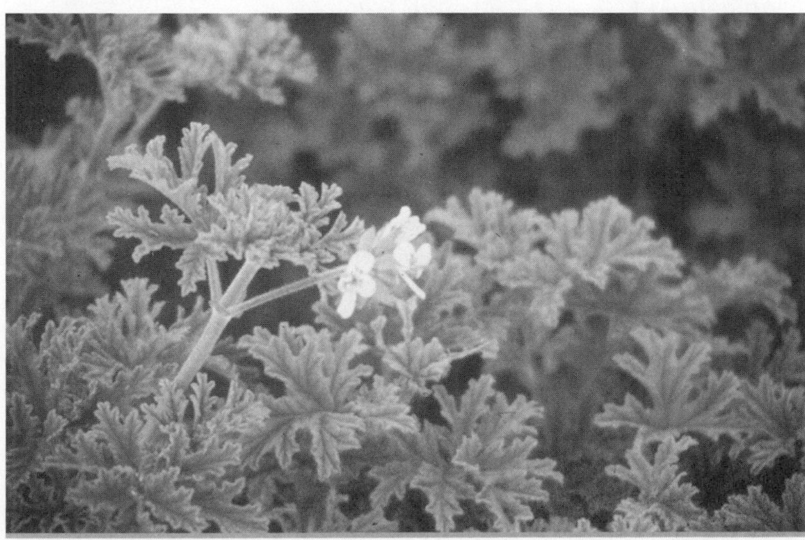

Figure 7-1 Geranium.

Grapefruit

Botanical Name: *Citrus paradisi*
Botanical Family: Rutaceae
Derived From: Fruit peel
Origin: Italy, USA
Cost: Low
Fragrance Character: Top note, fruit, low to moderate odor intensity
Blends Well With: Citruses, medicinal oils (tea tree, ravensare, eucalyptus), lavender, some florals, cedarwood
Application: Topical, inhalation, bath
Main Components: 95 percent (+)-limonene (monoterpene hydrocarbon); 2 percent aldehyde, coumarins, nootkatone

Therapeutic Uses

Properties: Antiseptic, purifier, diuretic
Medicinal Use: Antiviral, disinfectant
Skin, Hair & Body: General skin care, cellulite, acne
Mind/Emotions: Uplifting
Spiritual: Uplifting
Contraindications: None known

Helichrysum (Everlasting, Immortelle)

Botanical Name: *Helichrysum italicum*
Botanical Family: Asteraceae
Derived From: Leaves and flowers
Origin: Corsica, Bosnia
Cost: High
Fragrance Character: Middle note, dry, moderate to high odor intensity
Blends Well With: Lavender, German chamomile, geranium, Cape chamomile, cistus, vetiver
Application: Topical, use undiluted immediately: after injury, bath
Main Components: Esters (40 percent); sesquiterpenes (6 percent) italidione (diketone)

Therapeutic Uses

Properties: Anti-inflammatory, hematoma reduction, liver regeneration, cell regenerative

Medicinal Use: Inflammation, bruises, swelling, wound healing, liver decongestant
Skin, Hair & Body: General skin care, wound healing, inflamed skin conditions, atopic dermatitis, acne, psoriasis, scar reduction, wrinkle reduction, free radical scavenger
Mind/Emotions: Relaxing, balancing
Spiritual: Balancing
Contraindications: None known. Caution because of ketone content

Lavender

Botanical Name: *Lavandula angustifolia*
Botanical Family: Lamiaceae
Derived From: Flowers
Origin: France
Cost: Moderate
Fragrance Character: Middle note, floral, moderate odor intensity
Blends Well With: Works well with most oils, good blending oil
Application: Topical, inhalation, bath, shower
Main Components: Linalol (45 to 50 percent) and other monoterpenes (30 percent), linalyl acetate, coumarins and complex mixture of other compounds

Therapeutic Uses

Properties: Antiseptic, wound healing, regenerative, balance of central nervous system
Medicinal Use: Illness, burns, injury, migraine, spasm, all-purpose
Skin, Hair & Body: General all-purpose skin, hair and body care
Mind/Emotions: Reduce nervousness, tension, insomnia
Spiritual: Balancing
Contraindications: None known

Palmarosa

Botanical Name: *Cymbopogon martinii*
Botanical Family: Poaceae
Derived From: Grass

Origin: Brazil, Nepal
Cost: Low
Fragrance Character: Middle note, rose and geranium like, round, moderate odor intensity
Blends Well With: most oils especially with high content of terpene alcohols, esters and fruit oils
Application: Topical, bath
Main Components: Geraniol (75 percent) (monoterpene alcohol), geranyl formiate (10 percent) (ester)

Therapeutic Uses

Properties: Antiseptic, antiviral, antifungal, soothing
Medicinal Use: Antibacterial, viral and fungal infections
Skin, Hair & Body: General all-purpose skin care, acne, wounds
Mind/Emotions: Relaxing, Balancing
Spiritual: Balancing
Contraindications: None known

Peppermint

Botanical Name: *Menthax piperita*
Botanical Family: Lamiaceae
Derived From: Leaves
Origin: France, USA
Cost: Moderate
Fragrance Character: Middle and top note, mint, moderate to high odor intensity
Blends Well With: Lavender, geranium and other alcohol/ ester oils
Application: Topical, inhalation, with caution in bath
Main Components: Menthol (45 percent) (monoterpene alcohol), menthone (25 percent) (ketone)

Therapeutic Uses

Properties: Stimulant, cooling, digestive balance, liver tonic, antispasmodic
Medicinal Use: Stomach complaints, nausea, liver congestion, fevers, PMS, allergies, bad breath
Skin, Hair & Body: Acne, skin purifier and stimulant
Mind/Emotions: Energizing, mental stimulant
Spiritual: Clearing

Contraindications: Caution with small children (not to be used when under 30 months), Caution when used undiluted topically or in bath, because it reduces body temperature

Rose

Botanical Names: *Rosa damascena* and *Rosa centfolia*
Botanical Family: Rosaceae
Derived From: Flower petals (Distilled oil may be called "Rose Otto." The absolute is generally identified as "Rose Absolute.")
Origin: Bulgaria, Turkey, Egypt
Cost: High to very high
Fragrance Character: Middle note (though is considered to be self balanced with top/middle/base notes), beautiful floral, moderate odor intensity
Blends Well With: Blends well with herbs and spices, frankincense, myrrh and other exquisite florals (jasmine, tuberose, osmanthus)
Application: Topical, inhalation, bath
Main Components: Very complex with hundreds of known compounds that include monoterpene alcohols, rose oxide, esters, ethers, ketones, nitrogen structures and trace elements

Therapeutic Uses

Properties: "Cure all," antiseptic, cell regenerative, balancing, nerve tonic
Medicinal Use: Regulate liver and spleen, tonic
Skin, Hair & Body: General skin care, mature skin, wrinkles, scars
Mind/Emotions: Aphrodisiac, emotionally balancing, nervousness, self esteem, depression, anxiety
Spiritual: Stimulates heart and sexual charkas, meditation
Contraindications: None known

Rosemary Verbenone Type

Botanical Name: *Rosmarinus officinalis* CT *verbenone*
Botanical Family: Lamiaceae
Derived From: Blossoming plant

Origin: Corsica, France, South Africa
Cost: Moderate to high
Fragrance Character: Middle note, herbaceous and fresh, moderate odor intensity
Blends Well With: Medicinal oils (eucalyptus, tea tree, MQV), rose, lavender, geranium, helichrysum
Application: Topical, inhalation, bath
Main Components: Monoterpene hydrocarbons (40 percent); monoterpene alcohols (4 percent) verbenone (ketone)

Therapeutic Uses

Properties: Cell regeneration, respiratory balance, mucolytic, liver and gall bladder stimulant
Medicinal Use: Liver tonic, colds, flu, bronchitis
Skin, Hair & Body: General skin and scalp care, mature skin, wrinkle and scar reduction
Mind/Emotions: Balancing, uplifting
Spiritual: Balancing
Contraindications: None known

Tea Tree (Figure 7-2)

Botanical Name: *Melaleuca alternifolia*
Botanical Family: Myrtaceae
Derived From: Branches and leaves
Origin: Australia
Cost: Low to moderate
Fragrance Character: Top/middle note, eucalyptus-like, medicinal, moderate odor intensity
Blends Well With: Medicinal oils (eucalyptus, ravensare, thyme), lavender, Australian sandalwood
Application: Topical, inhalation, bath, shower
Main Components: Terpene alcohols (50 percent) including terpinen-4-ol; 1,8 cineole (oxide); monoterpene hydrocarbons (25 percent)

Therapeutic Uses

Properties: Very medicinal, expectorant, antiviral, antibacterial
Medicinal Use: Decongestant, colds, flu, inflammation
Skin, Hair & Body: Acne, general skin care, antiseptic, scalp cleanser, cellulite
Mind/Emotions: None specified

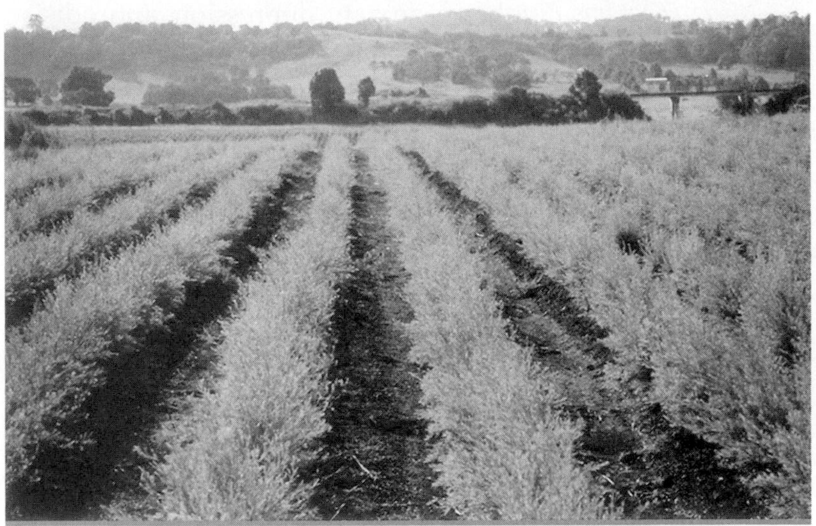

Figure 7-2 Tea tree farm, Australia.

Spiritual: None specified
Contraindications: May be irritating on sensitive or chapped skin

Ylang-Ylang

Botanical Name: *Cananga odorata*
Botanical Family: Annonaceae
Derived From: Flowers
Origin: Madagascar, Comores, Reunion, Philippines
Cost: Moderate
Fragrance Character: Middle note, floral and sweet
Blends Well With: Floral oil (rose, jasmine), resins (frankincense, myrrh), lavender, geranium, Australian sandalwood, cedarwood, vetiver
Application: Topical, inhalation, bath
Main Components: Terpene alcohols (55 percent) including linalool; farnesene (sesquiterpene); esters (15 percent)

Therapeutic Uses

Properties: Antiseptic, antispasmodic, nervous balance, sexual stimulant
Medicinal Use: Heart palpitations, cramps
Skin, Hair & Body: General skin care, scalp stimulant

Mind/Emotions: Euphoric, anxiety, depression, aphrodisiac
Spiritual: Uplifting, releasing
Contraindications: None known

FIVE ESSENTIAL OILS FOR INCREASED THERAPEUTIC ACTIVITY AND SPA APPLICATION

The previous list of thirteen essential oils provides a solid knowledge base of a collection of oils for complete therapeutic work. This next list of five essential oils increases the therapeutic potential of your collection of essential oils.

Bay Laurel

Botanical Name: *Laurus nobilis*
Botanical Family: Lauraceae
Derived From: Leaves
Origin: France, Corsica, Croatia, Slovenia
Cost: Moderate
Fragrance Character: Middle note, spicy, moderate odor intensity
Blends Well With: Medicinal oils (tea tree, ravensare, eucalyptus), lavender, lemon and other lemon fragrance oils, cedarwood
Application: Topical, inhalation, bath, shower (apply over lymph nodes during shower or sauna – not to be used more than 6 days straight)
Main Components: Cineole (oxide) (40 percent); euganol (phenylpropanoid) – (20 to 30 percent); terpene alcohols (10 percent); sesquiterpene lactones (5 percent); monoterpene hydrocarbons

Therapeutic Uses

Properties: Immune support, antibacterial, antiviral, detoxification, expectorant
Medicinal Use: Lymphatic drainage, sinus decongestant, general illness
Skin, Hair & Body: Acne, general skin care, detoxify and stimulate facial lymph, cellulite

Mind/Emotions: Balancing
Spiritual: Uplifting, balancing
Contraindications: None known

Cypress

Botanical Name: *Cupressus sempervirens*
Botanical Family: Cupressaceae
Derived From: Needles and cones
Origin: France, Italy
Cost: Low to moderate
Fragrance Character: Top/middle note, clean, light woody, airy, low to moderate odor intensity
Blends Well With: Citruses, medicinal oils (tea tree, ravensare, eucalyptus), lavender, other needle oil, Australian sandalwood
Application: Topical, inhalation
Main Components: Monoterpene hydrocarbons (50 percent); sesquiterpenes (including cedrol); diterpenes

Therapeutic Uses

Properties: Decongestant, antiviral, astringent, tonifying, stimulant, vasoconstrictor (constriction of capillaries)
Medicinal Use: Respiratory ailments, kidney support, sore throat, varicose veins, energizing
Skin, Hair & Body: Acne, cellulite, oily skin, scalp cleanser
Mind/Emotions: Uplifting, stimulant, clarity
Spiritual: Uplifting, aura cleansing
Contraindications: None known

Eucalyptus Citriodora

Botanical Name: *Eucalyptus citriodora*
Botanical Family: Myrtaceae
Derived From: Branches and leaves
Origin: Zanzibar, China, Tanzania, Brazil
Cost: Low
Fragrance Character: Top note, very lemony, moderate to high odor intensity
Blends Well With: Citruses, medicinal oils (tea tree, ravensare, other eucalyptus), lavender, Helichrysum italicum, melissa, Australian sandalwood
Application: Topical, inhalation

Main Components: Citronellal (aldehyde) (70 percent); monoterpene alcohol (20 percent)

Therapeutic Uses

Properties: Antiviral, anti-inflammatory, relaxing
Medicinal Use: Muscle pain, joint pain
Skin, Hair & Body: Acne, general skin care, cellulite
Mind/Emotions: Sedative, hypertension
Spiritual: None specified
Contraindications: None known

Lemon

Botanical Name: *Citrus limon*
Botanical Family: Rutaceae
Derived From: Fruit peel
Origin: Italy, USA, Argentina
Cost: Low to moderate
Fragrance Character: Top note, lemony
Blends Well With: Citruses, tea tree, eucalyptus globulus and radiata, lavender, needle oils
Application: Topical, inhalation
Main Components: Limonene (70 percent) (monoterpene hydrocarbon); citral (5 percent) (aldehyde); coumarin (2 percent)

Therapeutic Uses

Properties: Antiviral, antiseptic, relaxing, stimulating, diuretic, detoxifier
Medicinal Use: Disinfectant, liver detox, viral infection
Skin, Hair & Body: Skin purifier, cellulite, puffiness, water retention
Mind/Emotions: Relaxing, uplifting
Spiritual: Cleansing
Contraindications: Potential skin irritant

Niaouli/MQV

Botanical Name: *Melaleuca quinquenervia viridiflora*
Botanical Family: Myrtaceae
Derived From: Branches and leaves
Origin: Madagascar (referred to as MQV), New Caledonia (referred to as Niaouli)

Cost: Moderate
Fragrance Character: Middle note, medicinal, tea tree-eucalyptus-like, moderate odor intensity
Blends Well With: Tea tree, eucalyptus oils, medicinal herbal oils (thyme, oregano, rosemary) lavender, needle oils
Application: Topical, inhalation
Main Components: Oxide (55 percent); monoterpene and sesquiterpene alcohols; over 110 components

Therapeutic Uses

Properties: Antiviral, antiseptic, immune stimulant, expectorant, hormone balancing, antibacterial, antiviral
Medicinal Use: Immune deficiency, infection, respiratory ailments, hormone imbalance
Skin, Hair & Body: Skin purifier, cellulite, acne, infection, immune support
Mind/Emotions: Balancing
Spiritual: None specified
Contraindications: None known

OILS OF SPECIAL CONSIDERATION

Many excellent oils could be listed for special consideration. The essential oils included on this next list are ones that either have a very specific therapeutic use or are often considered for their superior benefits.

Bergamot

Botanical Name: *Citrus bergamia*
Botanical Family: Rutaceae
Derived From: Fruit peel
Origin: Sicily
Cost: Moderate
Fragrance Character: Top/middle note, citrus, "green" note, light to moderate odor intensity
Blends Well With: Citrus, ester/alcohol oils, jasmine, vetiver
Application: Topical, inhalation
Main Components: Esters (30 percent); monoterpenes (60 percent); coumarins

Therapeutic Uses

Properties: Calming, relaxing, astringent, antiseptic, digestive stimulant
Medicinal Use: Digestive cramping, nausea, infection
Skin, Hair & Body: Acne, atopic dermatitis, oily skin
Mind/Emotions: Anxiety, uplifting emotions
Spiritual: Uplifting
Contraindications: Possibly the most photosensitive essential oil. Avoid exposure to sun or UV lamps after application to the skin. Discolors the skin

German Chamomile

Botanical Name: *Matricaria recutita*
Botanical Family: Asteraceae
Derived From: Flowers
Origin: Germany (Bavarian is best), Hungary, Egypt
Cost: Moderate to high
Fragrance Character: Middle note, hay-like, dry, strong odor intensity
Blends Well With: Lavender, helichrysum, Roman chamomile
Application: Topical
Main Components: Chamazulene (sesquiterpene hydrocarbons); (-) alpha-bisabolol (sesquiterpene alcohol)

Therapeutic Uses

Properties: Anti-inflammatory, antiallergic, liver regenerative
Medicinal Use: Inflammation (wounds, muscles, infection), burns, reduce fever (foot wrap method), liver stagnation
Skin, Hair & Body: Inflamed skin conditions, hives (urticaria), acne, atopic dermatitis, psoriasis, rosacea, general skin care
Mind/Emotions: Relaxing
Spiritual: Throat chakra
Contraindications: None known

Roman Chamomile

Botanical Name: *Anthemis nobilis*
Botanical Family: Asteraceae
Derived From: Flowers

Origin: France, Chile, Germany, Italy
Cost: High
Fragrance Character: Middle note, apple-like or fruity, round, moderate to high odor intensity
Blends Well With: Lavender, florals, orange, mandarin, helichrysum, German chamomile
Application: Topical, inhalation
Main Components: Esters

Therapeutic Uses

Properties: Antidepressant, antianxiety, antispasmodic
Medicinal Use: Muscle tension, cramps, spasm, migraine, asthma
Skin, Hair & Body: Nervous skin conditions, atopic dermatitis, acne, rosacea, general skin care
Mind/Emotions: Powerful anxiety and tension release, depression, nervousness, fear
Spiritual: Relaxing, meditation
Contraindications: None known

Clary Sage

Botanical Name: *Salvia sclarea*
Botanical Family: Lamiaceae
Derived From: Leaves and flowers
Origin: France, Russia, Bulgaria, Germany, Australia
Cost: Moderate
Fragrance Character: Middle note, sweet floral, somewhat fruity, moderate to strong odor intensity
Blends Well With: Lavender, geranium and other ester/alcohol containing oils, vitex
Application: Topical, inhalation
Main Components: Linalyl acetate and other esters; linalool (monoterpene alcohol), sclareol (sesquiterpene alcohol), complex structure with many trace elements

Therapeutic Uses

Properties: Antidepressant, euphoric, antispasmodic, phyto-estrogen, hormone balance, regulates seborrhea
Medicinal Use: Muscle tension, cramps, spasm, migraine, PMS, hormonal imbalance, menopause

Skin, Hair & Body: General skin care, balance sebum for oily to dry skin and hair, soothing, mature skin, hormonal acne, scalp stimulant
Mind/Emotions: Depression, nervousness, tension, post-natal depression
Spiritual: Euphoric
Contraindications: None known. May be overly relaxing and sedating. Avoid during pregnancy.

Cistus (Rockrose) (Figure 7-3)

Botanical Name: *Cistus ladaniferus*
Botanical Family: Cistaceae
Derived From: Leaves and flowers
Origin: Spain, Portugal, France, Morocco
Cost: Moderate to high
Fragrance Character: Base/middle note, deep, warm, somewhat woody, dry, moderate to strong odor intensity
Blends Well With: Citrus oils, herbal, woods, resins, florals and spices
Application: Topical, inhalation
Main Components: Complex mixture, 45 percent pinene with other monoterpenes; 2 percent ketones

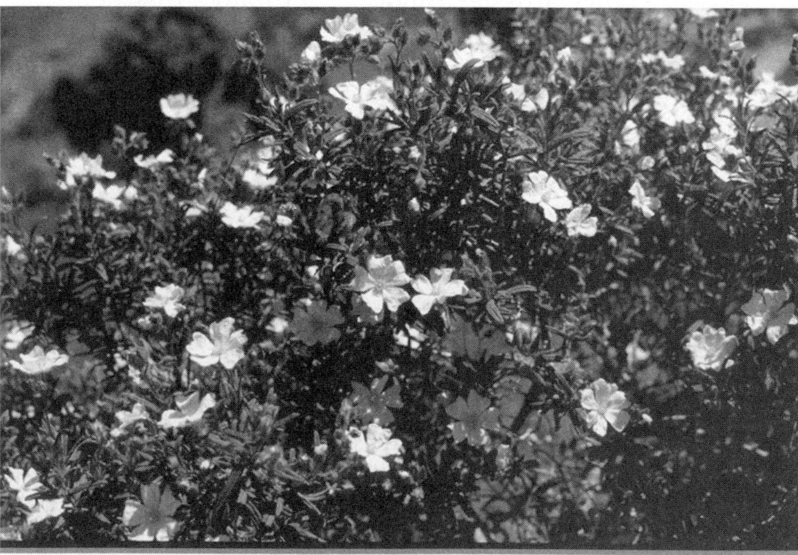

Figure 7-3 Cistus.

Therapeutic Uses

Properties: Antiviral, anti-infectious, wound healing, stops bleeding
Medicinal Use: Useful for many ailments and infection, excessive bleeding
Skin, Hair & Body: General skin care, wounds, bleeding, antiseptic, wrinkles and mature skin
Mind/Emotions: Comforting, balancing
Spiritual: Meditation, centering
Contraindications: None known

Frankincense

Botanical Name: *Boswellia carteri*
Botanical Family: Burseraceae
Derived From: Resin
Origin: Oman, Somalia
Cost: Moderate to high
Fragrance Character: Base/middle note, resinous, smoky, dry, "spiritual," moderate odor intensity
Blends Well With: Other resins (elemi, galbanum, myrrh), citrus, florals (jasmine, rose)
Application: Topical, inhalation, bath
Main Components: Monoterpenes (30 percent); sesquiterpenes; sesquiterpene alcohol

Therapeutic Uses

Properties: Strengthens immunity, cell regenerative, respiratory support
Medicinal Use: Bronchitis, immune deficiency
Skin, Hair & Body: General skin care, wrinkles, mature skin, dry skin, strengthening
Mind/Emotions: Fortifying
Spiritual: Meditation, spiritual practice and ritual use, stimulate third eye
Contraindications: None known

Jasmine (Absolute)

Botanical Name: *Jasminum grandiflorum*
Botanical Family: Oleaceae
Derived From: Flowers – hexane extraction
Origin: Egypt, India
Cost: High

Fragrance Character: Contains complete fragrance notes, sweet and exquisite floral, moderate to strong odor
Blends Well With: Most florals, orange, mandarin, lavender, vanilla, balsams, resins
Application: Topical, in dilution
Main Components: Very complex, containing benzyl acetate, linalool, cis-jasmone, indole, and many other compounds

Therapeutic Uses

Properties: Antidepressant, euphoric, aphrodisiac, soothing
Medicinal Use: Frigidity, impotence
Skin, Hair & Body: General skin care, soothing, mature skin, hormonal acne, scalp stimulant
Mind/Emotions: Depression, nervousness, tension, sexual stimulation, self-confidence
Spiritual: Euphoric
Contraindications: Use topically only. Caution because of solvent extraction. Both pure quality and synthetic varieties found in the marketplace.

Lavandin (*Lavandin grosso*)

This plant is a lavender hybrid, created by crossing *Lavandula angustifolia* with *Lavandula latifolia*. Lavandin is often sold as lavender or used to adulterate true lavenders. Though lavandin is much simpler than lavender in its composition, it is still a valued essential oil and beneficial as an inexpensive lavender replacement in blends. Along with the lavandin grosso, there are other varieties including super, reydovan, and abrialis.

Botanical Name: *Lavandin hybrida grosso*
Botanical Family: Lamiaceae
Derived From: Flowers
Origin: France
Cost: Low to moderate
Fragrance Character: Middle note, floral lavender-like, moderate odor intensity
Blends Well With: Blends well with most essential oils
Application: Topical, inhalation, bath
Main Components: A simplified lavender composition, mostly linalyl acetate and linalool

Therapeutic Uses

Properties: Calming, central nervous system balance, regenerative
Medicinal Use: Wound healing, headache, muscle spasm
Skin, Hair & Body: General skin care, wound healing
Mind/Emotions: Balancing, sedative, anxiety, tension, insomnia
Spiritual: Balancing
Contraindications: None known

Myrrh

Botanical Name: *Commiphora molmol*
Botanical Family: Burseraceae
Derived From: Resin
Origin: Oman, Somalia
Cost: Moderate to high
Fragrance Character: Base/middle note, resinous, earthy, moderate odor intensity
Blends Well With: Other resins, lavender, rose, jasmine, Australian sandalwood
Application: Topical
Main Components: Sesquiterpenes (50 percent); monoterpene hydrocarbons; ketones; aldehydes

Therapeutic Uses

Properties: Regenerative, analgesic, anti-inflammatory, immune modulator, antifungal
Medicinal Use: Coughs, reduce pain
Skin, Hair & Body: General skin care, wound healing, fungal infection, inflammatory skin conditions, ulcers, strengthens nails
Mind/Emotions: Emotionally fortifying
Spiritual: Meditation, spiritual practice, third eye and crown chakra
Contraindications: None known

Neroli

Botanical Name: *Citrus aurantium*
Botanical Family: Rutaceae
Derived From: Flower blossoms of the orange tree
Origin: Spain (Seville), France, Tunisia

Cost: High
Fragrance Character: Top note, fresh citrus like floral, low to moderate odor intensity
Blends Well With: Other citrus oils, cedarwood, jasmine, frankincense, myrrh, rose
Application: Topical (neat or diluted), inhalation, bath
Main Components: Monoterpene alcohols (30 percent); monoterpene hydrocarbons (20 percent); esters (20 percent)

Therapeutic Uses

Properties: Sedating, hypotensor, spasmolytic, antiviral, antibacterial, cell regenerative, aphrodisiac, circulatory tonic
Medicinal Use: Balance blood pressure, calm digestive tension (nervous stomach)
Skin, Hair & Body: Atopic dermatitis, stretch marks, balance skin condition, general skin care
Mind/Emotions: Depression, anxiety, uplifting, relaxing, insomnia
Spiritual: Aids all spiritual work, reconnects to higher self
Contraindications: None known

Orange

Botanical Name: *Citrus aurantium*
Botanical Family: Rutaceae
Derived From: Fruit peel
Origin: Italy, Spain, USA
Cost: Low
Fragrance Character: Top note, orange, low to moderate odor intensity
Blends Well With: Other citrus oils, cedarwood, lavender, chamomiles
Application: Topical, inhalation, bath
Main Components: Limonene (90 percent) (monoterpene hydrocarbon), linalool (5 percent), esters (2 percent)

Therapeutic Uses

Properties: Calming, antiviral, diuretic
Medicinal Use: Measles, chicken pox, edema
Skin, Hair & Body: Cellulite, purifying, acne
Mind/Emotions: Depression, sadness, uplifting, relaxing
Spiritual: Balancing
Contraindications: None known

Patchouli

Botanical Name: *Pogostemon cablin*
Botanical Family: Lamiaceae
Derived From: Leaves
Origin: India, Indonesia
Cost: Moderate
Fragrance Character: Base/middle note, earthy, musty, moderate to medium high odor intensity
Blends Well With: Citrus oils, resins, lavender, geranium
Application: Topical, inhalation, bath
Main Components: Sesquiterpene hydrocarbons (45 percent); 40 percent sesquiterpene alcohols

Therapeutic Uses

Properties: Antifungal, anti-inflammatory, regenerative, decongestant, vein tonic
Medicinal Use: Hemorrhoids
Skin, Hair & Body: Atopic dermatitis, psoriasis, acne, general skin care, dry and mature skin, dandruff
Mind/Emotions: Sedative at low dosage, stimulant at high dosage, balancing
Spiritual: Clarifying
Contraindications: None known

Pine (Common)

Botanical Name: *Pinus syvestris*
Botanical Family: Abiaceae
Derived From: Needles
Origin: Canada, France
Cost: Low to moderate
Fragrance Character: Middle/top note, pine, woody green, low to moderate odor intensity
Blends Well With: Other needle oils, resins, cedarwood, citrus, eucalyptus, Australian sandalwood
Application: Topical, inhalation, bath
Main Components: Monoterpene hydrocarbons (80 percent); esters; monoterpene alcohols

Therapeutic Uses

Properties: Antiviral, antiseptic, respiratory, tonic for glandular and nervous systems

Medicinal Use: Adrenal support and stimulation, respiratory ailments, viral infection, lymphatic drainage
Skin, Hair & Body: Lymphatic drainage
Mind/Emotions: Uplifting, clearing
Spiritual: Clarifying
Contraindications: None known

Thyme Linalool Type

Botanical Name: *Thymus vulgaris* CT *linalool*
Botanical Family: Lamiaceae
Derived From: Whole herb
Origin: France
Cost: High
Fragrance Character: Middle note, herbaceous, moderate odor intensity
Blends Well With: Other herbs and medicinal oils (eucalyptus, oregano, tea tree, ravensare)
Application: Topical, inhalation, bath
Main Components: Monoterpene alcohols (40 to 80 percent) (can be up to 78 percent linalool); esters, traces of sesquiterpenes, monoterpenes and phenols

Therapeutic Uses

Properties: Antimicrobial, antibacterial, antispasmodic, antifungal (Candida), anti-viral, neurotonic
Medicinal Use: Candida (yeast) infection, cleans and stimulates genito-urinary system, immune deficiency, respiratory ailments and infection, sprains and injury
Skin, Hair & Body: Acne, atopic dermatitis, psoriasis, all skin care, wounds, warts
Mind/Emotions: Calming, relaxing, nervous exhaustion
Spiritual: Clarifying, uplifting
Contraindications: None known

THE SANDALWOOD STORY

Sandalwood enjoys worldwide popularity as a fragrance, incense, and essential oil. It has a common use in skin care, spa, and aromatherapy products. Unfortunately, most of the sandalwood sold is synthetic. Sandalwood, extracted from the *Santalum album* species of Mysore, India, has historically been the primary source of sandalwood oil. The methods used to harvest the wood are destructive, because trees are uprooted, putting this species in danger of extinction. The sandalwood trees have been under government protection since the early part of the twentieth century. The government put a cap on exportation of sandalwood, the wood and the oil, and also sponsored the development of a synthetic replacement for the oil. This synthetic is the oil that most people are using for aromatherapy, skin care, and incense. Sustainable farms have been developed and are now producing authentic sandalwood oil. This oil is very expensive and reaches very few areas of the marketplace. The chance of a sustainable and plentiful source of the oil becoming available is still remote. An authentic *Santalum album* essential oil is purportedly being produced in Indonesia. Many issues, such as the use of slave labor, make this potential source of sandalwood a less than desirable alternative to the Mysore sandalwood. You can safely assume that any sandalwood oil sold and claimed to be from the Indian Mysore region is either synthetic, highly adulterated, or from a questionable Indonesian source.

The Sandalwood Solution

The solution to the sandalwood problem comes from Australia. On that continent is a sandalwood tree, *Santalum spicatum*, which is offered as a sustainable and authentic alternative to the Indian sandalwood oil. *Santalum spicatum* is a different species and therefore has a slightly different composition and fragrance. This oil is not a replacement for the rich woody sandalwood fragrance one gets from a genuine Mysore sandalwood. The Australian sandalwood has a softer and somewhat lighter fragrance. According to many aromatherapists who have worked with the Australian sandalwood, it does provide the necessary and expected sandalwood activity. Most likely, though, these same therapists were unsuspectingly using synthetic Indian sandalwood in the past. So how would they know how Australian compares to the Mysore sandalwood? Australian sandalwood is protected by the Australian government, is ecologically farmed, and will remain a sustainable source. Good quality, genuine, and authentic oils are available, because it is being produced mainly for the aromatherapy market.

Australian Sandalwood (Figure 7-4)

Botanical Name: *Santalum spicatum*
Botanical Family: Santalaceae
Derived From: Wood

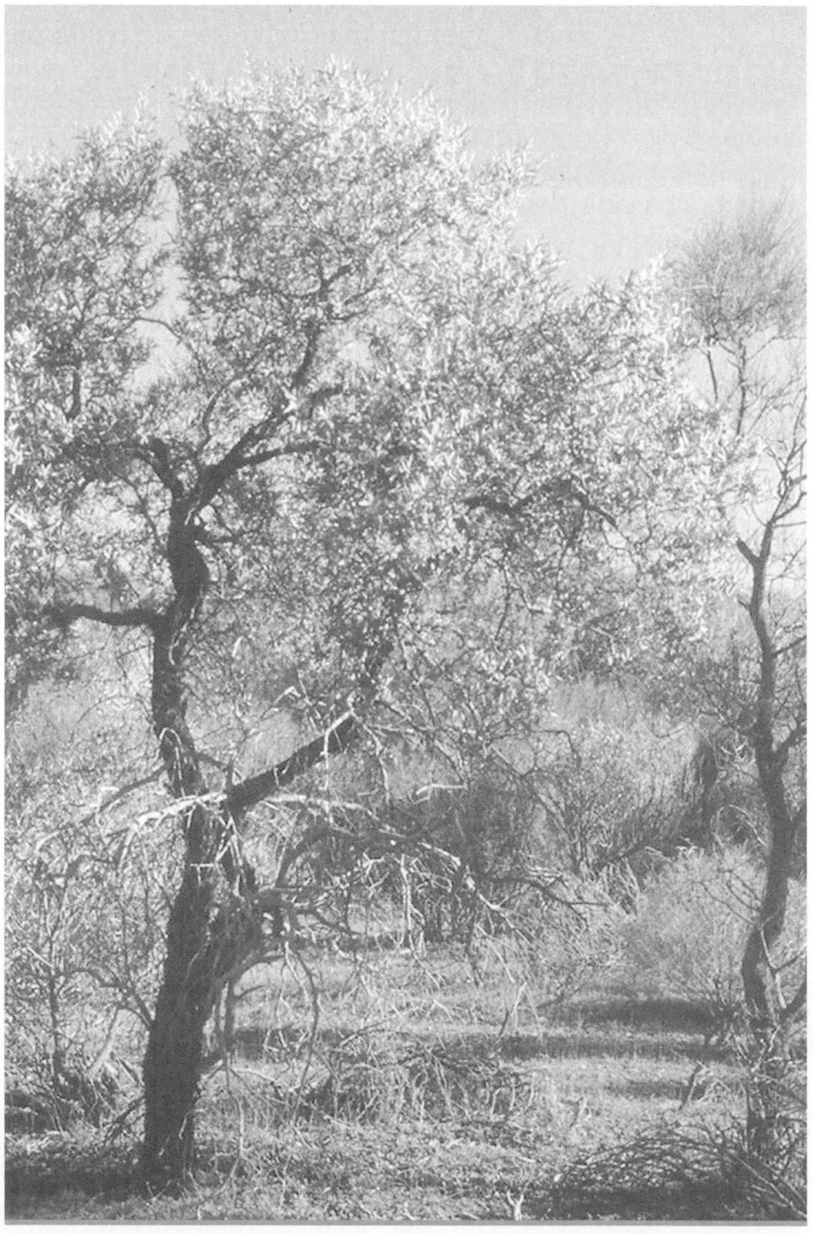

Figure 7-4 Australian sandalwood.

Origin: Australia
Cost: Moderate to high
Fragrance Character: Base/middle note, woody, warm, with sweet and fruity top notes, soft to moderate odor intensity
Blends Well With: Citrus, resins, spices and florals
Application: Topical, inhalation, bath
Main Components: Santalol and other sesquiterpene alcohols

Therapeutic Uses

Properties: Anti-inflammatory, antibacterial, immune stimulant, antiseptic, antifungal
Medicinal Use: Respiratory ailments, infection,
Skin, Hair & Body: General skin care, dry and mature skin, sunburn, atopic dermatitis, capillary strength
Mind/Emotions: Balancing, anxiety, nervous tension, stress, grief
Spiritual: Opening, meditation, ritual, opening third eye and crown chakra
Contraindications: None known

AUTHOR'S **NOTE**

DISCOVERING A NEW OIL

Random essential oil discoveries can be an exciting moment, especially for an aromatherapy enthusiast (or geek) like myself. In the mail today I received a couple of unexpected samples from an Australian supplier. There were two new sandalwood essential oils. I never knew either one existed. The first one is Yasi Sandalwood (*Santalum yasi*). This one has a very distinctive "sandalwood" fragrance, even more so than the Australian sandalwood. My immediate experience tells me this is an oil worth having and is almost certain to be added to my collection. My sense is that it will provide the qualities expected of sandalwood, and be useful in skin care, meditation, and yoga practice. This is my immediate impression. I know and trust this distributor, so I do not anticipate any adulteration.

Continued

The next step is to do some research. First is a simple internet search. This search pulls pages that describe the tree from the agricultural aspect but does not find any details about the oil's composition. If I know the composition, I can more accurately anticipate uses and expected results. As I'm writing this section, the fragrance is adamantly adhering to my olfactory bulb. It's pretty delicious. It's absolutely "sandalwood" with a lingering "cocoa" twist. That's fun. Yasi sandalwood is harvested from Tonga and Fiji. There are sustainability issues according to the letter accompanying the oils and also from information I have gathered from the internet. Fiji has poor control of harvesting. Tonga is well managed by the Royal Family. I assume that the one I received is from Tonga.

The second oil is from Vanuatu. I had to pull out the internet maps to find this place. It is a group of islands just north of Fiji and northeast of Australia. The oil, called Pacific Sandalwood (*Santalum austrocaledonicum*), is quite different from Yasi oil. A mix of components is blending into the typical woody santalol scent. It is its own unique sandalwood oil. There are some especially interesting notes in this oil. I can't put a name to them. This oil is also a potential addition to my collection.

I decided to have this experience and document it here to give you a sense of discovering a new oil. If you are an aromatherapy novice, you are about to have quite a few of these experiences, even with oils from familiar herbs and spices like black pepper, coriander, ginger and thyme. Enjoy it.

CHOOSING ESSENTIAL OILS FOR SPECIFIC CONDITIONS

In this section we'll look at a specific condition and select those essential oils that will best treat the condition based on chemistry (Chapter 5) and the properties of essential oils (Chapter 6). This exercise will familiarize you with a process that can be used to select essential oils for effective treatment. Oil selection and formulating are further developed in upcoming chapters.

Acne

An acneic skin condition is the model for this example. Acne is caused by inflammation within the follicles.[1] Based on this fact, we know that to correct and prevent an acneic condition the inflammation must be addressed. Inflammation may also be a symptom of an underlying condition that must be evaluated. If an underlying condition is discovered, appropriate essential oils are chosen to alleviate these causative conditions.

The mechanisms that cause acne lesions and inflammation are as follows: keratinized cells, the corneocytes of the stratum corneum within the follicle walls do not exfoliate properly (**retention hyperkeratosis**) and, it is believed that when the retained cells mix with sebum they become a sticky, viscous substance that clogs the follicle and eventually attracts bacterial infection. The acneic eruption is caused by the accumulation and engorgement of trapped debris within the follicle.

A more recent explanation notes that the cytokine interleukin-1, when triggered by stress, diet, or other factors, generates inflammation that causes corneocytes to become sticky. This event initiates the process that leads to clogged pores.[2] This explanation reveals that acne is an inflammatory condition caused by a combined imbalance in the nervous, immune, and endocrine systems.[3] Inflammation in this scenario is a cause and not just a symptom of the condition.

Finding Your Focus

To select essential oils to effectively treat acne, first identify the conditions to be addressed with the essential oils. They become the "focus" of the treatment. Always begin a treatment by creating a therapeutic focus. You don't know which direction to take if you don't know where you are going. The focus in treating acneic skin centers on these concerns:

- inflammation
- stress and anxiety
- infection
- congestion, debris, hardened sebum
- hormonal balance
- inflammatory diet and lifestyle

Essential Oil Compounds for Effective Treatment of Acne

The next step is to review the compounds from the chemical groupings that are most effective in treating the underlying conditions causing acne or those that are most effective in dealing with your therapeutic focus. The compounds can be selected as a group, having the required action, such as esters or monoterpene hydrocarbons; or they can be selected as individual molecules, like linalool from the monoterpene alcohol group or the sesquiterpene hydrocarbon, chamazulene. Essential oils are then selected that contain the chosen compounds. For instance, stress relief is included as a therapeutic focus to treat acne. A functional group that includes compounds known to effectively treat stress is the ester group. By reviewing Chapter 5 you will find that lavender, clary sage, geranium, and neroli all contain esters. These oils, or any others that contain higher amounts of esters, are recommended for stress. Once essential oils have been identified to contain the appropriate compounds, such as selected ester-containing oils, they can then be added to a list of potential oils to treat acne.

As you go through this process for each condition, or therapeutic focus, you will find that some essential oils are repeated, because they contain two or more of the compounds that have been selected for therapeutic use. This principle can be demonstrated with conditions of stress and inflammation. For stress, the ester group has been selected. Inflammation may best be treated using the sesquiterpene hydrocarbon group. Cape chamomile contains both esters and sesquiterpene hydrocarbons. Therefore, instead of using two oils, you could use only one, Cape chamomile, to fulfill the activity of two different compounds.

Choosing Essential Oils for Their Properties

Selecting essential oils based on the properties of the compounds they contain is one way to decide which essential oils to use. You can also select oils based on the known properties of the essential oil itself, which is the more common way to choose essential oils for therapeutic work. Matching essential oil properties to treat the defined therapeutic purpose is similar to the exercise of selecting compounds based on their properties. Helichrysum and German chamomile both contain anti-inflammatory properties; therefore, they are suitable to treat inflammation associated with acne. MQV and tea tree oil are well known for their antibacterial properties so both can be used when anti-infectious properties are needed. It is not necessary to write down every essential oil you find that may be used for a specific condition. In practice, you will list only those oils you feel are most appropriate, and if your collection is small, only those oils that are immediately available to you.

Using Experience to Choose Essential Oils

A seasoned aromatherapist often makes essential oil choices based on familiarity with oils and past experience. A beginner needs to rely on an essential oil reference guide by checking the properties and compounds of essential oils. (See Chapters 5, 6, and 7.)

Your Completed List of Essential Oils for Treatment

Through this exercise, you now have a list of compounds (see Table 7-1) and essential oils (Table 7-2) to choose from that address the symptoms and conditions of acneic skin. To complete this process, you will choose 4–7 final oils to be used in a treatment blend. Table 7-3 gives an example of a final blend. Formulation and blending is further discussed in Chapter 8.

Table 7-1 Choosing Compounds for Acneic Skin

This is an example list you may create when selecting the compounds that would best treat acneic skin.

Condition	Therapeutic Choice
Inflammation	Compounds – Aldehydes, sesquiterpene hydrocarbons
Stress/Anxiety	Compounds – Cedrol, esters, linalool, aldehydes,
Infection	Compounds – Mono and sesquiterpene alcohols, oxides
Congestion/Debris/Sebum	Compounds – Monoterpene hydro-carbons, oxides
Hormonal Balance	Compounds – Anethole, citral, sclareol

Table 7-2 Choosing Essential Oils for Acneic Skin

This is an example list you may create when selecting the essential oils based on their known properties that would best treat acneic skin.

Condition	Therapeutic Choice
Inflammation	Essential Oils: Helichrysum, Cape chamomile, German chamomile, *Eucalyptus globulus,* tea tree, myrrh
Stress/Anxiety	Essential Oils: Cape chamomile, cedarwood, clary sage, bergamot, geranium, lavender, neroli, rose
Infection	Essential Oils: *Eucalyptus globulus* and *radiata,* lavender, MQV, thyme linalool, tea tree
Congestion/Debris/Sebum	Essential Oils: *Eucalyptus globulus* and *radiata,* grapefruit, lemon, MQV, tea tree
Hormonal Balance	Essential Oils: Clary sage, fennel, geranium, lavender, MQV, sage, vitex

Table 7-3 Essential Oils Chosen for an Acne Treatment Formula

A blend can be fromulated from the following selection of oils. This list is extracted from a longer list compiled based on the properties of compounds and the individual essential oils for the therapeutic focus of acneic skin. This list includes the oil's main compounds that would best address the symptoms of acneic skin as well as the properties of the oil that result from its overall structure. You will learn how to blend and apply these oils in Chapter 8.

Common Name	Botanical Name	Contents	Properties
Lavender	*Lavandula angustifolia*	linalool, esters, coumarins	Soothing, general skin tonic, cell regenerative, anti-infectious, stress reduction

Table 7-3 *(Continued)*

Common Name	Botanical Name	Contents	Properties
MQV	*Melaleuca quinquenervia viridiflora*	terpene alcohols, sequiterpene alcohols	Immune stimulant, detoxifying, anti-infectious
Cape Chamomile	*Eriocephalus punctulatus*	sequiterpenes, esters	Anti-inflammatory, stress reduction, calming
Cedarwood	*Cedrus atlantica*	sequiterpene alcohols; cedrol	Gentle circulatory stimulant, autonomic nervous system balance

CHAPTER SUMMARY

Aromatherapy is based on skill and knowledge of essential oils. The seasoned aromatherapist becomes familiar with essential oils through the experience of working with oils. The novice can become familiar with the oils by beginning to work with just a few essential oils. Using the list included in this chapter will provide a good starting point for reference and oil selections.

To select oils for a specified condition begin by developing a therapeutic focus (a list of symptoms or possible causes that relate to the condition). To select appropriate essential oils, one then determines which compounds and essential oils contain properties that address the condition, symptoms and causes. Finally narrow the list to a few selected essential oils to develop a specific therapeutic formula or recipe.

REVIEW QUESTIONS

1. What is the best way to begin learning about individual essential oils?
2. How many essential oils do most aromatherapists work with?

3. How will working with recipes or formulas assist the beginner aromatherapist?
4. What is it about the sandalwood oil from Mysore, India that you should be aware of?
5. How should you begin to select oils to treat a specific condition?
6. Once you have a therapeutic "focus," what three steps are necessary to select essential oils needed to treat a specific condition?

CHAPTER REFERENCES

1. Jones, D. (2005). "The potential immunological effects of topical retinoids." *Dermatology Online Journal 11* (1); 3.
2. Ingham, E., Walters, C. E., Eady, E. A., Cove, J. H., Kearney, J. N. & Cunliffe W. J. (1998). "Inflammation in acne vulgaris: Failure of skin micro-organisms to modulate keratinocyte interleukin 1 production in vitro." *Dermatology 196* (1); 86–88.
3. Perricone, N. (2003). *The Acne Prescription*. New York, NY: HarperCollins.

Blending and Methods of Application

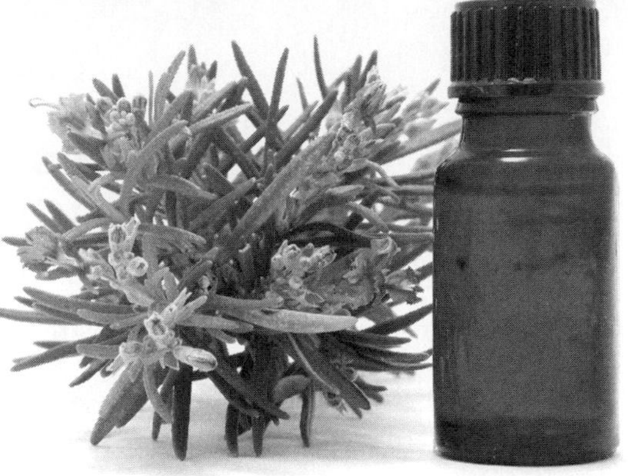

CHAPTER 8

One becomes two, two becomes three, and by means of the third and fourth achieves unity; thus two are but one . . .

–Maria the Jewess

LEARNING OBJECTIVES

1. Gain sufficient knowledge to create aromatherapy blends as part of a creative, artistic, and scientific craft.
2. Expand aromatherapy skills through the use of essential oil synergy, thereby using the combined effect of two or more essential oils.
3. Learn simple introductory methods of application and formulation for precise therapeutic treatment to create powerful therapeutic synergies.
4. Discover the basics of developing well balanced and pleasingly fragrant essential oil blends.

DIVERSITY OF ESSENTIAL OIL APPLICATION

One of the unique qualities of essential oil use is the diversity of application methods. A single oil or blend of two or more oils may be applied topically in a variety of methods that includes massage, skin and body care, perfumes, baths, showers, body wraps, or poultices. Each of these topical application methods includes a number of formulation techniques and choices. Essential oils can be inhaled using diffusers, candles, or steam or by inhaling the oil from a tissue or directly from a bottle. In medical treatment, oils may be prescribed and administered orally or through suppositories.

This flexibility in application methods not only enables precision in aromatherapy treatment but also permits the practitioner or user to select methods for specific reasons that include ease of application, availability of supplies, time constraints, and even mood. Table 8-1 demonstrates the versatility of application methods used in an aromatherapy treatment.

Table 8-1 Methods of Essential Oil Application

Method	How applied
External	in a carrier oil base or neat
Bath/Soak	in water
Shower	either neat or in carrier
Inhalation	in steaming water, candles, and diffusers
Personal care	in skin care, lotion, or spray preparations
Spa	in masks, sprays, wraps, and lotions
Nose	inhaled from tissue placed in nose
Internal	taken in capsules, in liquid, with honey, or dropped directly into mouth
Suppositories	in cocoa butter

BLENDING ESSENTIAL OILS

This chapter is a review of essential oil blending and formulation. It is not always necessary to create a blend of essential oils. An aromatherapy treatment may be complete with just one essential oil or formulated with a synergistic blend of three or more oils. A single oil may be a complete therapeutic treatment. No rule dictates whether one oil or a blend of oils is more appropriate. Experience will guide you in this area.

Art, Science, and Scent of Blending

Blending essential oils is a scientific venture, as well as an artistic one. The science of aromatherapy relies on understanding and incorporating chemistry, research, and clinical studies to develop precise therapeutic formulations. The art reflects intuitiveness, spontaneity, and inspiration to select essential oils. The aromatherapy enthusiast will also develop a *nose,* the talent associated with a perfumer, for fragrance blending. Fragrance, in relation to the sense of smell discussed in Chapter 3, is important to the therapeutic result in aromatherapy. The most effective formulations and blends are created using a balance of art, science, and scent.

ESSENTIAL OIL SYNERGY

Synergy occurs when two or more agents, organs, or organisms work and cooperate with each other to produce a sum, or result, greater than the total effects of each agent operating by itself.[1] The process of emerging properties was introduced in Chapter 5. In emerging properties, the result is greater than the sum of the individual units, as when cells become organs with a function that overrides and cannot be fully understood by the function of the individual cells. In aromatherapy, synergy describes the resulting emergent properties that develop from the molecular composition of an individual oil or from a blend of oils. The unique character and the properties of oils are a consequence of the combined synergistic activity of its molecular structure. Essential oils can have properties that go beyond the described properties of the functional groups that compose the oil. This synergy becomes evident when analyzing the properties of individual oils listed in Chapter 7 in comparison with the listed components. One finds the expected properties as defined by the molecular components, but additional properties that result from synergism are also evident.

In aromatherapy, the term *synergy* is more commonly used to describe the resulting character of a blend of essential oils. When essential oils are blended, the formula may have an enhanced character that cannot be explained by the properties of the individual parts. Another aspect to the art of aromatherapy is to formulate effective therapeutic and fragrance synergies.

Synergy of Essential Oil Molecular Components

A compound synergy can be fashioned to enhance a desired therapeutic effect. For example, if the desired result of the blend is sedation, this effect can be formulated by using the sedative properties of ester compounds. An *ester synergy* is formed when two or more essential oils that contain large amounts of ester compounds are combined or blended (Table 8-2). The resulting synergy enhances the sedative and anti-anxiety properties of the blended ester compounds. This compounded effect leads to a synergistic increase in the antispasmodic and antifungal properties of the esters as well. Ester synergies are very useful for skin conditions that result from high stress and anxiety. If the synergy arises from large amounts of sesquiterpene hydrocarbon compounds, the result will enhance the anti-inflammatory properties of these compounds. Expectorant action can be increased with a 1,8 oxide synergy, and wound healing is improved through a ketone synergy.

Table 8-2 Oils for an Ester Synergy

Essential oils that may be used in an ester synergy are:
Roman chamomile (*Anthemis nobilis*)
Cape chamomile (*Eriocephalus punctulatus*)
Clary sage (*Salvia sclarea*)
Geranium (*Pelargonium asperum*)
Lavender (*Lavandula angustifolia*)
Mandarin petitgrain (*Citrus reticula*)
Neroli (*Citrus aurantium*)

Holistic Synergy

Synergy is sometimes used to explain the holistic therapeutic healing action of essential oils and their ability to harmonize or support body systems. The action of essential oils is the result of their molecular synergy interacting with cells and functions of the body. Add to this an antimicrobial effect and you can understand how an oil such as *Eucalyptus polybractea,* which contains the expectorant properties of 1,8 cineole, the anti-inflammatory effects of phellandral, mucolytic ketones, and antimicrobial terpene alcohols is capable of full spectrum healing because of its synergistic composition.[2] This synergistic action can be mimicked by thoughtfully combining essential oils according to their known components. The more complex an essential oil blend, the more diverse the activity may be within the body. Increasing the complexity of a blend allows for therapeutic diversity that may holistically address more functions of the body and the cells. This relationship between complexity and spectrum of action should not be seen as meaning that the potential of an oil or blend that is simpler in its composition is limited. Keep in mind that a single oil, like the *Eucalyptus polybractea,* is capable of great holistic synergistic action.

DOSAGES

Discussion is ongoing among aromatherapists to determine standard dosage recommendations. There can be a wide disparity of opinion about what constitutes safe and effective dosage amounts. Most authorities agree that essential oils deliver therapeutic efficacy at "low dosages," though what either low or high dosage means is never satisfactorily defined or explained. For this text, we accept the most common recommendations and ranges for several application methods.

Specific Dosages and Lower Concentrations

When essential oils enter the body, they react with the systems and specific receptors of the cells.[3] **Receptors** are cell components that interact with hormones, drugs, and chemical mediators in the body that trigger a response in the cell. The receptor relationship with all chemical mediators, such as hormones, neuropeptides, and drugs is similar to that of a lock and key, meaning that the essential oil, a chemical mediator, must be the correct shape to fit the receptor. This relationship is designed to influence specific functions within the cell. **Specific effects** of essential oils are defined by the interaction with receptors and the interaction many oils have with physiological systems. Specific effects are often noted at lower rather than higher concentrations.

Studies show that essential oil compounds with sedative effects have their strongest efficacy at lower dosages and that the effect diminishes as dosages are increased.[4] Expectorant and sedative actions are specific effects of essential oils. Essential oils used in low concentrations for inhalation showed positive effect, and that effect was minimized at higher concentrations.[5] A higher concentration for inhalation is determined to be the level at which the inhaled air has a slight noticeable aroma.

Non-Specific Dosages and Higher Dosages

Non-specific effects are apparent at higher dosages, that is, more than one undiluted drop of essential oil. Non-specific effects are mediated by the oil's ability to connect to the cell membrane and other fatty components of the body. For acute conditions, high dosage formulations are often used. This practice is especially apparent with internal or undiluted topical use. Higher dosages are most effective for antiviral activity that is associated with the lipophilic nature (an affinity for fats) of essential oils.

Other Dosage Considerations Knowing specific and non-specific essential oil functions may assist you to determine dosages. Other considerations for dosage quantity include application method, area of body, individual sensitivity, oil contraindications, and the person's constitution and overall health. A person in a relatively weak state is commonly started at lower dosages.

DOSAGES FOR BASIC ESSENTIAL OIL BLENDING

Essential oils are combined to become a percentage of the total formula when added to a cream, oil, or perfume blend. The percentage tells you how much essential oil is used; the **dilution** amount in the entire product or blend. The basic guidelines to follow are shown in Table 8-3.

Table 8-3 Essential Oil Dilution Percentages

0.5 percent – 1 percent Blend	For use in "subtle" aromatherapy, children, people with weak immunity or weak constitutions, and people who are overly sensitive.
1.5 percent – 2.5 percent	This concentration is the most common blending percentage. Most formulas are between 2 percent – 2.5 percent of essential oils.
2.5 percent – 5 percent	Used to increase fragrance balance or for increased physical therapeutic activity. Higher percentages are used for larger parts of the body, such as legs and buttocks, and for cellulite reduction.
5 percent – 10 percent	This concentration of essential oils is used for specific areas, such as the abdomen, lower back, or large muscle areas; use when a deeper concentration of oils is desired.
10 percent – 50 percent	A high percentage of essential oils is used for physical conditions that require deeper or more aggressive therapeutic activity. Arthritis and joint pain, some lower back pain, and parasitic infections are situations in which a high concentration is applicable. Skin care seldom, if ever, requires such a high concentration. When blending at this percentage, note that potential irritation or sensitivity may be encountered.

Measurement in "Drops"

An interesting attribute to aromatherapy is the common measurement in drops. Drops are an unscientific method of calculating the amount of essential oil used in formulation. This is not a precise form of measurement because of differences in essential oil viscosity. One drop of lavender is not the same weight or volume as a drop of myrrh. There is also variance in the size

Table 8-4	Approximate Conversion of Essential Oil Drop to Weight and Volume
Approximately 20 drops = 1 gram (g).	
Approximately 20 drops = 1 milliliter (mL).	

of the dropping apparatus, such as pipettes, droppers, or **orifice reducers,** a fitting inside the neck of a bottle that allows drops to be extracted. This variety means that identical lavender oils, dropped from two different bottles with different orifice reducers, can vary in the volume contained in each drop. Though these conditions make drops an inaccurate form of measurement, it remains the standard measurement used in aromatherapy. This form of measurement gives the impression that aromatherapy can be approached casually, without the tension of precision attached. The drops method is valid so long as basic guidelines and application contraindications for certain oils are followed. For more precise formulation, the essential oils must be measured by weight or liquid volume. Keep in mind that if you measure in weight, the weight of the entire formula must be calculated. Measurement in volume must also remain consistent throughout the entire formulation. See Table 8-4 to approximate the weight or volume of a drop of essential oil.

CALCULATING FOR A BASIC ESSENTIAL OIL BLEND

Calculating the number of drops needed in a formula requires some basic math. A simple formula to calculate a 2.5 percent dilution of essential oils is computed by noting the bottle size in milliliters (30 mL is approximately 1 ounce). Divide this number by 2; this amount equals the total number of essential oil drops needed for a 2.5 percent concentration for the final blend. See this formula in Table 8-5.

This formula can be used to calculate other percentage dosages. Simply double your final number of drops, and you have a 5 percent formula; double again, and the formula specifies the

Table 8-5	Calculation to Determine a 2.5 percent Essential Oil Dilution
Number of mL ÷ 2 = total number of essential oil drops.	

number of drops for a 10 percent dilution of essential oils. For a lower percentage of essential oils in a blend, divide the number of drops used to create the original 2.5 percent dilution in half, for a 1.25 percent solution. See formulating examples in Table 8-6.

Table 8-6 Dilution Example Using a One-Ounce (30 mL) Bottle or Jar

Dilution Formula: 30 mL ÷ 2 = 15 drops
Fifteen (15) drops of essential oil are used in a 30 mL bottle for a 2.5 percent concentration. If the formula requires four oils, the following distribution may be used:
3 drops cedarwood
4 drops lavender
5 drops orange
3 drops ylang-ylang
Total: 15 drops for a 2.5 percent dilution
The remaining 97.5 percent of this blend consists of carrier oils (see Chapter 9). This blend of oils may be added to 30 mL of an unscented base formula such as a cream or shampoo.
To create a 5 percent dilution of essential oils, this formula is doubled:
In a 30-mL (1-ounce) bottle or jar:
6 drops cedarwood
8 drops lavender
10 drops orange
6 drops ylang-ylang
Total: 30 drops for a 5 percent dilution
Double it again, and you have a 10 percent dilution of essential oils:
In a 30-mL bottle or jar:
12 drops cedarwood
16 drops lavender
20 drops orange
12 drops ylang-ylang
Total: 60 drops for a 10 percent dilution

Table 8-7 Reformulate a 2.5 percent to a 1.25 percent Essential Oil Dilution (30-mL Bottle)	
Begin with the formulation and number of drops in the 2.5 percent dilution in Table 8-6.	
1.5 percent Dilution	Recalculate to whole number
1.5 drops cedarwood	recalculate to 1 drop cedarwood
2 drops lavender	2 drops lavender
2.5 drops orange	recalculate to 2 drops orange
1.5 drops ylang-ylang	recalculate to 1 drop ylang-ylang
Total: 6 drops for a 1.25 percent dilution (approximate)	

Note that in the examples provided in Table 8-6, not all blends will fit accurately within this formula. If you are using a half-ounce (15 mL) bottle or jar, the formula requires using 7.5 drops of essential oil (15 mL ÷ 2 = 7.5 drops). In this case, because there are no half drops, the formula can be made using either 7 drops or 8 drops. The aromatherapist decides whether to use 7 or 8 drops.

To create a lower concentration aromatherapy dilution, you need to reduce the formula. The sample in Table 8-7 is an example of a 1.25 percent dilution created by dividing the previous formula, for a 2.5 percent dilution, in half. This example refers to half drops, so simply recalculate and use a whole number of drops.

Note that in the Table 8-7 example, the recalculation lowers the number of drops in half, to their next lowest whole number. For subtle aromatherapy, lower doses are preferred. It would be equally correct to recalculate the drop amount to the next highest whole number, or mix them up, with some higher, and some lower. The resulting percentage will not be exactly 1.25 percent, but an approximation of that percentage.

Precise Calculations and Measurement

For more precise calculations and dilution measurements, formulas are calculated using percentages of weight or volume. A 1-ounce bottle or jar holds approximately 30 grams (± 2 g) of ingredients by weight. A 2 percent dilution of essential oils in a 1-ounce container is approximately 0.6 grams total of essential oils. A measurement of liquid volume, assuming that a container holds a total of 30 mL of liquid ingredients, totals 0.6 mL of essential oils for a 2 percent dilution. These measurements are used when accurate calculations are desired for scientific research, for clinical studies, and for manufacturing purposes.

"NEAT" ESSENTIAL OILS

The term for undiluted essential oils is *neat.* Although it is often recommended that essential oils never be used neat on the skin, at times doing so is appropriate, and at times it is the easiest and quickest method of application. It is best to use oils neat only when you are familiar with their actions. If you are new to aromatherapy and lack experience, it is better to be very cautious. Generally, aromatherapists avoid neat application of essential oils. It is best, and highly recommended, not to use neat essential oils with children, during pregnancy, and on sensitive individuals.

The main precaution for neat application is to know which essential oils are potential irritants. Oil of cinnamon will irritate the skin if applied neat. A 0.5 percent dilution of cinnamon has a lesser chance of irritating the skin or mucous membranes. Other essential oils may irritate some skin but not others when applied undiluted; this potential varies from person to person. Essential oils are very concentrated, so using them undiluted on the skin is generally not necessary.

Effective Use of High Dosage, Neat Essential Oil Application

Medical aromatherapy often uses large amounts of oils neat on the skin. A number of techniques using neat oils poured directly onto the body are especially effective for difficult conditions. One treatment reported to have profound healing benefits involves the neat formulation and application of known irritants and may include cinnamon, clove, thyme thymol type, oregano, *Eucalyptus smithii*, and others. The clinical use of neat essential oils, including antimicrobial oils that are potential irritants, are within the highly successful repertoire of Dr. Daniel Pénoël. Only experienced aromatherapists should apply known sensitizing oils neat. In some countries or states, use of neat oils may require proper licensing.

A Review of Potential Safety and Sensitivity Issues for Neat Application of Oils

Oils with the greatest amounts of terpene alcohols are the safest to use directly on the skin. These oils include lavender, tea tree, geranium, and MQV. Tea tree oil has shown irritant potential in some studies, however, especially when applied neat.[6,7] Interestingly enough, some studies acknowledge the anti-inflammatory action of tea tree oil.[8,9] The findings of irritation could have been caused by using oil that was not genuine and authentic or was applied to a sensitized skin. Any neat oil can be uncomfortable on the skin. Use caution, experience, and common sense if applying oils neat.

BLENDING FOR MASSAGE

A basic essential oil massage blend can be created by using a 2.5 percent dilution formula. Essential oils are added to a carrier oil (see Chapter 1), most often a vegetable or fruit oil. Typical carriers are grapeseed, sunflower, avocado, or olive oils. (See Table 8-5 for the 2.5 percent dilution calculation.) Using organic carrier oils is important; also note whether the client has sensitivities to any of the nut oils. For example, sensitivity to hazelnuts is common.

Massage Lotions and Creams

Essential oils for massage can also be added to a cream or lotion base, depending on the preferences of the therapist and client. Lotions and creams are a preferred carrier for foot massage, sport injuries, and deep tissue massage. Chapter 10 provides information about the ingredients used to make creams and lotions. Essential oils are added to unscented cream and lotion bases using similar percentages as those used with carrier oil bases.

ADDING ESSENTIAL OILS TO A CARRIER OIL, CREAM, OR LOTION BASE

Adding essential oils to a base oil or cream is relatively easy. Several methods are used for blending, and techniques depend on a practitioner's personal experience and research. Learn several methods from alternate sources and then select or create one that works best for you.

Basic Massage Oil Blending Technique

Compute the amount of oil to use from the calculation method described in Table 8-6. In an empty bottle or jar, add the total number of essential oil drops calculated for the formula. If using a pre-blended essential oil formula that contains *only* essential oils, simply add the total amount of drops calculated for the size container you are using. If the container holds 30 mL, and your desired formula is a 2.5 percent dilution, the total number of drops is 15. Add one oil at a time until you have the desired amount of essential oil in the container; then roll the bottle slowly between your hands. This technique is used to combine the essential oils as a blend before diluting them with the other ingredients. (If you use pre-blended oil, rolling is not necessary.) The advantage of a pre-blended essential oil, whether purchased or pre-blended by you ahead of time, is that the essential oils have time to bond and synergize. After adding and rolling the essential oil blend in your hands, add the remaining ingredients (see Table 8-8).

Alternate Blending Technique

There is no absolute rule to adding essential oils to a carrier. Adding the essential oil before the other ingredients, and rolling the bottle between the hands, is not a required method. Adding the essential oils to base ingredients already in the container is fine. This method is especially appropriate when you are adding essential oils to an unscented base you purchase specifically for use with essential oils. The important point for best results is to be sure that your essential oils are mixed well into your carrier.

Some chemists report that rolling a blend in one's hands, or shaking the blend, disrupts the oils, either from the heat created or by allowing the lighter monoterpene compounds to evaporate. A warning such as this may be valid if precision is required for research or clinical studies. However, the rolling technique has been performed by aromatherapists and natural fragrance perfumers for decades without disrupting essential oil quality or therapeutic integrity.

BLENDING FOR SKIN CARE

Follow the same instructions as those for a massage blend when blending essential oils for skin care. A 0.5 percent to 2 percent

Table 8-8 Blending Essential Oils to an Empty Bottle

Step 1.	Choose the oils for the blend. Write out your formula and keep it in your client's file and in a recipe file. (See Figure 8-1.) 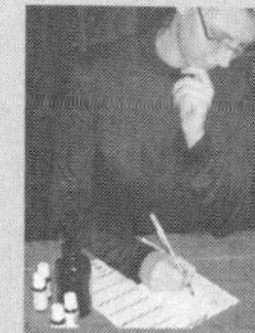 **Figure 8-1** Following your selection of essential oils for blending or formulation, it is very important to write down the recipe and the anticipated application. It is common for aromatherapists to tell tales of the ideal blend that "got away' due to failure to document it.
Step 2.	Use the calculation method described in Table 8-5 for a 2.5 percent basic essential oil blend.
Step 3.	Add one oil to the container at a time. If you use a pre-blended formula, add the total drops. (See Figure 8-2.) 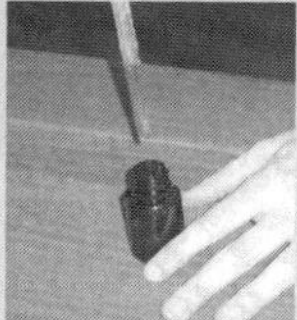 **Figure 8-2** Add essential oils by using a dropper, pipette or the orifice reducer in the bottle.
Step 4.	Record any changes you make to the essential oil formula.
Step 5.	Roll the bottle between your hands. (This step is not necessary with a pre-blended formula.)
Step 6.	Add the carrier oil or oils. If more than one carrier oil is used, record both oils and amounts. (See Figure 8-3.) 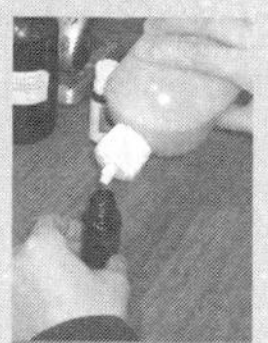 **Figure 8-3** Add the carrier oil to your blend of essential oils.
Step 7.	Roll the entire blend between your hands to mix the oils.

dilution is best for facial skin care. Essential oils for care of the face should generally not be more than a 2 percent dilution. Be especially cautious of essential oils that are designated as potential sensitizers, because the facial skin tends to be more delicate and susceptible to irritation than skin elsewhere on the body. Sensitizing oils are rarely used on the face and then only by skilled aromatherapists.

TRANS-DERMAL PENETRATION OF ESSENTIAL OILS

Application of essential oils topically will likely be your most common method of use. The efficacy and benefits of essential oils applied this way rely on penetration into the dermal layer of the skin. It would be advantageous to know how much of the oil applied is actually absorbed. Though debate exists in this area, there is enough evidence acknowledging the ability of essential oils to penetrate the dermis. To support this evidence, skin physiologist Dr. Peter Pugliese says "just about everything can, and will, penetrate the skin" and continues by explaining that it is a mechanical process with some chemistry involved.[10]

Essential oils are lipid soluble. The skin, which has a lipid barrier, readily absorbs essential oils. In test subjects, linalool and linalyl acetate, the two main constituents in lavender, were absorbed within 20 minutes.[11] The absorption rate and amount depend on the size of the molecule, its polarity, and other factors of chemistry. Some pharmaceutical companies use essential oil compounds in drug patches, such as eugenol (principal ingredient in clove oil) and limonene (derived from citrus rind), to carry larger pharmaceutical molecules into the body.[12] This ability of these compounds to carry these larger molecules into the bloodstream demonstrates the highly effective nature of their transdermal penetration. Fatty acids, such as linolenic acid and palmitic acid, found in vegetable and fruit fixed oils, are also used for this purpose.[13] Bear in mind that when these compounds are found within an oil, as complete structures, they have different penetration properties. Most studies have been performed on the individual components rather than the complete structure.

Many factors must be considered to predict the amounts of essential oils, or their compounds, that will actually be absorbed when applied topically. Some of the oil will evaporate before absorption occurs. Wrapping or covering the area helps prevent evaporation and is considered the most effective method for complete absorption into the skin. Penetration of the oils is also enhanced by friction, or massage, which causes the blood vessels in the dermis to dilate. Topical applications vary, and with each of these variations, the trans-dermal penetration differs. Elements that are known to increase penetration are heat, water, and damage to the skin. Vegetable and fruit oils slow the process of essential oils entering the dermis, and also slow the evaporation rate of the essential oils. To ensure that essential oils are absorbed, massage the blend completely into the skin.

BATH

Essential oils are very beneficial when added to a bath, especially considering that a bath includes two factors, heat and water, known to increase absorption. The amount of oil and dilutions that may be used vary widely. Essential oils may be added undiluted to bath water or diluted using unscented soap, alcohol (vodka is generally recommended), or whole milk as a carrier.

To prepare an aromatic bath, add 12 to 60 drops of an essential oil or blend to the running water just before getting into the bath. If diluting the oils, add them to a capful, approximately 1/8 to 1/4 ounce, of the chosen carrier, then add this mixture to the running bath water (see Table 8-9).

When oils are used undiluted in a bath, the same precautions apply as stated in the section Neat Essential Oils. Some oils may become more irritating when used in a bath, because heat and water enhance absorption. Use caution with neat oils in the bath and pay special attention to known irritants as well as the citrus, mint, and needle (pine and spruce) oils. Oils evaporate quickly from a bath when not diluted. When a person bathes in undiluted oils, the oils' evaporation permeates the air to create an inhalation. This inhalation is beneficial for a cold, flu, or other respiratory illness and also relieves stress and soothes or balances the emotions.

Jacuzzi and Whirlpool

Check with the manufacturer's manual before using essential oils in a Jacuzzi, whirlpool, or any other machine-operated

Table 8-9	Preparing an Aromatic Bath
Step 1.	Add essential oils to a capful of your selected carrier (unscented soap, vodka, or whole milk).
Step 2.	Mix with an orange stick or other thin utensil.
Step 3.	Add mixture to running bath water.

bath. Essential oils can dissolve plastic parts or have detrimental effects on metal parts. Be sure that the manufacturer specifically approves use of essential oils in their equipment.

SHOWER

Essential oils may be used in a steam or shower by simply rubbing a few drops over an already wet body. These oils are usually used undiluted, and penetration is quick, so obey appropriate precautions. Essential oils are used in showers to increase immunity (MQV) and stimulate lymphatic drainage (bay laurel). To prevent or eliminate viral infection, dosages of 30 drops are often used. Prolonged use of the same oil, more than 6 days in a row, can cause skin to become sensitized.

INHALATION

Inhaling essential oils is one of the easiest, and most effective, methods of aromatherapy application. Several techniques can be used for inhaling essential oils.

Electric or Ceramic Diffusers

A diffuser is anything that can disperse essential oils into the atmosphere. Many varieties of diffusers exist, including ceramic diffusers, electric pumps, and candles. Some diffusers require more oils than others, and some are more convenient to use. Selection of diffusers is based on individual preference and needs. Run a diffuser for 10 to 20 minutes and keep the fragrance at or below the level of perception. Do not run a diffuser system to the point where the odor is overwhelming.

Steam Inhalation

This is a simple method for a quick essential oil treatment. Add 5 drops of essential oil, one oil or a blend, to a bowl of steaming hot water (not boiling). Tent your head with a towel, lean over the bowl, and inhale. Be very careful as you lean over the steam; the essential oil evaporates quickly and may irritate the eyes and mucous membrane. This same technique is used for a homemade facial steam.

Tissue Method

The tissue has its place in aromatherapy treatment, though the oil evaporates quickly and the atmospheric concentration of the oil is not as sustained as that produced by a diffuser. Drop a chosen essential oil or blend on a tissue and place near the head while lying down. This technique is often used at bedtime to induce sleep, or in the spa for added therapy or relaxation.

Nostril Inhalation (Pütz Method)

This method is both cost effective and successful. It can be used as a preventive measure or as a treatment for sinus infections and other respiratory conditions. Place one drop of the desired blend or oil on the center of a 2-inch × 2-inch piece of soft paper towel or tissue. Roll it into a small rod shape and place in the nostril (repeat for second nostril) for 5 minutes. Observe caution for those oils that may cause irritation.

MEDICINAL OR MEDICAL APPLICATIONS

Modern aromatherapy originally developed as a medical practice. Internal application and the use of suppositories are both common medical methods and continue to be used in French aromamedicine (see Chapter 2). These methods are highly effective treatments when used properly.

Suppositories

In this method of application, the oils are absorbed into the veins through the tissue of the rectum, bypassing the liver. The process of making the suppositories involves melting 20 grams of cocoa butter in a double boiler and adding 10 mL of hazelnut oil to the melted butter. Sixty to seventy (60 to 70) drops of essential oils are then added. As the mixture cools, it is poured into molds.

Internal Use

A typical dosage for internal use of essential oils is 2 to 3 drops of essential oil used two or three times per day. The desired oil or blend is dropped into an empty capsule, along with an edible vegetable oil. This technique is very useful for those essential oils with powerful infection-fighting properties that tend to be the most irritating, such as the phenolic oils (thyme thymol, oregano) and cinnamon. These oils are generally well tolerated internally. Essential oils can also be added to water or honey for internal use. For small dosage and a time-release effect, useful for sore throats, essential oils are placed on a charcoal tablet and allowed to dissolve in the mouth.

Taste

Taste, in the practice of traditional Chinese medicine, is important to the healing quality of herbs and oils. Jeffrey Yuen, an 88th generation Taoist Master, explains that "understanding the taste quality can add tremendous insight to medical aromatherapy with the internal ingestion of certain oils." He says that "taste received by the taste buds will generate signals/reactions from the brain to direct gastric secretions toward the ingested substance."[14] According to Yuen, the flavor demonstrates a host of activity, such as the sweet tasting oils like peppermint that moisten dryness, soothe inflammation, strengthen immunity, and nourish the body, especially when one is very weak.

FRAGRANCE BLENDING

The art of blending embraces the ability to produce pleasingly aromatic blends. Fragrance is an element of a therapeutic blend that inspires its use. Fragrance is a tool that has long been used in product manufacturing and marketing. People are fragrance oriented and tend to use a product or an aromatherapy formula for skin or for health if they like the way it smells. Fragrance blending is an art that develops through practice. Some guidelines that may help you to build this talent are described in the next sections.

Top, Middle, and Base Note

Fragrance blending is like creating a piece of music. The descriptive language used reflects this similarity. In fragrance blending, the goal is to produce a balance of top, middle, and base notes. *Top, middle,* and *base* are the words used to describe the fragrance character of single essential oils. Though you will find that different authors classify individual oils differently, the classification into notes is the closest thing to a standard that can be found. Use this method as a guide only. There is no absolutely right way to accomplish a fragrance blend. Experiment and be creative.

Top Notes

Top note oils tend to be the most volatile oils and evaporate the quickest. In a blend, they are the first fragrance to meet your nose. Top notes create the first impression and are generally the main component that identifies the fragrance. Some top notes include:

- citrus oils
- needle oils
- mints
- cinnamon and other sharp spices

The fruit oils can be used liberally in a blend to cover or fix an "off" fragrance in your blends. Some top notes, like cinnamon and other spices, may overpower a blend if too much is used.

Middle Notes

These are the oils that create the "body" of the blend. In fact, this is another way to visualize your blend: top is the head, middle is the body, and base is the legs and feet. The middle fills out the fragrance and usually is the main component of the blend. The middle notes round out sharp fragrances in a blend. Middle notes include:

- lavender
- geranium
- palmarosa
- petitgrain
- chamomile

Base Notes

The heavier, more viscous oils are the base notes. These oils evaporate slowly. It is this quality that makes them a base note, as they "hold down" the fragrance. As the other notes, especially the top notes, combine with the base notes, their ability to evaporate is reduced. So a base note helps to create a more even fragrance as the blend holds together and the notes tend to "hit" the nose more evenly. For this reason, base notes are called *fixatives*. Base notes are usually the smallest percentage in a blend and are generally faint when the blend is smelled from the bottle. When it is applied to the skin, the base note becomes more apparent. A base note also helps to hold the total fragrance longer on the skin. There is a real art to blending with a good base note. *Jitterbug Perfume* by Tom Robbins (1990) is a great story that involves the search for an elusive base note. Base note oils are:

- cedarwood
- cistus
- balsam
- frankincense
- patchouli

AUTHOR'S **NOTE**

BUY THE OILS AND USE THEM

In the Introduction to this book, I stated that essential oils are simple and you need only buy them and use them to get benefit from them. Well, each chapter has been one step further away from simple. In Chapter 4, I turned the simple task of buying oils into a tremendous adventure of knowing what to look for in an essential oil. The chemistry of essential oils is simple. Not! In this chapter, the blending of essential oils has become a good deal more involved than just "use them."

The information learned in this text combined with years of experience will turn aromatherapy into a simple art for you. You will, with confidence, simply buy them from people you have learned to trust. You will simply apply them, using any one of the many methods you have learned and practiced over the years.

I usually carry a pocketful of essential oils with me. I don't know if it's part of normal conversation or if I inspire this, but a health condition always seems to enter my dialogue with people. It's funny how I almost always have the remedy for whatever condition they bring up. This comes from carrying a few, or more, essential oils that will provide me with a wide array of therapeutic properties. It's worth mentioning that my pocketful of brown bottles comes with a certain entertainment value, if I choose to work it that way, and I usually do.

Continued

I've had my moments of entertaining circumstances. Early in my career as an aromatherapist, I created a company called Rock & Roll Aromatherapy. I was a touring musician for years and maintained my associations in the entertainment industry. After giving up the road, I continued to work with bands as a stylist and skin care consultant. When I discovered essential oils, it seemed like a natural transition to present them as a provider of health for touring musicians; fatigue, colds, laryngitis, and other conditions were common on the road. I acquired many tales — but little else — from what is best described as an attempt to bring alternative health to rock and roll. It was a premature endeavor, because the awareness of alternative healing is more prevalent today and is now accepted by many musicians.

Doing what one commonly does in the music industry, I attended lots of parties, concerts, and events. With a pocketful of essential oils, I was ready and willing to present the remedy of the moment. This had the potential to be pretty amusing, as it was when I was backstage before the show of a mid-nineties "hair band." I was talking with the band's road manager, who was visibly exhausted from being awakened to deal with an incident at 3 A.M. The soundman and another member of the stage crew were also present. It seemed that exhaustion was a theme for the backstage crew that evening.

I reached into my pocket and presented a bottle of basil essential oil. I put a couple of drops on a tissue and told each to hold it beneath his nose and just breathe it in. Basil is an excellent mental stimulant. A whiff of clear-headed stimulation was an especially wise thing for the soundman, the person responsible for the quality of the band's sound. He, or she, can make or break an evening's performance.

Curiosity wafted through the area and soon I had about eight people, mostly crew members, surrounding me. Within the next few minutes, several people were walking around the backstage area with a tissue held intently to the nose. Some were forcibly swaying their heads back with each inhalation, an action that may be suitable with the use of other substances but is not necessary for essential oils. I sat back to watch the scene I had created. It was rock and roll at its most unusual.

Basil on a tissue is aromatherapy in the simplest form. I had an essential oil and used it. This simple aromatherapy treatment was effective — and extremely entertaining.

CHAPTER SUMMARY

Essential oils are applied in a variety of ways and dosages. This variety provides flexibility in applying the oils that not only enables precise aromatherapy treatment but also permits the practitioner or user to select methods for specific reasons that include ease of application, availability of supplies, time constraints, and even adjustments according to mood. Blended essential oils create a synergy that produces something greater than the sum of the individual parts.

Essential oils are used in dilution with some form of carrier, such as a vegetable oil or unscented cream base. The essential oils can be blended at any percentage, which is generally determined by the area, the health condition, and the person to be treated. A simple formula can be used to calculate a typical 2.5 percent dilution and can be altered to calculate higher or lower percentages of essential oil. A system of top, middle, and base notes of essential oils is used to develop a fragrance blend.

REVIEW QUESTIONS

1. What is synergy, and how does it relate to essential oils?
2. What results are achieved through an essential oil compound synergy?
3. What dosage is best used for sedative effects?
4. What is the most common blending percentage of essential oil?
5. What is the calculation formula used to produce a 2.5 percent dilution of essential oils?
6. What does the term "neat" mean in applying essential oils?

CHAPTER REFERENCES

1. Venes, D. (Ed.) (1997). *Tabor's Cyclopedic Medical Dictionary* (18th edition). Philadelphia, PA: F. A. Davis Company.
2. Schnaubelt, K. (1985). *The Aromatherapy Course.* San Rafael, CA: Pacific Institute of Aromatherapy.
3. Schnaubelt, K. (2004). *Aromatherapy Lifestyles.* San Rafael, CA: Terra Linda Scent and Image.
4. Kennedy, D. O., Wake, G., Savelev, S., Tildesly, N. T. J., Perry, E. K., Wesnes, K. A. & Scholey, A. B. (2003). "Modulation of mood and cognitive performance

following acute administration of single doses of *Melissa officinalis* (lemon balm) with human CNS nicotine and muscarinic receptor-binding properties." *Neuropsychopharmacology 28* (10); 1871–1881.

5. Boyd, E. M. & Sheppard, E. P. (1968). "The effect of steam inhalation of volatile oils on the output and composition of respiratory tract fluid." *Journal of Pharmacology and Experimental Therapeutics 163* (1); 250– 256.
6. Rubel, D. M., Freeman, S. & Southwell, I. A. (1998). "Tea tree oil allergy: what is the offending agent? Report of three cases of tea tree oil allergy and review of the literature." *The Australasian Journal of Dermatology; 39* (4); 244–247.
7. Fritz, T. M., Burg, G. & Krasovec, M. (2001). "Allergic contact dermatitis to cosmetics containing *Melaleuca alternifolia* (tea tree oil)." *Annales de dermatologie et de vénéréologie, 128* (2); 123–126.
8. Brand, C., Grimbaldston, M. A., Gamble, J. R., Drew, J., Finlay-Jones, J. J. & Hart, P. H. (2002). "Tea tree oil reduces the swelling associated with the efferent phase of a contact hypersensitivity response." *Inflammation Resource 51* (5); 236–244.
9. Khalil, Z., Pearce, A. L., Satkunanathan, N., Storer, E., Finlay-Jones, J. J. & Hart, P. H. (2004). "Regulation of wheal and flare by tea tree oil: Complimentary human and rodent studies." *Journal of Investigative Dermatology 123* (4); 683–690.
10. Pugliese, P. (2005). *Advanced Professional Skin Care: Medical Edition.* Bernville, PA: The Topical Agent, LC.
11. Buckle, J. (2003). *Clinical Aromatherapy Essential Oils in Practice.* Philadelphia, PA: Churchill Livingstone.
12. Zhao, K. & Singh, J. (1998). "Mechanisms of percutaneous absorption of tamoxifen by terpenes: Eugenol, D-limonene and menthone." *Journal of Control Release 55* (2–3); 253–260.
13. Bhatia, K. S. & Singh, J. (1999). "Effect of linolenic acid/ethanol or limonene/ethanol and iontophoresis on the in vitro percutaneous absorption of LHRH and ultrastructure of human epidermis." *International Journal of Pharmacy 180* (2); 235–250.
14. Schnaubelt, K. (ed.). & Yuen, J. C. (2002, October). *Essential Oils and Chinese Medicine.* Essential Oils East West: Proceedings of the 5th Scientific Wholistic Aromatherapy Conference.

Therapeutic and Topical Use of Carrier Oils

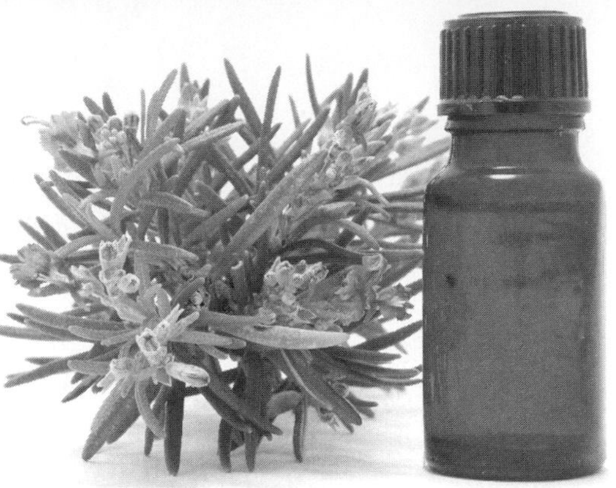

CHAPTER 9

If olive oil comes from olives, where does baby oil come from?

–Stephen Wright

LEARNING OBJECTIVES

1. Discover the therapeutic value of carriers, such as olive and hazelnut oils, used to dilute and blend essential oils.
2. Review fatty acid chemistry to better understand the topical application of carrier oils.
3. Recognize the skin conditioning and healing benefits of carrier oils.
4. Enhance blends and treatments by learning to synergize the essential oil activity with the therapeutic properties contained in the carrier oils.

FIXED, OR CARRIER, OILS USED IN AROMATHERAPY APPLICATIONS

The most common ingredient used to dilute essential oils is a fixed oil, a botanically derived and non-volatile oil (see Chapter 2) that does not evaporate. Fixed oils are called carrier oils (see Chapters 1 and 8) when they are used to dilute essential oils. Several oils are used as carriers, mainly vegetable seed, fruit seed, or nut oils.

Base and Carrier

Base is another term used in reference to a carrier oil or carrier oil blend. A base can also be a cream, which usually consists of fixed oils, an emulsifier, and water. Some definitions make a distinction between the terms *base* and *carrier.* A carrier is simply an oil used to dilute and spread, or carry, an essential oil or essential oil blend. A base is a fixed oil or combination of oils, with therapeutic value of its own, which is used in therapeutic synergy with the oils.

Avoiding Synthetics and Petrochemicals

This text assumes that all the ingredients used with essential oils are natural, pure, and are not petrochemicals or other petroleum derivatives. **Petrochemicals** are substances that are created or processed using petroleum. Petrochemicals such as mineral oil and propylene glycol are often used in cosmetics and are considered **inert,** meaning they are inactive and have a limited ability to react with the body or other ingredients in a formula. Although inert petrochemicals can be used as essential oil carriers, using them violates the standards of purity and therapeutic value that should be expected from aromatherapy formulations.

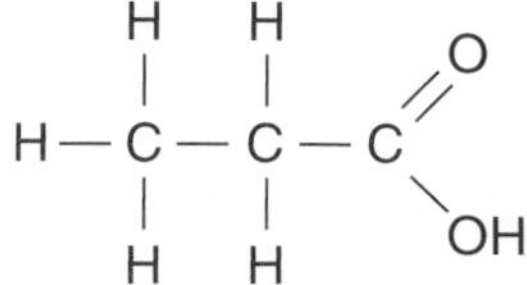

Figure 9-1 A carboxyl group attached to a hydrocarbon chain to form a fatty acid.

Fatty Acids

A **fatty acid** is a hydrocarbon chain with one of the hydrogen atoms replaced by a carboxyl group (COOH) (Figure 9-1). Fatty acids are classified as saturated, monounsaturated, or polyunsaturated (Table 9-1).

Table 9-1 Fatty Acids

Saturated	No double bonds	Stearic acid, Palmitic acid
Monounsaturated	One double bond	Oleic acid (Omega-9)
Polyunsaturated	Two or more double bonds	Linoleic acid (Omega-6) Linolenic acid (Omega-3)

Carrier and Base Oils: Composed of Fatty Acids

Vegetable and other carrier oils are composed of fatty acids. Oils also contain **triglycerides,** a saturated structure comprising three fatty acid chains attached to a glycerol molecule. All fatty acids have some benefit in skin care. The saturated oils tend to have the most **slip,** or ability to glide along the skin. This makes oils such as coconut, palm, and cacao butter good choices for a massage base. Saturated oils are absorbed into the skin at a slower rate. This feature may provide a barrier to temporarily protect the epidermis. Carrier oils comprising mainly monounsaturated fatty acids (olive, hazelnut, and sunflower) provide adequate slip and penetration. These fatty acids also provide therapeutic benefits that include the cancer-fighting capability of oleic acid.[1] The most beneficial fatty acids for skin health are the polyunsaturated **essential fatty acids,** omega-6 and omega-3. Essential fatty acids are vital for many functions of the body in addition to the strength and structure of cells. The body does not manufacture essential fatty acids; therefore, they must be provided through a healthy diet. Topical application of oils containing essential fatty acids has been shown to benefit the skin and assist in healing wounds.[2] See Table 9-2 for a listing of properties associated with the topical application of saturated, monounsaturated, and polyunsaturated oils.

Trans-Dermal Penetration of Fatty Acids

The topical transdermal penetration of essential oils is discussed in Chapter 8. Both beneficial and toxic molecules can penetrate the skin.[3] Penetration may be enhanced if the skin's lipid barrier function is compromised. Like essential oils,

Table 9-2 Properties of Saturated, Monounsaturated, and Polyunsaturated Oils
Lipid barrier protection
Anti-inflammatory
Moisture retention/Transepidermal water loss reducer
Skin conditioning emollient
Assists wound healing
Photoprotection

essential fatty acids harmonize with the skin's lipid barrier and are readily absorbed into the epidermal layers of the skin. The ability of essential fatty acids and essential oils to carry other compounds into the epidermis and bloodstream is evident in their use as carriers for pharmaceutical patches.[4]

Aromatherapy literature generally reports that carrier oils enhance the transdermal penetration of essential oils; however, some studies report both an enhanced and a diminished effect on the dermal penetration of essential oils in a carrier. The enhancement can be understood from the ability of both to harmonize with the lipids of the skin barrier. It is assumed that saturated oils are less likely, or slower, to penetrate the epidermis. The monounsaturated oils have a moderate absorption rate, whereas polyunsaturated oils penetrate the epidermal layers readily.

As you begin to work with carrier oils, research and follow formulas and seek advice from those who have worked with the essential oils and carriers you want to use. Experience will help you adjust formulas for the most effective use of carrier oils in aromatherapy.

Gamma-Linoleic (Omega-6) and Alpha-Linolenic (Omega-3) Polyunsaturated Fatty Acids

Polyunsaturated oils, those high in omega-3 and omega-6 fatty acids, are very active in their ability to protect and benefit the skin.[5] These polyunsaturated fats may provide an excellent topical remedy for a compromised lipid barrier function of the skin.[6]

When the lipid barrier is compromised, many skin disorders may occur, including atopic dermatitis and dehydration. Carrier oils containing omega-6, omega-3, and monounsaturated omega-9 (oleic acid) are extremely beneficial for repairing the lipid barrier function.[7] These fatty acids that temporarily mimic the lipid barrier help regenerate the skin's natural lipid barrier.

CARRIER OILS

Many seed, fruit, and nut oils are excellent therapeutic choices when used in combination with essential oils. Initially, experiment with a few carriers, then expand to incorporate other oils. Use available recipes and formulas from this book or any one of several aromatherapy recipe books to select carrier oils and blends.

Oils from organically grown sources are highly recommended. If organic oils are not available, be sure that the oils you use are pure and natural and have no added oils or synthetics. Also consider the extraction process when selecting carrier oils. Avoid oils that have been extracted using hexane or any other solvent. Look for expeller-pressed rather than cold-pressed oils. Cold pressing is an ideal process, but because the term is not regulated, oils with this labeling can actually be hexane or solvent extracted. Vegetable and fruit oils are often refined to remove color and odor. Use carrier oils that have not been deodorized, bleached, chemically washed, or **degummed** (a process that removes phosphorous-containing lipids). This kind of product is called RBD: refined, bleached, and deodorized. These oils may be missing compounds that have therapeutic benefit, such as antioxidants, lecithin, chlorophyll, phytosterols, and skin-enhancing lipids.[8] Not all oils are available unrefined, and some compromises must be made when selecting specific oils. If an oil choice, such as meadowfoam (*Limnanthes alba*), is available only as a refined oil, be sure that it is pure and solvent-free.

Carrier Oils' Shelf Life

Carrier oils have a limited shelf life and will become **rancid,** a state caused by partial decomposition of a fatty acid, after a time. Essential oils, when blended with carrier oils, prolong the carrier's shelf life. Once blended, the entire composition has a limited time before the carrier goes rancid. This time is generally anywhere from 3 to 12 months, depending on the essential oils, the carrier, how often the bottle is opened, and how often it is exposed to temperature changes. Oils that are exposed to high temperatures or to frequent temperature changes go rancid more rapidly than those kept at a constant, cool, refrigerated temperature.

Useful Carrier Oils for Aromatherapy

Some common aromatherapy carrier oils, their main compositions, and their properties are listed below. This information will guide you in selecting a carrier for almost any therapeutic application. The shelf life noted for each is the length of time the unblended oil can be stored before becoming rancid. The asterisk denotes that the listed shelf life is approximated and depends on storage, quality of the oil, production date (when the oil was pressed), and temperature. The temperature should be cool, or refrigerated, and steady. Avoid drastic temperature changes. Keep carrier oils out of direct light.

Sweet Almond Oil

Botanical name: *Prunus dulcis*
Contains: Oleic acid (main component), alpha-linoleic acid
Shelf life: 6 to 10 months
Almond is a light-textured oil, easily absorbed by skin. It has a subtle odor that does not affect essential oil fragrance blends. It has a light gold color. Almond oil also has good slip for massage and is beneficial for all skin types. When used topically, sweet almond oil will relieve dryness, itching, and burns. It has a moderate shelf life.

Castor Oil

Botanical name: *Ricinus communis*
Contains: Several unsaturated fatty acids, lecithin, ricinoleic acid
Shelf life: 1 year *

This oil is not commonly used in aromatherapy massage. When added to a blend, it should be about 10 percent of the total base blend. Castor oil has healing benefits that combine well with those of other essential oils for therapeutic use. It has the ability to dissolve cysts, warts, and corns[9] and boosts the immune system. Castor oil is very good for children when used as packs for congestion of the chest and digestive system. It is easily absorbed through the epidermis and dermis layers of the skin and thereby into the body.

Coconut Oil

Botanical name: *Cocos nucifera*
Contains: Rich fatty acid composition with palmitic acid, lauric acid, oleic and linoleic acids
Shelf life: 1 year or longer
Coconut is highly recommended as an emollient face and body oil. It is a dense (heavy) oil with a moderate penetration rate. Coconut oil is very stable, and most tests indicate no signs of rancidity after a year's storage at room temperature.[10]
Coconut becomes solid at room temperature and must be melted before being added to a blend. Coconut RBD is widely available but lacks the truly luscious fragrance of the pure oil. Use non-RBD virgin coconut oil in your blends for the added tropical fragrance in addition to the more pronounced therapeutic benefits. Coconut provides antimicrobial and antioxidant skin protection.[11]
Coconut oil is appropriate to use for dryer, sensitive, and compromised skin and is ideal for all skin types. Coconut oil is an exceptional and healthy food with nutritive benefits that include anti-inflammatory[12] and weight loss effects.[13]

Grapeseed Oil

Botanical name: *Vitis vinifera*
Contains: Linoleic acid, oleic acid, palmitic acid, stearic acid
Shelf life: 1 year to 14 months
Grapeseed oil is relatively inexpensive and has very good slip. This explains why it is one of the most common carriers used in massage. It penetrates the skin quickly, leaving a non-greasy feel following massage. When used in a facial blend, a 15 to 25 percent concentration is recommended. Grapeseed is relatively odorless and does not affect the fragrance of essential oil blends. The refined oil is a pale yellow color, and unrefined grapeseed oil is a deeper green with a light fruit odor.

Hazelnut Oil

Botanical name: *Corylus avellana*
Contains: Oleic acid, linoleic acid, palmitic acid, vitamins C and E
Shelf life: 6 months to 1 year
Hazelnut is an emollient and a nourishing oil for the skin. It is easily absorbed and has an astringent quality. This oil is very good for all skin conditions, especially dry and damaged, and can effectively be used in blends for acne and oily skin. Hazelnut is a good blending oil that harmonizes well with other oils, such as jojoba. It is expensive to use for full body massage but can be very beneficial if the body is dry or in need of conditioning.

Jojoba Oil

Botanical name: *Simmondsia chinensis*
Contains: A "liquid wax" (a fatty acid attached to a long chain alcohol); also contains some fats and minerals
Shelf life: Indefinite
Jojoba is a liquid wax from the bean of a North American desert plant. It is very similar to the natural sebum of the skin. Jojoba is an emollient and contains skin nutrients. It is ideal for aging and dry skin. It's an excellent scalp tonic and can be used as a conditioner for dry and damaged hair. It is also used to control wiry or frizzy hair.
Jojoba does not go rancid, so it is an excellent carrier for perfume blends or blends that are used up gradually over time.

Meadowfoam Seed Oil

Botanical name: *Limnanthes alba*
Contains: Over 90 percent long-chain fatty acids and triglycerides
Shelf life: 1 year *
This oil is recognized for outstanding stability in cosmetic products. It has over 98 percent fatty acids, with a higher quality triglyceride level than other oils. Meadowfoam is an excellent moisturizer that rejuvenates skin cells and provides good barrier protection. This oil is good for all skin types but is especially nourishing for damaged skin and psoriasis. It may be too heavy to use as the only carrier and may need to be blended with lighter carrier oils.

Olive Oil

Botanical name: *Olea europaea*
Contains: Oleic acid, linoleic acid, palmitic acid, stearic acid, polyphenols, minerals
Shelf life: 1 year to 14 months
Olive oil is the Mediterranean answer to beautiful skin. Its ***polyphenol*** content provides powerful antioxidant and anti-inflammatory properties. Polyphenols are therapeutic molecules that contain a phenolic ring. Topical and internal use of olive oil results in radiantly healthy skin. Olive oil is a rich emollient conditioner and has photoprotective qualities.[14] Olive oil does smell like olives, and the fragrance may be detectable if this oil is used full strength as a carrier. It can easily be blended with other oils to diminish its odor to an undetectable level.

Pumpkin Seed Oil

Botanical name: *Cucurbita pepo*
Content: Oleic acid, linoleic acid, alpha-linoleic acid, amino acids
Shelf life: 1 year*
Pumpkin seed oil has a therapeutic balance between omega-6 and omega-3 fatty acids. Pumpkin seed oil is anti-inflammatory, cell rejuvenating, and anti-oxidant.[15] It is excellent for all skin types, especially good for mature, damaged, and problem skin. Pumpkin seed oil is used at about 10 to 15 percent of a carrier blend.

Sesame Seed Oil

Botanical name: *Sesamum indicum*
Contents: Oleic acid, alpha-linoleic acid, linolenic acid, palmitoleic acid, stearic acid, vitamin E
Shelf life: 4 months to 1 year*
Sesame seed oil is a healing and balancing oil that is recommended in Ayurvedic medicine for daily self-massage to nourish and detoxify.[16] It is often listed among those oils that offer UV protection. Sesame has a nutty odor and penetrates skin slowly. This quality may present some problems with topical application of essential oils. Experiment with sesame oil to determine optimal blending amounts. Some skin absorbs it more rapidly than others.

AUTHOR'S **NOTE**

FINDING STUDIES TO SUPPORT CLAIMS

I use many sources to research claims for and potential uses of my ingredients, as well as to find new uses. Many resources are available online; some require membership fees or charge per download. I recommend two free sites that will provide you with valuable information. One is http://www.pubmed.com. This site is operated by the National Institutes of Health's National Library of Medicine. Go to this site, type your keywords into the search field, and you will be provided with the available studies. These studies are peer reviewed scientific studies and are not always easily translated without a scientific background. Every so often, you may have to pay for a study you would like to read.

Here's an example: I just typed in a search for "jojoba oil UV" and got no results. Bad example; I'll have to find that information somewhere else. I'll go with the general search "jojoba oil." This search will tell me what's available on jojoba without asking for a specific claim. The search provides 22 studies, most of which are irrelevant to my work. A few are very interesting because they are essential oil studies using jojoba as a carrier. This result is good; I'll save these studies for later use. I find a study regarding anti-inflammatory properties of jojoba. I read through it to see how it relates to topical application. This article could be helpful in using jojoba in future formulations. This web site has been a valuable source of information. I can randomly search an ingredient to see what research is available or try to research a specific claim regarding the substance. If you read through my references regarding the claims in this book, you'll see I did much better than the search I made here for the UV protective qualities of jojoba.

The other site I recommend is http://www.ars-grin.gov/duke. This site, run by the US Department of Agriculture, is pre-eminent herbalist Dr. James Duke's detailed analysis of an extremely long list of herbs. It includes many of the oils on this chapter's carrier oil list. I used this site to support my descriptions of the carrier oils and their contents. I cross-reference most of my information, so I may not always give this website resource credit.

I use this site when I'm interested in learning more about specific oils. I do this by going to the site and, for example, selecting "Chemicals and activities" under Plant Searches. The Plant choices - Phytochemical Databases page asks you to make other selections and then to type in name of the plant. If you type "almond," for example, it takes you to a list of the components in almond. This page lists all the components in the plant and identifies the part of the plant where the compound is found. You will need to know what part of the plant extract you're interested in. For example, almond oil is pressed from the almond seed, so you will refer to the seed components that are listed, such as alpha-linoleic acid and stearic acid. This part gets a little tricky, because (as in this example) a few items in the plant part may not be pressed into the oil. These items include components, such as selenium and other minerals, that are not fatty acids. For some plants, the site lists oil or EO (essential oil) as the plant part that contains the component, making guesswork unnecessary. On this site you can further research compounds by clicking on them to find a listing of their therapeutic activity. A thorough search on this web site will provide you with valuable knowledge regarding the use of oils.

Now you know what I do for a good time on a Friday night.

CARRIER OILS FOR THERAPEUTIC SKIN CARE

This list contains vegetable, fruit, and nut oils that have pronounced therapeutic effects. They are identified by their specific therapeutic properties that offer therapeutic synergy with essential oils. These oils are used primarily for facial care but are also useful for full body treatments if the skin needs special attention. The oils included on this list are generally blended with other oils to create synergistic bases with specific therapeutic focus. Most of these oils are used in 5 to 15 percent concentrations.

Apricot Kernel Oil

Botanical name: *Prunus armeniaca*
Contents: Oleic acid, palmitic acid, linoleic acid, minerals
Shelf life: 6 months to 1 year
Apricot oil is light and easily absorbed and has a nice, silky texture. Apricot kernel oil blends well with most oils and is generally used in formulas for dry, sensitive, inflamed, or aging skin. This oil has a soft, fatty fragrance that is not usually detectable in a blend.

Avocado Oil

Botanical name: *Persea americana*
Contains: Oleic acid, linoleic acid, linolenic acid, vitamins A, B-6, C, E and D; minerals, protein, palmitic acid, stearic acid, and lecithin
Shelf life: 8 months to 1 year
Avocado produces oil from the pulp of the fruit, which has restorative properties because of its high vitamin content, high mono- and polyunsaturated fatty acids content, and other skin-nourishing compounds. It is a desirable addition to skin care, particularly for eczema, parasitic skin damage, and dry, mature, or scaling skin.[17] Avocado is a viscous oil but one that is easily absorbed by the skin. It is dark green and may have a detectable nutty odor in a blend. The refined oil has less fragrance and a lighter color, and it is also less therapeutic.

Borage Oil

Botanical name: *Borago officinalis*
Contains: Gamma-linoleic acid, linolenic acid, palmitic acid, some vitamins and minerals
Shelf life: 4 to 8 months
Borage is one of the more popular oils that contains large amounts of the omega-6, gamma linoleic acid (GLA). Borage oil is used to promote healthy skin and reduce the effects of aging on the skin. It's also recommended for treating eczema, psoriasis, and drab (lifeless-looking) skin.[18] Use a 3 to 5 percent concentration of borage for oil-based blends.

Calophyllum (Tamanu or Kamanu) Oil

Botanical name: *Calophyllum inophyllum*
Contains: Saturated, mono- and polyunsaturated fats, vitamin F, and terpene compounds
Shelf life: 1 year *
Calophyllum is often included on essential oils lists, though technically its fatty acid structure classifies it as a fixed oil. The Polynesians, whose name for it is tamanu, have traditionally used this oil for health and skin care. It is used in wound healing and for problem skin. Calophyllum has also been used, with very positive results, to treat shingles.[19]
Calophyllum has a very strong, nutty odor and a deep green color. It is viscous (sticky) oil that is readily absorbed into the skin. It can be used in drops in the essential oil formulas or added as a smaller percentage (0.5 to 5 percent) of a blend percent.
Shingles Formula: 50 percent calophyllum with 50 percent ravensare aromatica essential oil.

Cranberry Seed Oil

Botanical name: *Vaccinium macrocarpon*
Contains: Linoleic acid, linolenic acid, oleic acid, palmitic acid, vitamins, minerals, phytosterols
Shelf life: 1 to 2 years; a very stable oil
Cranberry seed, with its high content of essential fatty acids, is a beneficial addition to skin care products. It was introduced into the supplement industry and is considered unique because of its 1:1 ratio of omega-6 to omega-3 fatty acids. Cranberry seed contains 70 percent essential fatty acids, making it a superb emollient, lubricant, and conditioner for the skin. It is an excellent skin, hair, lip, and baby care oil. Cranberry seed oil contributes to the lipid barrier protection of the skin, is UV protective, and assists in retaining moisture. It is used in 2 to 10 percent dilutions. Cranberry, a pale yellow- to red-colored oil, is readily absorbed. It has a moderate viscosity and a grassy, raspberry-like odor.

Evening Primrose Oil

Botanical name: *Oenothera biennis*
Contains: Several forms of linoleic and linolenic acids, oleic acid, glutamic acid, vitamins, minerals
Shelf life: 3 to 8 months
Evening primrose is very rich in omega-6 (linoleic) and omega-3 (linolenic) fatty acids, especially in gamma-linoleic acid. Evening primrose oil is similar to borage and is often used in combination with it. Evening primrose oil is used to treat dry or aging skin, wrinkles, scarring, psoriasis, fragile or stressed skin, as well as skin problems that are related to hormone imbalance including menstruation and menopause.[20] This oil is used internally for menstrual and menopausal imbalance, the cardiovascular system and cystic breast disease. It is also used to treat weight problems and is reported to assist in nutritional weight loss programs. The oil is absorbed readily through the skin, and has a slight odor.

Red Raspberry Seed Oil

Botanical name: *Rubus idaeus*
Contains: Linoleic acid, linolenic acid, oleic acid, palmitic acid, vitamin E, phytosterols
Shelf life: 1 year to 18 months; a very stable oil
Raspberry seed oil, like cranberry seed oil, is a new addition to the list of available oils that contain essential fatty acids. It comprises 54 percent omega-6 and 29 percent omega-3 essential fatty acids. Raspberry seed oil is emollient, lubricating, and conditioning; it provides lipid barrier protection and moisture retention for the skin. This oil has UV absorptive properties beneficial for photoprotection. It has the expected raspberry fruit fragrance and taste. The oil is pale yellow and easily absorbed into the skin. A red raspberry carrier blend is effective in a 2 to 10 percent dilution.

Rose Hip Seed Oil (Rosa Mosqueta)

Botanical name: *Rosa rubiginosa* or *Rosa canina*
Contains: Glycosides, linoleic and linolenic acids, polyphenols, vitamin C, carotenes (including zeaxanthin)
Shelf life: 6 to 11 months
Rose hip oil, high in omega-6 fatty acids, is extremely beneficial for skin maintenance and for repairing damaged skin.

It has cell regenerative properties and reduces wrinkles, fine lines, stretch marks, scars, and sun damage.[21] It slows the aging process of the skin when used daily. This oil is a very important addition to any skin care program. It is easily absorbed; it is reddish-gold and has a moderately strong, nutty odor.

Wheat Germ

Botanical name: *Triticum aestivum*
Contains: Vitamin E, minerals, B vitamins, linoleic and other fatty acids
Shelf life: 6 months *
Wheat germ oil is a rich source of vitamin E. It is a superb antioxidant and promotes skin elasticity. It is recommended for psoriasis, eczema, and inflamed skin. Wheat germ oil is used as a stabilizing antioxidant for other oils to prolong their shelf life; however, its use is limited because of its strong odor. Also, wheat germ's dark orange color and rich, thick, viscous texture make it a difficult addition to skin care products.

AUTHOR'S **NOTE**

HOW DO I SELECT CARRIER OILS?

Three things primarily guide my carrier oil selection. These considerations include:

- What is readily available?
- What are the necessary therapeutic properties?
- How will the fragrance and the texture blend in with the essential oils and application?

When I select a carrier oil, I should have it on hand, so question one is answered by common sense. The trick is to buy, and have on hand, vegetable and fruit oils you will use in a timely manner, before they go rancid. I have a collection of carrier oils that I use in almost every blend. I generally buy small amounts of the oils I am experimenting with or use only periodically, especially those with a short shelf life. When they go rancid, I throw them out and don't feel that I have wasted too much money.

I use two standard carrier blends.

For massage I use sunflower seed oil (45 percent), coconut oil (35 percent), and jojoba oil (20 percent) as a

Continued

basic carrier blend. This recipe can be made flexible to create a different feel to the carrier by, for example, dropping the coconut content to 25 percent and increasing the sunflower content to 55 percent.

My facial care blends, though they tend to fluctuate and are adjusted according to the skin condition, have a base of olive oil (45 percent), jojoba (25 percent), and a blend of berry oils I call Berryer Repair[22] (30 percent). This blend contains an assortment of berry oils that includes cranberry, blackberry and others, containing high amounts of omega-3 and 6 fatty acids as well as other compounds that help protect the skin from transdermal water loss[23] and mimic the skin's lipid barrier function. This is an especially beneficial blend for skin that has been compromised due to environmental damage, harsh cleansers or stress. An alternate to the berry blend, using oils that are easier to find, is hazelnut or coconut (15 percent), rose hip seed (10 percent), and evening primrose (5 percent).

I'll let you use the knowledge acquired so far in this text to determine my therapeutic focus and the fragrance/texture requirements of these sample carrier oil blends.

CHAPTER SUMMARY

Carrier oils are vegetable, fruit, and nut oils that are used to dilute essential oils. These oils contain fatty acids, triglycerides, and other nutrients and compounds that add therapeutic benefit to aromatherapy blends. Vegetable, fruit, and nut oils may contain fatty acids that are saturated, having no double bonds; monounsaturated, with one double bond; or polyunsaturated, with a fatty acid chain that has two or more double bonds. This quality of the carrier determines many of properties of the oil, such as slip (for ease of use in massage) and antioxidant and other therapeutic activity. Carriers can be blended for specific action and combined with essential oils for synergistic value.

REVIEW QUESTIONS

1. What is a fixed oil?
2. How are base oils used in aromatherapy?
3. What are the three classifications of fatty acids, and which group has the best slip for use in massage?

4. What are the two groups of essential fatty acids that are beneficial in skin care?
5. What is the best quality of fixed oil for use in aromatherapy?
6. What is rancidity, and how can you best protect your oils from it?

CHAPTER REFERENCES

1. Menendez, J.A., Lupu, R. (2006). "Mediterranean dietary traditions for the molecular treatment of human cancer: anti-oncogenic actions of the main olive oil's monounsaturated fatty acid oleic acid (18:1n-9)." *Current Pharmaceutical Biotechnology* 7 (6); 495–502.
2. Cardoso, C. R., Souza, M. A., Ferro, E. A., Favoreto Jr., S. & Pena, J. D. (2004). "Influence of topical administration of N-3 and N-6 essential and N-9 nonessential fatty acids on the healing of cutaneous wounds." *Wound Repair and Regeneration 12* (2); 235–243.
3. Pugliese, P. (2005). *Advanced Professional Skin Care: Medical Edition.* Bernville, PA: The Topical Agent, LC.
4. Rastogi, S. K. & Singh, J. (2005). "Effect of chemical penetration enhancer and iontophoresis on the in vitro percutaneous absorption enhancement of insulin through porcine epidermis." *Pharmaceutical Development and Technology 10* (1); 97–104.
5. Murray, M. T. (1996). *Encyclopedia of Nutritional Supplements.* Rocklin, CA: Prima Publishing.
6. Elias, P. M., Brown, B. E., Ziboh, V. A. (1980). "The permeability barrier in essential fatty acid deficiency: Evidence for a direct role for linoleic acid in barrier function." *Journal of Investigative Dermatology 74* (4); 230–233.
7. Yang, L., Mao-Qiang, M., Taljebini, M., Elias, P. M. & Feingold, K. R. (1995). "Topical stratum corneum lipids accelerate barrier repair after tape stripping, solvent treatment and some but not all types of detergent treatment." *British Journal of Dermatology 133* (5), 679–685.
8. Erasmus, U. "How Bad are Cooking Oils?" Accessed on August 5, 2007 at http://www.udoerasmus.com.
9. Sheppard-Hanger, S. (1995). *The Aromatherapy Practitioner Reference Manual.* Tampa, FL: Atlantic Institute of Aromatherapy.
10. Deal, G. A. (2005). "Coconut Oil is Better Than Olive Oil and Butter." Accessed on August 5, 2007 at http://www. sunsignyoga.com.

11. Holzapfel, C., Holzapfel, L. (2003). *Coconut Oil for Health and Beauty.* Summertown, TN: Book Publishing Company.
12. Sadeghi, S., Wallace, F. A. & Calder, P.C. (1999). "Dietary lipids modify the cytokine response to bacterial lipopolysaccharide in mice." *Immunology 96* (3); 404–410.
13. St-Onge, M. P., Ross, R., Parsons, W. D. & Jones, P. J. (2003). "Medium-chain triglycerides increase energy expenditure and decrease adiposity in overweight men." *Obesity Research 11* (3); 395–402.
14. The Olive Oil Source. (2006). Accessed on August 5, 2007 at http://www.theoliveoilsource.com.
15. Duke, J. Dr. Duke's Phytochemical and Ethnobotanical Databases. Accessed on August 5, 2007 at http://www.ars-grin.gov.
16. Swami, Sada, Shiva, Tirtha. (1998). *The Ayurveda Encyclopedia.* Bayville, NY: Ayurveda Holistic Center Press.
17. Harrison, J. (2003). *The Scientific and Therapeutic Use of Essential Oils.* Bellevue, WA: Phytotherapy Institute.
18. Kanehara, S., Ohtani, T., Uede, K., Furukawa, F. (2007). "Undershirts coated with borage oil alleviate the symptoms of atopic dermatitis in children. *European journal of dermatology.*" 17(5):448–449.
19. Franchomme, P. & Pénoël D. (1990). *L'aromathérapie exactement.* Limoges, France: Roger Jollois Editeur.
20. Balch, J., & Balch, P. (1997). *Prescriptions for Nutritional Healing: A Practical A to Z.* Garden City Park, NY: Avery Publishing Group.
21. Hampton, A. (1987). *Natural Organic Hair and Skin Care.* Tampa, FL: Organic Press.
22. Harrison, J. (2006). *Healthy Ingredients, Healthy Skin.* Bellevue, WA: Phytotherapy Institute.
23. Tanojo, H., Boelsma, E., Junginger, H.E., Ponec, M., Boddé, H.E. (1998). "In vivo human skin barrier modulation by topical application of fatty acids." *Skin Pharmacology and Applied Skin Physiology.* 11(2); 87–97.

Composition of Therapeutic Cosmetic Formulas and Spa Treatments

CHAPTER 10

As a cosmetic chemist my soul is in the woods.

–Aubrey Hampton

LEARNING OBJECTIVES

1. Learn to discriminate quality skin care products and differentiate between products and marketing programs.
2. Develop a useful definition of "natural" ingredients.
3. Develop an understanding of cosmetic ingredients and the skin care formulas used in clinical practice.
4. Describe functions of the ingredients used in specialized spa treatments and cosmetic formulations.

QUALITY SKIN CARE FORMULATIONS AND PRODUCTS

Think about how many different products are used daily for personal grooming or during a spa treatment. In personal daily skin care, two to six products are used, twice a day. In an esthetic or spa practice, at least three to six are used in each service, plus additional products in add-on services.

All of these products are a composition of many ingredients that include a variety of surfactants, emulsifiers, thickeners, conditioners, and preservatives. And as in creating the perfect steak, a memorable apple pie, or the most phenomenal wild and spicy salad, the quality of all the ingredients in the recipe and formula will matter. If you use the juiciest, tastiest organic apples in your pie recipe and top it off with a foul tasting synthetic cinnamon, the flavor is diminished by the inferiority of the cinnamon. Quality is determined by the synergy of all the ingredients. A skin care formula with an inferior, or possibly toxic, ingredient is not recognized through taste. But one bad ingredient in an otherwise excellent formula can be recognized through an off-odor or irritation. With experience, one begins to recognize quality through texture, appearance, scent and, especially, results. Your recognition of individual ingredients listed on a label will become your best tool to distinguish quality skin care formulations.

Quality Counts

Quality is an ongoing theme in this book. By now, you understand that the quality of the essential oils and fixed oils used, along with the quality of your work, has an overriding effect on the therapeutic outcome. The most relaxing facial technique will not be beneficial if the products contain inferior-grade ingredients that cause sensitivity or leave an unpleasant residue on the skin. The outcome of all treatments, services, and daily regimens is more beneficial and successful when attention is given to the overall ingredient quality and formulation of the products.

Quality Formulation and Manufacture

Cosmetic quality does not end with ingredients. Recipe formulation and manufacturing standards are equally important when producing functional and effective skin care preparations.[1] Skin care products that contain fresh, organic herbs and botanicals that do not harmonize well can become ineffective or have adverse effects. By comparison, it is possible to develop a product formulated primarily with inexpensive inert ingredients, combined with just the right balance of a few active cosmeceuticals (see Increasing Therapeutic Activity with Nutrients in this chapter) that may have profoundly beneficial skin care results. A poorly made formula may be too acidic or too alkaline, which could cause irritation even if the overall quality of the ingredients is good.

AROMATHERAPY AND SKIN CARE PRODUCTS

Essential oils interact or synergize with the skin and whatever else is on it. For this reason, it is important to know the quality of ingredients and the manufacturing practice for all products used with essential oils. Quality has an effect, whether subtle or evident, on aroma-therapeutic results. The possible negative effects include irritation, rash, breakouts, or a lessening of the expected benefits from essential oils.

AUTHOR'S NOTE

WORKING WITH MANUFACTURERS

Over the years, I've worked in varied positions with several personal care and cosmetic companies. I worked the trade shows, talked the talk, and developed product knowledge for spa and salon training programs. This work was a great learning experience. What I learned, more than anything else, was how to sell an idea. The more I learned about ingredients, the more I learned how ideas, not ingredients, are sold. This is not to say that there aren't ingredients or formulations that live up to the sales pitch. There are. But a product isn't always what it says it is, either.

As with any other product, there is art to the selling and marketing of skin care. "Create a need and fulfill it" is the

Continued

common philosophy of sales. In a crowded market place, it takes skill to garner attention and convince the consumer why your product is the best. I found it especially amusing, and not necessarily artful, when a sales rep would eat the product to demonstrate how natural it is, a result of fulfilling the need for natural ingredients. I've seen what people are willing to eat, so a sales rep who regularly eats a synthetic food diet should find a synthetic cosmetic very similar. To actually chow down on a chunk of D&C Yellow No. 5, Quaternium 22, PEG 40 stearate, or DMDM Hydantoin would be a bit of a stomach churner. Some of the products I saw people eat did contain menthol for that minty taste, and panthenol, a B vitamin, which I suppose contributes some nutrient value. The ingredients in the sales reps' snacks will be defined later in this chapter.

I, like all of you, base a product on its performance and results. My purpose in writing anything that would appear negative about products, companies, or marketing isn't to create fear. I do it to raise the bar on what is expected of the performance and the results of skin care products. My experience tells me that a lot can be achieved through high quality ingredients. I have worked directly in product research and development for skin care manufacturers, which put me in the position of researching ingredients to find the studies that will support their use and results, ingredient resourcing to seek the most sociologically and environmentally sustainable quality ingredients, consulting on formulations, developing the training for sales brokers and staff, and outlining the marketing material. A good portion of this text is written from this experience. Part of my job has been to look at what other product companies are doing. The ones with a focus on quality and integrity, and they are out there, perform better and create products that result in healthier skin.

In Dr. Wayne Dyer's book, *Intention*, he quotes this line from the John Keats' poem *Ode on a Grecian Urn*, "Beauty is truth, truth beauty, that is all ye know on earth, and all ye need to know." Reading "beauty is truth" strongly resonated with me. It takes truth to get to beauty. It's truth in the skin care that will produce beauty. I know this may sound a bit lame, but it can be demonstrated, and it has been, over and over again. When the truth, not the marketing, not the idea and not the sales pitch, but the truth of quality and integrity, is in your skin care, the result is true beauty. True beauty is healthy beauty.

Philosophy and Methods Used in Manufacturing a Skin Care Program

Becoming attentive to the methods and philosophies of skin care cosmetic formulation can be an enlightening and informative experience. Asking, "Why?" is a means of probing deeper into a product formulation and manufacturing practice. The more attention an esthetician gives to the philosophy and science (the why) behind the use of particular ingredients and methods of formulation or particular processes of manufacture, the more effective he or she will be when using that product to obtain specific results. Therefore, you need to understand the use of organic botanicals, aromatherapy, nutritional supplements, the latest cosmeceuticals, and mainstream cosmetic chemistry relative to the influence they have on outcome or results.

Many formulating philosophies may also be used, such as Ayurveda, traditional herbalism, alchemy, or the latest cosmetic scientific technology. The formulating philosophy provides a basis for selecting ingredients, followed by the methodology, which involves preparation and formulation of the final composition. Where a product is produced, from the handmade cosmetic kitchen to a high-tech laboratory, is considered part of manufacturing philosophy. Manufacturers use the value of their formulating philosophies as marketing tools to advertise or disclose to the consumer how their products "are handcrafted by indigenous peoples of . . ." [or] " intensified using laser technology to . . . " Your own preference, whether created through experience or from research, will determine the value, or quality, you place on these formulating philosophies and methods. Learn to recognize what is hype and what is valid and useful.

Choosing Skin Care Products

A well-defined desired result assists the esthetician to determine which skin care products to choose. This selection may change according to the specific condition being treated. For personal care or in professional practice, the process of product selection requires research, time, and study to fully understand product formulation and ingredient choices. The effort involved is worthwhile, because understanding product ingredients and formulating methods will result in precision and expertise in applying them.

Concerns and Contraindications

Another important factor in ingredient and formulating knowledge has to do with contraindications and safety. The safety of many commonly used cosmetic ingredients has been questioned.[2, 3] When skin irritation is present, a diverse knowledge of ingredients will help you determine if a specific ingredient contained in a product is the potential cause. Irritation and dermatitis may or may not be caused by specific ingredients that are known irritants. Sensitivities can be caused by individual allergic reactions, as you learned in Chapter 6. In some situations, the cause of a product irritation is elusive. In these cases, the formulation and the synergy created by the ingredients may cause the irritation, rather than one or two specific ingredients. Learn about as many product and ingredient contraindications as possible.

DIFFERENTIATING BETWEEN QUALITY AND MARKETING HYPE

Thorough research concerning ingredients is a useful method to determine differences between a marketing campaign and results that may be derived from an ingredient. Ingredient knowledge helps clarify differences between what can be achieved, given the quality of ingredients, and the claims of the manufacturer's marketing campaign.

In the world of marketing, it is necessary to identify a need. The product, or service, is then marketed and sold to fill that need. Product ingredients are used in marketing to fulfill needs, such as alpha lipoic acid to reduce wrinkles, tea tree oil to eliminate acne, alpha hydroxy acid (AHA) for a youthful complexion, or herbal fragrance to produce an ecstatic experience in the shower. Often, new "advanced" ingredients are created and introduced as being able to produce some miraculous result never before achieved. The new ingredient could be nothing more than an advanced new marketing campaign that lacks any actual benefit to the skin.[4] You can protect yourself from marketing techniques that mask poor product quality by looking for evidence to support marketing claims.

Researching Marketing Claims

Marketing claims of therapeutic efficacy regarding product formulas and ingredients should always be suspect until you have researched the available data. Do not depend on information from the manufacturer. Work proactively to become savvy in unveiling the difference between quality products and marketing strategies. Not all products and ingredients have test results to support their healing claims. To complicate matters, some tests provide conflicting results or outcomes. One way to sidestep this situation is to have personal experience with the product and ingredient. It also helps to become familiar with the product manufacturer's integrity rather than just their marketing skills.

Marketing Natural Ingredients

The current trend in skin care, fueled by consumer demand, includes the use of natural and organic ingredients. To satisfy this desire for natural ingredients, marketing now promotes the use of herbs, essential oils, and other botanical ingredients. Phrases such as *naturally rejuvenating* are used to promote products that may or may not contain natural ingredients. This language could be the closest thing to "natural" contained in the product. Although some products do contain good quality natural and organic ingredients, a large number of available skin care products contain only traces, or synthetic versions of natural ingredients. The quality of the natural ingredients could be so poor that the therapeutic result is minimal. The challenge to the consumer and the practitioner is to become knowledgeable enough about cosmetic formulation and natural ingredients to be able to tell when a product's function is really coming from natural ingredients contained in it. You must also be able to discern whether the "natural" ingredient is actually natural.

Natural Scents or Synthetic Fragrance?

Skin care products often promote "natural" or "aromatherapy" fragrances. This is an area in which deceit is very common and easily accomplished, given the lack of regulation within the cosmetic industry. A product advertising the natural smell of fresh strawberries, using strawberry essential oils, should send up a red flag. There is no essential oil of strawberry. Such an oil does not exist in the plant or fruit; the so-called natural strawberry essence can only be synthetically created. If you compared the fragrance of a handful of fresh herbs to most "herbal" fragrances, you would suspect them to be nothing more than synthetic blends. The experience you acquire from using and smelling true essential oils will help you to easily recognize a synthetic fragrance.

Natural Truth

Detecting the truth behind other natural ingredients, such as herbs, botanical oils, and naturally derived nutrients, may prove to be more problematic. Labeling regulations allow manufacturers to list an extract without mentioning the actual amount of the plant material in the extract. Ingredient labels are required to list ingredients from the most abundant in the product to the least. If the first ingredient is "aqueous extract of chamomile," the product appears to contain chamomile in the highest proportion. Without a listing of the actual percentage of chamomile in the aqueous solution, it is impossible to know what the actual amount of chamomile is. The solution could contain 99.999 percent water and just 0.001 percent of chamomile. If this water, or aqueous extract of chamomile, is 50 percent of the total formula, the amount of active chamomile in the product is 0.0005 percent. This is not an active amount of chamomile. It will not always be the case that an extract is so heavily diluted, but consumers and practitioners must be aware of this possibility. This practice redefines the idea of reading labels and, again, is a situation that calls for trust and awareness of the manufacturer and their practices.

SYNTHETIC VERSUS NATURAL

Are natural ingredients better than synthetic ingredients? This question is the basis for an ongoing debate that each practitioner must decide. Aromatherapy and the use of essential oils is a practice focused on using ingredients from nature, rather than manmade synthetics. In holistic therapy, natural botanicals, such as essential oils, are preferred over synthetics. In holistic aromatherapy, the use of natural ingredients will override the use of synthetics, although under special circumstances some synthetics have a place in holistic formulations. In cosmetic manufacturing, some very gentle, semi-synthetic surfactants are used, such as the hydrolyzed soy and oat proteins. Nutritional additions to a cosmetic formula may also be synthetic compounds. Alpha lipoic acid and MSM are not easily derived from natural sources, so synthetic copies are more common. Esterified C is synthetic ascorbic acid that is esterified in a fashion that does not occur in nature (see Ascorbyl Palmitate in this chapter).

The identity and definition of "natural" is not always clear; thus, the question of which is better, synthetic or natural, is difficult to answer in absolute terms. This text focuses on ingredients that are derived from nature and are used in their naturally extracted state, without any additives or further processing.

What Is Natural?

What defines a natural ingredient? What defines a synthetic ingredient? Ask ten skin care chemists to answer these questions, and you will likely get ten different answers. The word *natural* lacks a standardized meaning in relation to cosmetics and is over-used to the point of being meaningless. Dissect the concept of natural to its basic elements, and you may be able to develop your own definitions, understandings, and personal distinctions regarding what is natural and what is synthetic.

What Is Organic?

Organic, as a modern definition and a standard, is explained by the methods, practices, and substances used in producing food crops. Unlike *natural*, *organic* is well defined, with a precise meaning, because international standards have been developed. The USDA Organic standard and the California Organic Food Act of 1979, along with other state-by-state standards, identify the qualifications for growing and labeling organic food or botanical ingredients[5] in the U.S. The EU-Eco-regulation in the European Union and other standards of organic certification that have been developed worldwide.

Identifying organic-certified farming practices became necessary because of the development of industrial and high-tech farming. A main advantage to organic farming is that it avoids harmful industrial pesticides and fertilizers, some of which are endocrine disrupters, substances known to throw hormones out of balance in humans and other animals and cause neurological damage that includes hyperactivity and attention deficit.[6] Organic farming improves, rather than depletes, farmland and is all-around better for the environment.

Back to Basics

A simple way to understand the terms *organic* and *natural* is to imagine what it may have been like to live in 800 B.C. a time when agriculture had been fully developed, but chemical industrialization was years in the future. How would food and herbs have been grown, picked, processed, and stored? Plants would have been grown without the manipulation of industrial chemicals, pesticides, and fertilizers. The absence of modern technology would have assured a plant or plant extract to be clean of synthetics and rich in naturally occurring compounds. The herbs, unguents, hennas, and other materials used by Cleopatra during her Egyptian reign would today be considered organic ingredients. What were the processes used by the Egyptians in 45 B.C. to create cosmetics from plant-based materials? Cleopatra had her trusted alchemists mixing and blending in ways similar to uses of essential oils, clay, and botanicals discussed in this book; she had no chemists in labs combining or breaking down molecules with expensive scientific machinery. Don't misunderstand: there are, and were in her time, potentially hazardous plant-based extracts used in cosmetics or for beauty purposes, such as the Egyptian henbane extract, atropine, which Cleopatra used to dilate her pupils to appear more alluring.[7]

Technology such as genetic modification to make foods and herbs "better" and more abundant, or farming practice "easier" and more profitable, was non-existent at this time in history. Industrial chemical manipulation and synthetic manufacturing could not be performed without the technology available today. The food and cosmetic process was much simpler in those times. Alchemists, the potion makers of long ago, were able to manipulate chemical reactions, and farmers were cross breeding to produce new agricultural genetics with nature's cooperation, but not on the scale that is accomplished today. A definition of organic helps us to maintain a respect for growing and using plants that was established well before humans entered the planet and provides perspective in defining what is natural.

Identifying a Natural Ingredient

To simplify the complications encountered when defining the term *natural*, let's review two types of ingredients that could easily be identified as natural ingredients.

- The most inarguable form of a natural ingredient is one that is totally unaltered from its original form. This unaltered natural ingredient is derived from a plant or other substance that grows or occurs naturally (organically) in nature and is not extracted or picked using any chemical means, which includes water, oil, and alcohol. It is used in its unaltered, complete form; not isolated, chemically treated, heated, cooked, or changed in any way. Examples of this kind of natural ingredient would be dried herbs and expeller-pressed vegetable and fruit oils (not hexane or solvent extracted). Salts and minerals acquired through a non-chemical process, such as sea salt obtained by evaporating seawater, are also in this category of natural ingredients.
- The next category of natural ingredients is where defining *natural* begins to get tricky, because in this category the original substance has been altered through an extraction process. These substances are still ingredients derived from plants or other substances that grow or occur organically. What makes them different from the previous group is that these ingredients are derived using "natural process," a process that can be described as one using non-petroleum or non–man-made chemical substances to extract the desired portion of the plant. The natural substances that are used to produce extracts are water, oil, or alcohol. The plant material is no longer whole. The substance used to extract the desired portion of the plant will extract only the compounds in the plant with which it is compatible. A cup of herbal tea is a water extract. When the leaf or herb is placed in hot water, only water-soluble compounds from the plant will be extracted into the water. The compounds that are extracted will not be altered from their extracted state, so this product is still considered a natural extract. Essential oils and **herbal tinctures,** alcohol derived herbal extracts, are examples of naturally derived ingredients.

From this point on, the definition of *natural* becomes fuzzy. Extracts derived from a plant source may be further manipulated or broken down. Isolated active molecules may be extracted from a plant or essential oil; an example would be the menthol isolated from peppermint as flavor or included in muscle soothing rubs. It is still a natural derivative, unchanged by any other chemical means or mechanical manipulation.

When does a natural become a synthetic? Many materials are constructed of isolated compounds derived from a natural source and combined to create something new, a substance that does not naturally occur in nature. The process of adulterating essential oils, as explained in Chapter 4, is where the intervention of human science begins to create what may be considered a synthetic, even though the adulteration is performed using molecules produced in nature. Where is the line that is crossed when a substance composed of natural compounds is defined as either a natural or synthetic?

ISOLATES

An **isolate** is a compound that is isolated from the substance that contains it. The menthol from peppermint is an example of an isolate. The use of isolates is very common in nutritional and pharmaceutical medicine. Many vitamins are isolated compounds, such as ascorbic acid (vitamin C) and d-tocopherol (vitamin E). Isolates have value as vitamin nutrients, but they may also cause irritation and imbalance in body systems. This potential has become evident as more and more people supplement with high doses of vitamins. An unusually high amount of a vitamin that is not normally available in these dosages through diet may cause imbalance, such as the nerve toxicity that occurs from high levels of vitamin B_6.[8]

Much of the focus in contemporary pharmacology is on the activity of a specific molecular compound, such as acetylsalicylic acid, also known as aspirin. Acetylsalicylic acid is a headache relieving and anti-inflammatory compound, originally extracted from willow bark as salicin. After some chemical manipulation, this compound becomes salicylic acid. The salicylic acid has a specific activity and function; in this case, it is analgesic. In an isolated form, however, salicylic acid has negative effects on the digestive tract. Adding an acetyl component to the salicylic acid to reduce the digestive problems altered the chemical isolate. The created compound is now acetylsalicylic acid. This process was perfected in 1899 by a German chemist assigned by the Bayer Company to find a way to reduce the negative digestive action. The ulcerative properties are still present with acetylsalicylic acid, however. The chances of digestive ulcers occurring are nonexistent when the whole willow bark extract is used. Using a whole plant extract remains the safest method of use, preferred over the use of isolated active compounds and their "improved" synthetic versions.

Understanding Isolates and Their Therapeutic Benefits

In the quest for acceptance by the medical mainstream, some alternative researchers and clinicians have focused on the properties of specific isolated compounds. This narrow focus may create unnecessary fear of beneficial oils or herbs containing extracts that, when isolated, have valid contraindications. This misperception occurred with tea tree oil, whose 1,8 cineole component has been found in certain studies to be an irritant.[9] Tea tree oil in its whole form is a proven anti-inflammatory.[10] Another well-known irritant is carvacrol, isolated from oregano. Used as an isolated compound, carvacrol has powerful antibacterial properties but severe irritating effects. In the whole essential oil of oregano, the carvacrol is balanced by the naturally occurring anti-inflammatory property of the oil's sesquiterpene content. This molecule tempers the irritating effects of carvacrol and allows oregano to be used with proper precautions.

The natural balance gives value to using the whole plant or whole extract with a significant therapeutic advantage. The antispasmodic activity of the esters in lavender is supported and enhanced by the presence of the trace element coumarin. At times, a plant compound believed to give a therapeutic result fails a clinical study when the research is performed using only the isolated compound. The compound may not be as effective without the presence of the other components contained in the whole plant or extract. In other words, the therapeutic effect is a consequence of the synergistic structure rather than being caused by just one specific compound.

Balancing Isolated Ingredients

Isolated molecules are often used in cosmetics and skin care. The cosmeceuticals and other nutrients, such as alpha lipoic acid, vitamins A, C, and E, and hyaluronic acid, have received high praise for their corrective and protective action in skin care. When formulating using isolated and synthetic compounds, it becomes the art of the cosmetic chemist to combine the ingredients in a non-irritating balance meant to mimic the natural balance that nature may provide. The art of the natural ingredient formulator is to combine the complex natural activity of botanicals into a harmonious and balanced formula. Many synthetics are inert, having no activity or interaction with the function of the skin, and are used as functional ingredients that assist in creating attractive products for consumer appeal.

INGREDIENTS AND THE SKIN

The role of a cosmetic is to either maintain or regenerate healthy skin. Cosmetics should restore balance to skin conditions and help retain moisture and lipid content. For cosmetics to have any benefit. the ingredients must interact with the metabolic functions and harmonize with the epidermal layer. The surface skin is protected by the hydrolipid layer, which consists of free fatty acids, phospholipids, triglycerides, and cholesterol. A cosmetic that contains similar constituents would seem to be ideal for skin health and dermal penetration of nutrients. Essential oils and carrier oils certainly fulfill the role of active and harmonious ingredients for skin care.

Opinions and attitudes about skin active ingredients differ widely among cosmetic chemists and manufacturers. Some believe that a few active ingredients within an inert formulation are sufficient, while others attempt to use only those ingredients that provide active value to the skin. Qualifying ingredients for their benefit to skin health becomes a philosophical consideration as much as a functional one. The holistic approach prefers the most harmonious and balancing ingredients. This preference includes ingredients derived from nature and containing those properties of biological familiarity mentioned in Chapter 3. Ingredients that fall into this classification contain saturated and unsaturated fats, terpenoid compounds, vitamins, enzymes, carbohydrates, phospholipids, and proteins.

Consumer-Friendly Ingredients

The packaging of a product dominates in the appeal of mass marketed skin care products. Color, texture, and fragrance are all important marketing elements. The use of natural and active ingredients complicates the process of producing attractive, consumer-friendly cosmetics. Natural substances tend to add colors, such as browns and yellows. A whole food cosmetic is not always capable of staying **emulsified**, when substances that are not mutually soluble have an ability to mix together, which may give the product a runny or separated appearance. Synthetic ingredients have been developed to impart texture, color, and ease of use to cosmetics to make them acceptable to the mainstream buyer. These synthetic ingredients, such as emulsifiers and pearlizers, provide only the consumer-friendly appearance and ease of use to the product. They do not serve any purpose to benefit skin health. The debate over natural and synthetic ingredients is influenced by the marketability of the end product.

PRECAUTION FOR USING ESSENTIAL OILS IN FORMULATIONS

A unique precaution should be acknowledged when using essential oils in skin care, especially when the product contains synthetic or isolated compounds. Several essential oil molecules have been noted for their ability to pull larger molecules into the blood stream. In Chapter 9, you read how they are currently being used in topical pharmaceutical patches as carriers to help drugs penetrate into the bloodstream. This example underscores the ability of essential oils to carry a variety of molecules into the body. Knowing the potential irritation or toxicity of all ingredients contained in an essential oil formula is important. The essential oil may attach to one compound contained in an otherwise balanced synthetic formula. Though the compound may not be irritating in the balanced formula, it may become an irritant if the essential oil carries it into the skin. Ask questions of the manufacturer as well as do your own research to be sure that all the ingredients are safe for penetration. If the formula contains synthetics or isolates, consider whether, if the essential oil pulls even one of these synthetic compounds into the dermis or bloodstream, it raises a chance of potential irritation or other imbalance in the body. This exercise demonstrates the value of using as much unaltered, whole ingredients in skin care as possible, such as olive oil, berry oils, and herbs known for their harmony in skin care.

INGREDIENTS USED IN SKIN CARE AND COSMETIC FORMULAS

In a book with a primary focus on essential oils, it is consistent to concentrate on natural ingredient formulas. As a practitioner, you will develop your own ideas, philosophies, and motivations about product formulation and the quality of natural ingredients. Vast amounts of information are available, and both practitioners and consumers need to make informed choices about products.

Many reference books and manuals define and describe the variety and uses of popular skin care ingredients. Refer to as many of them as possible to get a balanced understanding. The Internet is a wonderful resource, but be cautious and wary of information extracted solely from the Internet that cannot be verified by support from scientific studies.

Emulsifiers

One rarely finds a commercial cosmetic product in today's marketplace that requires the consumer to mix, shake, or stir before use. This is quite a phenomenon, considering that most cosmetics are a blend of oil and water and, as you know, oil and water don't mix. To combine the water and oil ingredients, cosmetics use **emulsifiers**, compounds that have the ability to combine a fat or oil with water. This action creates a bridge, or bond, between the water and oil ingredients and keeps them from separating in a cosmetic cream or lotion. Emulsification permits the consumer to use the product without having to shake or stir it. Consumers are accustomed to shaking some products, as they do with a bottle of salad dressing that contains obviously separated oil and vinegar components. Consumers are not as relaxed about their cosmetics and feel there is something wrong with the product if the oil separates from the water. This feeling has been a challenge for natural cosmetic manufacturers, who have had a difficult time convincing consumers to stir products. The result is that synthetic emulsifiers have found their way into natural cosmetics. Polyethylene glycol (PEG) compounds are currently one of the most common synthetic emulsifiers used.

Most common cosmetic emulsifiers are synthetic and do not penetrate the skin. This may impede the skin's natural ability and function to absorb or eliminate. Natural emulsifiers, such as lecithin, vegetable glycerin, and vegetable emulsifying wax, work harmoniously with and may benefit the skin. These more natural emulsifiers are increasingly being used to replace PEGs in natural cosmetics.

Surfactants

The ability of a cleanser to lift dirt and debris from the skin comes from its surfactant content. In cosmetics, **surfactants** are used as emulsifying agents, cleansing agents, and foam boosters. Surfactants are necessary to effectively clean skin. Water alone is not an effective cleanser, because it cannot lift oily dirt from the skin. A surfactant loosens the dirt from the oil. Surfactants provide soap's familiar lather, but lather is an unnecessary function for a cosmetic and may mean that its surfactant is overly aggressive in its cleansing action. If the surfactant is too strong or aggressive, it will disrupt the skin's lipid barrier function, resulting in skin irritation and atopic dermatitis.[11] One of the most common synthetic surfactants used is sodium laurel sulfate. Within the category of natural surfactants is castile soap or saponified vegetable oils.

> For Your Information
>
> **Chlorine: A Precaution**
>
> According to Doris J. Rapp, MD, author of Is This Your Child's World? exposure to chlorine in tap water, showers, pool, laundry products, cleaning agents, food processing, sewage systems, and other sources can affect health by contributing to asthma, hay fever, anemia, bronchitis, circulatory collapse, confusion, delirium diabetes, dizziness, irritation of the eye, mouth, nose, throat, lung, skin, and stomach, heart disease, high blood pressure, and nausea. It is also a possible cause of cancer.[12] Even though you will not see chlorine in personal care products, it is important for you to be aware of the need to protect your skin when bathing and washing. Chlorine is very drying to the skin and should be suspected in any irritated skin conditions. Shower and water filters are highly recommended.

COMMON SYNTHETIC INGREDIENTS TO AVOID IN AROMATHERAPY

This section reviews the most common synthetic ingredients found in cosmetics, including some marketed as natural cosmetics. Some evidence indicates that some of these compounds may be toxic.[13] The cosmetics industry maintains that the amount of these ingredients used in cosmetics poses no real risk.[14] Nevertheless, questionable synthetic ingredients should be avoided in conjunction with essential oils.

Parabens (Methyl, Butyl, or Propyl)

Para-hydroxybenzoic acid esters (parabens) are synthetic, petrochemical preservatives used in most cosmetics. The parabens most commonly used are methyl-, ethyl-, and butyl-. The parabens are very effective, wide spectrum preservatives that are easily added to shampoos, lotions, and most other types of cosmetics. They are accepted for use in "natural" cosmetics and considered safe as used by the Cosmetic Ingredient Review. Controversy over the use of parabens in cosmetics was stimulated by a 2004 study that linked parabens to breast cancer.[15] This study had several flaws, and the connection is believed to be tenuous. Some reports relate parabens to allergic reaction and sensitivity,[16] and they are noted as endocrine disrupters, though whether this ability affects human health is speculative.[17]

Mineral Oil and Other Petroleum Products

Mineral oil is a petroleum ingredient commonly used as an emollient and lubricant on the skin. It, like other petroleum products, forms an **occlusive layer,** which physically blocks water loss from the skin. Mineral oil and petrolatum, or petroleum jelly, appeal to manufacturers because they are inexpensive and stable. The lubricant and occlusive nature of mineral oil, and its inert quality, are the benefits of using mineral oil in skin care. Some believe that petroleum-based products, especially lubricants such as mineral oil or petroleum jelly, disrupt the natural immune barrier of the skin and inhibit its ability to absorb nutrients and release toxins. Such a lubricant certainly would interfere with the penetration of essential oils and other therapeutic ingredients.

PEG (Polyethylene Glycol)

PEGs are polymers that are combined with other molecules to create emollients, surfactants, emulsifiers, and viscosity adjusters. This group includes PEG-8 myristate, PEG-18 palmitate, and PEG-25 PABA. A by-product, 1,4 dioxane, may be formed in the manufacture of the product and is a known carcinogen.[18] In other words, PEG compounds may be contaminated with dioxins.

Propylene Glycol (PG)

This substance is a cosmetic **humectant,** an agent that promotes moisture retention, and solvent. It is able to penetrate the skin and possibly act as a carrier for other ingredients. Its safety is much debated, and many cautions are associated with it. Studies have acknowledged it as a skin irritant, and it may be responsible for other health-related issues.[19]

Sodium Lauryl Sulfate (SLS) and Sodium Laureth Sulfate (SLES)

These compounds are used as surfactants in many skin and hair cleansers and toothpastes. SLS is a powerful degreaser. SLES, thought to be a less aggressive detergent, is created when SLS is converted by a process called ethoxylation. SLS and SLES are not natural ingredients, as many natural product manufacturers claim, even though their starting material is derived from coconut. The list of hazards for direct exposure to these detergents includes eye damage, depression, labored breathing, diarrhea, severe skin irritation, and inflammation. The Journal of the American College of Toxicology reports that "SLS may be damaging to the immune system, especially within the skin. Skin layers may separate and inflame due to its protein denaturing properties."[20] These compounds are possibly the most irritating of all ingredients in personal care products. Research has shown that SLS, when combined with other chemicals, can be transformed into nitrosamines, a potent class of carcinogens. These data, as well as results from other studies, pose serious questions regarding the potential health threat from the use of these surfactants in shampoos, cleansers, and toothpastes. SLES is considered a milder surfactant than SLS. The opinion of some cosmetic chemists is that SLS and SLES may contain warnings and safety precautions for chemists working with the pure ingredient in the lab but do not have the same effect when used in appropriate concentrations in finished products.[21]

DEA (diethanolamine) and TEA (triethanolamine)

DEA and TEA are usually listed on the ingredient label in conjunction with other compounds, having names like cocamide DEA and lauramide TEA. These compounds are thickeners commonly found in personal care products that foam, including bubble baths, body washes, shampoos, soaps, and facial cleansers. These ingredients are known to form cancer-causing nitrates and nitrosamines and have a high potential to cause certain cancers.[22]

FD&C Color Pigments

FD&C (Food, Drug & Cosmetic) colors are possible causes of allergies, skin sensitivity, and irritation. They are possible carcinogens.[23] A great deal of controversy exists about the use of FD&C colors, even though they are listed as safe by the FDA. Several FD&C dyes are used in cosmetics; some are safe, but others are considered to be harmful. Colors serve absolutely no purpose or benefit to the skin and are used solely for marketing.

Fragrance

Fragrances are very important in the manufacture and sale of cosmetics. Huge amounts of money are spent on creating the ideal scent, one that appeals to the largest consumer segment and triggers large sales volume. Consumers will buy a product because it smells good. Using this truth as a guide, manufacturers of consumer products, such as laundry detergent, toilet paper, and household cleaner, began modeling their fragrances after popular perfumes.[24] Many products, not just cosmetics, are developed and tested based on the power of scent. Millions of dollars are invested in creating and producing fragrance compounds, with new ones introduced on a yearly basis. It does not seem reasonable to think that these new and existing compounds are all tested for safety.

The word *fragrance* on a label can indicate the presence of up to 5,000 separate ingredients. It is possible that 95 percent of fragrance compounds used are developed in laboratories and are petroleum or coal tar-based synthetics.[25] Symptoms reported to the FDA related to exposure to synthetic fragrances have included headaches, dizziness, rashes, skin discoloration, violent coughing, vomiting, and allergic skin irritation.[26] Clinical observation by medical doctors have shown that exposure to fragrances can affect the central nervous system, causing depression, hyperactivity, irritability, inability to cope, and other behavioral changes. The population of people diagnosed with fragrance sensitivities is growing. This increase has triggered the growth of "fragrance free" zones, especially doctors' offices and hospitals that are beginning to show up across the United States. This trend poses a problem for the use of essential oils if they are defined as a fragrance.

Some compounds used in fragrance are isolated from essential oils. Commonly used essential oil isolates are linalyl acetate, linalool, farnesol, coumarins, and indole. Some studies report negative side effects or sensitivities with the use of these compounds.[27] Using isolates from essential oils is not aromatherapy, though many manufacturers would like the consumer to believe that isolates equate to the complete essential oil.

Essential oils are often labeled and used as a fragrance in cosmetics. Most cosmetics, even those that state they contain essential oils, likely use oils from the flavor and fragrance industries. These oils are commonly adulterated to ensure consistent scents from batch to batch and to lower the cost of otherwise expensive essential oils. Please be clear that authentic essential oils, as discussed in this book, are therapeutic ingredients, not a fragrance or fragrance compounds. An unscented product does not necessarily need to be free of essential oils, though this would be the common perception.

Diazolidinyl Urea (Germall II); DMDM Hydantoin; Imidazolidinyl Urea (Germall 115); Quaternium 15

These substances are preservatives that release formaldehyde (formaldehyde-donors). Formaldehyde is a known sensitizing agent that can cause dermatitis and itching. It is a suspected carcinogen, and exposure may lead to an immune response and irritation of the eyes, nose, and throat. It can also aggravate coughs and colds and trigger asthma.[28] Unlike Japan, Europe, and Thailand, the United States and the FDA do not regulate the content of formaldehyde or formaldehyde donor ingredients in cosmetics.[29] An article from the *Journal of Food and Drug Analysis* tested formaldehyde donor ingredients and reports that quaternium 15 liberated 58.80 percent formaldehyde; DMDM hydantoin liberated 17.12 percent; diazolidinyl gave up 15.43 percent, and imidazolidinyl gave 12.53 percent.

OTHER COMMON COSMETIC INGREDIENTS

The following primarily synthetic ingredients are found in natural and mainstream skin care preparations. These substances are generally regarded as safe though there are reports that may question their safety and may have a tendency to cause irritation.

Cetearyl Alcohol

This semi-synthetic mixture of stearyl and cetyl fatty alcohols is used as an emollient and emulsifier in cosmetics. Consumers have a tendency to confuse this material with the drying specially denatured (SD) alcohols. This ingredient is generally safe and suitable for use in natural cosmetics. There is no reported potential for irritation.

Cetrimonium Bromide or Chloride

These compounds are synthetic ammonium salts used as a preservatives and emulsifiers in cosmetics. Cetrimonium bromide and chloride do have toxicology warnings and irritation issues, though they are considered safe for use when they are used topically in rinse off products.[30] Due to the potential toxicity and irritation, it is best not to include essential oils in formulas that contain cetrimonium bromide or chloride.

Cocamidopropyl Betaine (also Coco Betaine)

This surfactant and foaming agent is used as a more gentle replacement for SLS and SLES. Some cautions exist, such as reports of sensitivity associated with this ingredient. More gentle surfactants are recommended in combination with essential oils.

NATURAL INGREDIENTS IN COSMETICS

The following ingredients are derived with the least amount of manipulation or chemical process and are useful in therapeutic skin care. No toxicology reports relate to any of these ingredients. Ingredients on this list should be acknowledged for individual sensitivities and allergies, however. This is an abbreviated list of possible naturally derived ingredients that have skin conditioning properties. Essential oils work in harmony and synergy with all the ingredients on this list. See Table 10-1 for formulating possibilities using natural ingredients for specific skin conditions.

Cocoa Butter

This fatty wax with a buttery texture is obtained from the seeds of the cacao bean. Cocoa butter is an excellent skin conditioner and softener with antioxidant properties.

Honey

Honey contains a large amount of potassium, which is responsible for its anti-bacterial properties. It's a good skin humectant and leaves the skin feeling soft. Honey conditions the skin and is a great addition to masks and wraps for the body.

Hydrosols (Hydrolates; Floral Waters)

Hydrosols are the by-product of essential oil distillation. They contain the water-soluble properties of the plant. Hydrosols contain sesquiterpene and monoterpene alcohols and very little, if any, of the potentially irritating terpene hydrocarbons. They are a subtle, somewhat homeopathic and gentler form of the essential oil.

Lecithin

Lecithin is used as an emulsifier in cosmetics and is usually extracted from soy. It contains phospholipids and phosphatidylcholine. The phospholipids are fatty acids with a phosphorus molecule, similar to those that compose the membrane that envelopes the cells of the body. Phosphatidycholine, also contained in the cells, stabilizes the natural skin barrier and provides protection from water loss. Lecithin provides moisturizing benefits to the skin because of its ability to mimic the phospholipids of the skin's lipid barrier. Lecithin that is derived from a non-GMO (genetically modified organism) soy source is best.

INCREASING THERAPEUTIC ACTIVITY WITH NUTRIENTS

Incorporating nutrients into a formula for topical use may increase the therapeutic activity of formulas. The following list is designed to help you understand the function of certain ingredients that may be found in prepared formulas containing nutrients, sometimes called **cosmeceuticals** or **nutraceuticals**. All of the nutrients listed here are also available, and first were popularized, as health-giving and therapeutic dietary supplements. The cosmeceuticals listed here are vitamin and nutrient isolates. It is difficult, or impossible, to extract some of these substances from a natural source, so they are developed in a laboratory as synthetic-identicals, vitamins and nutrients that are manmade to mimic the molecular structure of the natural. From a purist's perspective, this is not an ideal situation. The logic is similar to adding supplements to a healthy diet. In our high-stress and environmentally toxic culture it is necessary to support a healthy diet or natural skin care with a stronger emphasis on antioxidants and anti-inflammatory nutrients. The isolated compounds on this list will provide this needed support.

Alpha Lipoic Acid

This is a very powerful antioxidant with anti-inflammatory action.[31] It assists in healing and protecting the skin and has the potential to reverse damage caused by aging and sun exposure. It is used in formulas designed to reduce wrinkles, fine lines, and scarring. This effect may arise from its ability to prevent the breakdown of proteins caused by sugar binding, called **glycation.**[32] Studies have shown that alpha lipoic acid is effectively absorbed and used by the cells when topically applied. One of its special features is its ability to be absorbed and used in both the water portion and the fat portion of the cells, giving it a unique ability to provide the cells with complete antioxidant protection. Alpha lipoic acid is manufactured in cells and plays an important role in the production of cellular energy (ATP). It is difficult to extract from a natural source, so it is primarily available as a synthetic for use in supplements and as a cosmeceutical. R-lipoic acid and R-dihydro-lipoic acid are the forms that occur naturally in the body. The R-lipoic acid is used more effectively by the cells and may be the preferred form to use.[33]

Benefits of Alpha Lipoic Acid

- Protects from free radical damage
- Reduces inflammation

- Prevents glycation (glycation occurs when sugar molecules bond to proteins. These compounds become advanced glycation end-products, which interfere with the function and shape of the protein. Glycation stiffens the collagen proteins, causing crosslinking and the formation of wrinkles.)

Astaxanthin

Astaxanthin, because it is a supercritical extract (CO_2), an extraction method disussed in Chapter 4, fits better in the essential oils category. It is included here because it is primarily sold as an internal nutritional supplement and has recently been introduced for use as a topical cosmeceutical. This complex, derived from the Hawaiian algae *Haematococcus pluvialis*, is abundant in naturally occurring carotenoids. Astaxanthin is excellent in topical skin care, because it protects the skin from free radical damage,[34] provides UV protection (as an "SPF booster"),[35,36] is an anti-inflammatory,[37] suppresses hyperpigmentation, and is a skin-brightener. It is used in very small concentrations in formulas. It is an extremely bright red/orange color, which is capable of staining clothing, making it difficult to work with but well worth the formulating difficulties. Any formula that contains astaxanthin will have a red color to it.

Benefits of Astaxanthin

- Protects against free radical damage
- Reduces inflammation
- Provides UV protection
- Reduces hyperpigmentation

DMAE (Dimethylaminoethanol)

DMAE is a nutrient that provides anti-inflammatory relief and helps to create a firmer facial tone and reduce sagging. DMAE is a nutrient found in fish and is known to increase brain function. DMAE is one of the reasons that fish is considered "brain food."[38] When used topically, it protects skin cells and tones the facial muscles. The skin firming activity comes from DMAE's ability to stimulate acetylcholine from the nerves, stimulating facial muscles. In clinical studies, skin was instantaneously made "firmer, less lined and smoother" when DMAE was applied topically.[39] Skin firming results are also seen with daily consumption of a portion of wild Alaskan salmon, a fish high in DMAE content.

Benefits of DMAE

- Protects against free radical damage
- Reduces inflammation
- Firms and tones skin

MSM (Methylsulfonylmethane)

MSM is a skin-strengthening and -protecting compound. It enhances collagen and elastin production for a youthful, smooth, and radiant complexion.[40] MSM is readily absorbed and used by the dermal tissue. MSM is a biologically active source of sulfur and a building block for the amino acids cysteine and methionine. These amino acids are important in forming connective tissue (collagen), hair, nails, and the keratinized skin cells of the epidermal layer. It reduces scar tissue and keloids by normalizing the cross-linking of collagen.[41] MSM is a nutrient found in many foods, including milk, coffee, tomatoes, and beer.

Benefits of MSM

- Protects against free radical damage
- Reduces inflammation
- Strengthens skin cells
- Promotes healthy collagen and elastin

Vitamins A (Carotenes, Retinyl Esters, Retinol, Retin-A™)

Products containing vitamin A, especially Retin-A, have been popular since the mid 1970s and are often recommended by dermatologists for acneic skin conditions. Vitamin A, an umbrella term used for several fat-soluble retinoids, is well known for its antioxidant properties and support of skin cell regeneration. The popular Retin-A has been used successfully for skin conditions but does have some minor side effects that include peeling, redness, and sun sensitivity.

Using carotenoids such as beta-carotene, astaxanthene, and naturally occurring plant oils such as carrot oil, sea buckthorn, and astaxanthin is a more holistic and natural method of supplying vitamin A to the skin. Carotenoids are the precursors to vitamin A and can be applied without the risk of side effects. The use of a vitamin A isolate, such as retinol, may be necessary to treat severe skin conditions.

Benefits of Vitamins A

- Protects against free radical damage
- Reduces inflammation
- Treats acneic conditions

Vitamin C (Ascorbic Acid and Ascorbyl Palmitate)

Vitamin C is a popular antioxidant and nutrient necessary for overall health and wellness. Vitamin C is a water soluble compound, called L-ascorbic acid. Vitamin C, as a dietary nutrient, has an impressive list of health-giving rewards. It protects and supports many of the vital functions of the body, including the cardiovascular, nervous, and immune systems, along with being a necessary nutrient for collagen production.

Ascorbic acid has been used in skin care for many years, though it is not very stable and is believed to break down quickly in a cosmetic formulation, meaning it will have very little activity by the time it is used on the skin. Even if it were stable, its benefit would be questionable, because it is water-soluble and does not penetrate the lipid barrier easily. It also has the potential to irritate skin. The solution to using the bioactive properties of vitamin C topically is **vitamin C ester,** a fat-soluble form that was developed to stabilize the vitamin and make it soluble in lipids, or the skin. **Ascorbyl palmitate** is a vitamin C ester formed by combining L-ascorbic acid with the fatty acids of palm oil. The skin derives antioxidant protection through the use of ascorbyl palmitate. It also promotes the development of healthy collagen

Benefits of Vitamin C

- Protects against free radical damage
- Reduces inflammation
- Promotes healthy collagen and elastin

Vitamin E and Tocotrienol

There are eight naturally occurring forms of vitamin E, each with its own biological activity. The most familiar and commonly used in skincare is the d-alpha-tocopherol. This form of vitamin E was thought to be best in protecting against lipid peroxidation. Recently another form of the vitamin E, tocotrienol, was found to have a higher antioxidant capability than the alpha-tocopherol when applied to the skin. Alpha-tocotrienol has 40 to 60 times greater antioxidant potency than the more commonly used alpha-tocopherol. Tocotrienols penetrate the skin quickly and provide superior protection against UV-light–induced oxidative stress and damage. Using both nutrients provides more complete antioxidant action and lipid protection of skin cells. Controversy exists over the choice and effectiveness of the synthetic form of E, dl-tocopherol. In the context of holistic health and skin care, natural derivatives are always preferred.

Benefits of Vitamin E and Tocotrienol

- Protect against free radical damage
- Reduce inflammation
- Provide UV protection
- Promote wound healing

HERBS IN SYNERGISTIC ESSENTIAL OIL FORMULAS

Herbal medicine, known as herbology, is a specialized practice. Aromatherapy has a special harmony with herbal medicine. Herbs offer a full range of therapeutic activity, similar to that of essential oils, for the health and well-being of humans. Their properties are extracted using water, oil, or alcohol. Each method of extraction differs depending on the medium used. Many herbs do not contain a volatile oil that can produce a usable essential oil.

Herbs are used dry and in tinctures, infusions, or decoctions. Infusions and decoctions are water extracts. Infusions are like a tea: boiling water is poured over the herb, which is allowed to steep for a specified time. Placing the herb in water, then bringing the mixture to a boil, is how a decoction is made. This method is used for woods, barks, and roots. A tincture is made by placing the herb into alcohol, glycerine, vinegar, oil, or syrup, and allowing the properties to be absorbed before removing the herb. Tinctures are made in different strengths. Tinctures tend to work best in aromatherapy preparations, because water-based products cannot mix with the oils. Dried herbs can also be put into capsules as a medicinal or supplement.

Following is a description of five herbs that work synergistically with essential oils in topical formulations for skin care. These herbs do not produce essential oil, but they have a synergistic activity and relation to skin care when combined with essential oils.

Aloe Vera

Botanical name: *Aloe vera*

The juice from the aloe is extracted by squeezing it from the leaf of the plant. Aloe has a historic and familiar employment as a wound healing plant. It conditions the skin and is a soothing agent for irritation. Aloe juice is an ideal digestive aid and when swallowed has many other healing advantages.

Aloe is added to many essential oil formulas. It synergizes with the cell-regenerative properties of essential oils and speeds recovery after burns or wounds. Aloe is a soothing choice for skin conditions such psoriasis and eczema. Aloe vera naturally contains large amounts of water. Because water and oil don't mix, aloe cannot be blended with essential oils or base oils. Use aloe in skin cream preparations that contain emulsifiers. Aloe can be added to a water-based spray formula with essential oils; these mixtures must be shaken before each use.

Aloe comes out of the plant as a watery liquid. Aloe gel products that are more viscous contain a thickening agent, usually a seaweed extract called carrageenan.

Benefits of Aloe Vera

- Protects from free radical damage
- Reduces inflammation
- Promotes wound healing
- Soothes irritated skin and atopic dermatitis

Calendula (Marigold)

Botanical name: *Calendula officinalis*

Calendula is on the A list of herbs to use for general skin care, inflammation, wounds, and any other skin condition. It contains carotenoids, saponins, flavanoids, and sterols, all of which are compounds that combine to yield a variety of healing properties. In skin treatments, calendula may be used for bruises, burns, cuts, insect bites, slow-healing wounds and ulcers, fungal infections, and bleeding.[42] Calendula is available as a CO_2 extract.

Benefits of Calendula

- Promotes wound healing
- Reduces inflammation
- Treats fungal infections

Comfrey

Botanical name: *Symphytum officinale*

Comfrey is an impressive wound healing herb with extreme benefit to the skin. It has an impressive biochemical makeup that includes allantoin. Allantoin is a compound often used as an isolate in cosmetic formulas. It contains **keratolytic** properties, which promote desquamation or exfoliation, which is the shedding of the horny outer layer of skin. Allantoin also increases cell regeneration by precipitating, or building, proteins on the skin. These properties of allantoin are also properties of comfrey. Comfrey benefits the skin in its quick healing of wounds, preventing the formation of scar tissue.

Caution must be used if comfrey is used internally for ulcers,[43] because it can cause liver damage.[44]

Benefits of Comfrey

- Promotes wound healing
- Increases cell regeneration
- Prevents scarring

Red Clover

Botanical name: *Trifolium pratense*

Red clover is safe to use for children's skin disorders, which makes it an excellent treatment for eczema, psoriasis, and other chronic childhood skin conditions. It is also useful for adult skin disorders. It contains coumarins and, like essential oils containing the same compound, has anti-spasmodic properties.

Benefits of Red Clover

- Soothes irritated skin
- Treats psoriasis and atopic dermatitis

Green Tea

Botanical name: *Camellia sinensis*

As a beverage, green tea has a long list of health benefits. Drinking at least one cup of green tea a day is recommended. Therapeutic activity includes anti-oxidant properties, cancer protection, and immune support. Green tea also promotes weight loss. This is an impressive array of benefits coming from something so enjoyable to drink. Green tea's polyphenol catechin content provides much of its therapeutic benefits.

Used topically, green tea is an impressive skin conditioner. It protects against UV damage and tumors by its antioxidant action and photoprotection effects.[45] Green tea is produced in tinctures suitable for topical use in aromatherapy formulas.

Benefits of Green Tea

- Protects against free radical damage
- Reduces inflammation
- Provides UV protection
- Improves skin tone

Sea Buckthorn

Botanical name: *Hippophae rhamnoides*

The fruit, or berry, from this plant has been a traditionally used medicinal material in Europe and Asia for centuries. It has recently gained popularity in skin care and as a nutritional supplement for its high EFA, vitamin C, and carotenoid content. The oil from the pulp and seeds is difficult to press, so it is commonly extracted in an oil, such as olive, or extracted through supercritical carbon dioxide (CO_2). Sea buckthorn is an ideal source of the omega-7 fatty acids. These are a rarely found group of fatty acids that protect, nourish, replenish, and restore the skin and the delicate membranes of the digestive tract.[46]

Sea buckthorn oil assists in regenerating and repairing the skin. Its benefits include the healing of atopic dermatitis,[47,48] rosacea, burns, wounds,[49] and sun damage. Sea buckthorn oil contains large amounts of fatty acids (oleic, linoleic, pentadecenoic, palmitoleic, linolenic, and others), carotenes (alpha- and beta-carotenes, lycopene, cryptoxanthin, zeaxanthin, taraxanthin, and phytofluin), tocopherols, and phytosterols, all important compounds for maintaining healthy skin. The EFA content of sea buckthorn oil extract is 80 to 95 percent.

Benefits of Sea Buckthorn

- Speeds healing of wounds and burns
- Supplies high EFA content to condition and moisturize the skin
- Treats atopic dermatitis and rosacea
- Provides antioxidant protection of skin cells

AUTHOR'S **NOTE**

BIOLOGICALLY FAMILIAR

I began using the term **biologically familiar** to describe the preferred quality of ingredients used in skin care. This term refers to those ingredients that exist in nature as plants, animals, and minerals, or the compounds extracted from them. Chapter 5 discusses the evolutionary connection between humans and essential oils. Through the process of evolution, humans have developed a harmony or aversion to the compounds that exist on this planet. Only recently in our existence have we been exposed to synthetic compounds developed by humans. The compounds we have co-existed with for millennia are those that our bodies will recognize as being either beneficial or harmful. These compounds are the biologically familiar ones that are best suited for our use, whether in food, personal care, clothing, or building materials.

Synthetics do not have this same harmony with the human body. Compounds that the body does not recognize may be stored in the tissues, with unknown effects to the body. This fact, demonstrated by the finding of parabens[50] in cancerous breast tissue, led me to define ingredients by their biological familiarity. The idea was to work with compounds that the body recognizes and will know how to handle, primarily to support health. If a biologically familiar ingredient, like an essential oil, is not harmonious with the person using it, irritation or allergic reaction occurs. A natural material will, most of the time, let you know that the human should not be using it. In an extreme case, such as an overdose of belladonna or drowning in water, a biologically familiar compound causes death. For example, the parabens build up in the body, as do many other toxic and unfamiliar synthetic compounds. Sometimes the damage this buildup does is known, such as the carcinogenic risk of pesticide residue[51] and sometimes it is not; for example, paraben buildup has unknown negative effects.

Just this week I received a notice from the environmental group, Friends of the Earth, warning of the possible damage nanoparticles may wreak on the heart, liver, and cell mitochondria. **Nanoparticles** are manufactured particles that are less than 100 nanometers in size; they include nanoized zinc oxide and titanium oxide, which are used extensively in sunscreens and cosmetics.[52] These nanoparticles, which are substances that have been artificially altered from their natural state, are not biologically familiar.

Essential oils are natural and biologically familiar ingredients used in skin care. Extracted herbs, pressed vegetable oils, and clays are also natural and biologically familiar ingredients. Biologically familiar, as a definition, becomes helpful when analyzing nutrients such as alpha-lipoic acid and methylsulfonylmethane (MSM), both nutrients that occur in nature. These compounds must be synthetically made, because they cannot be extracted from a natural source. The question is, are they natural? They are biologically familiar because both compounds are created in nature and necessary to the human body. When used in supplement form or for topical use, these compounds have excellent benefits to the human body, as already defined in this chapter, but they are synthetic. Rather than defending their naturalness, it makes more sense to accept the fact that they must be synthetically created. They are beneficial compounds found within the human body and in edible plants; that is, they are biologically familiar.

When choosing ingredients, I always look for the whole ingredient, such as dried herbs, or whole extracts like unrefined (non-RBD) vegetable and fruit oils. These ingredients are in their most biologically familiar form. When extracts are altered, or compounds are isolated, they are removed from the biologically familiar state. At this point, natural becomes more

Continued

potentially dangerous, as with the highly irritating quality of alpha hydroxy acids or of eugenol, an extract of clove used in fragrances and other topical applications. I do at times break away from my purist ethic, as in my preference for a select group of isolated nutrients, like vitamins E and C, MSM, and other substances. I do so when I feel that increased benefit can be obtained with no negative effects. Given a choice, I always select the naturally extracted nutrient if available. In the case of alpha lipoic acid, I use the more biologically familiar form, R-lipoic acid.

I can only share my knowledge and experience with you. You must decide, based on educated evaluation, what ingredients are right for you and your clients.

Table 10-1 Natural Ingredients for Specific Skin Conditions

There are a variety of formulating possibilities when using essential oils. These possibilities range from simple carrier-oil–based formulas to complex cosmetic formulations that use ingredients discussed in this chapter, and many more. Here is a very brief sample listing of natural ingredients that can be included in formulations for certain skin conditions.

Dry Skin
Sunflower seed oil
Olive oil
Aloe vera gel
Cocoa butter
Lavender essential oil
Geranium essential oil
Rose hydrosol
Sensitive Skin
Safflower oil
Rice bran oil
Avocado oil
Cocoa butter
Roman chamomile essential oil
German chamomile essential oil
Comfrey

Lavender hydrosol
Sea buckthorn CO_2 extract
Psoriasis/Eczema
Shea butter
Neem oil
Helichrysum italicum essential oil
Borage oil
Evening primrose oil
Hemp oil
Calendula extract
Red clover extract
MSM
Arnica hydrosol
Helichrysum hydrosol
Mature Skin/Wrinkles
Shea butter
Rose hip seed oil
Cranberry seed oil
Olive oil
Raspberry seed oil
Rose otto essential oil
Rosemary verbenone essential oil
Calendula extract
Alpha lipoic acid
Rose hydrosol
Inflammation
Shea butter
Neem oil
Raspberry seed oil
Arnica extract
Calendula extract
Helichrysum italicum essential oil
Tanacetum annuum essential oil
Eucalyptus globulus (Corsica) essential oil
Arnica hydrosol

RECIPES FOR SKIN AND SPA

These are sample recipes for skin care and spa treatments, combing essential oils, other natural ingredients, and cosmeceuticals.

Scars, Wrinkles, and Stretch Marks

Formulation type: 2 percent essential oils in a carrier blend
Container: 30-mL (approx. 1 ounce) bottle, preferably with a treatment pump
Application: Massage into the area 3 to 6 times per day until results are achieved. Useful for wounds or following surgery (allow tissue to heal before applying) to prevent scarring.

Formula:

7 drops *Helichrysum italicum* essential oil (EO)

7 drops Rosemary verbenone type EO

(This essential oil combination is slightly more than 2 percent)

3 mL rose hip seed oil

3 mL jojoba oil

2.5 mL cranberry seed oil

0.5 mL d-alpha-tocopherol or mixed vitamin E. (You may use the contents of one or two vitamin E capsules.)

20 mL hazelnut oil or olive oil

Cellulite, Detoxification, and Lymphatic Drainage

Formulation type: 5 percent essential oils in a carrier blend
Container: 30-mL (approx. 1 ounce) bottle
Application: Massage into the area 1 to 6 times per day until results are achieved. This is a great spa treatment

or massage blend. It will help detoxify the tissues and reduce water retention. Can be applied before or after a shower or a steam.

Formula:

4 drops bay laurel EO

4 drops cedarwood EO

4 drops cypress EO

4 drops *Eucalyptus globulus* EO

7 drops grapefruit EO

3 drops lemon EO

4 drops MQV EO

0.5 mL d-alpha-Tocopherol or mixed vitamin E. (You may use the contents of one or two vitamin E capsules.)

25 mL sunflower oil

5 mL olive oil

A spray mist containing MSM and lavender hydrosol may be used as an adjunct to the essential oil formula.

Formulation type: 5 percent MSM in a hydrosol base
Container: 4-oz bottle with spray (atomizer) top
Application: Shake bottle and spray over body, focusing on legs, belly, and buttocks

Formula:

6 mL powdered MSM (methylsulfonylmethane)

70 mL distilled water

20 mL organic grape alcohol (preferred) or organic grain alcohol or vodka – do NOT use denatured SD-alcohol.

25 mL lavender hydrosol

AUTHOR'S **NOTE**

THE HYDROSOL FORMULA

I didn't include this formulation method in Chapter 9, so I will give you an overview of how to work with hydrosols and MSM. When working with hydrosols, you can blend whatever amount suits your needs mixed in with whatever liquids fit your purpose. Hydrosols can be used at percentages of 2 percent to 100 percent. Use your own judgment and creative impulses. I have suggested lavender hydrosol in this formula because it is one of the easier ones to find in the quality expected. Other good choices for this blend would be any fruit hydrosol, cistus, geranium, rose, or a needle tree (pine, spruce, juniper) hydrosol.

Remember, hydrosols are water. Because water grows algae and bacteria, hydrosols have a limited shelf life: three months to a year, on average. Pure grain alcohol is often used as a preservative. My recommendation is to buy smaller amounts that can be used before they go "off." If you buy in large amounts, the suggested percentage of alcohol to use for preservation is 2 to 10 percent.

This hydrosol formula is excellent to treat the skin of the entire body. MSM is used in this case to strengthen the keratin structure and collagen of the skin. Be sure to dissolve, by stirring or shaking, the powdered MSM completely into the formula. MSM is water soluble, which is why a hydrosol blend is more appropriate than an oil blend. Powdered MSM is available at most health and nutrition stores. Use pure organic grape alcohol in this formula for best results. It may be difficult to find, so the next best choice would be organic grain. If vodka is your only choice, fine.

Combine the ingredients and shake. That's all there is to it. You now have an excellent skin conditioning spray. You may find that the sprayers become clogged with crystallized MSM. If this becomes a persistent problem, simply pour a small amount of the solution into the palm of the hand and massage it into the desired areas. If you use a 100 mL Euro-bottle (usually amber or cobalt blue, with a DIN-18 size cap and Euro-dropper; the common bottle set-up used for essential oils), you may drop the solution out rather than pouring it.

Stressed Skin (Soothing)

Formulation type: 2 percent essential oils in an unscented cream base
Container: 15mL (approx. 1/2 ounce) cup or jar
Application: Massage entire body in treatment or as desired for home use. Used to soothe the nerves and calm the skin. This formulation can also be used as a facial moisturizer.

Formula:

Step 1. Pre-blend this recipe into a separate bottle (5 mL to 15 mL) with a dropper (orifice reducer).

8 drops cape chamomile EO

3 drops Australian sandalwood EO

2 drops frankincense EO

4 drops population lavender EO

7 drops neroli EO

2 drops vetiver EO

4 drops palmarosa EO

Step 2. Add 5 drops of this formula to an unscented cream base in a small (15 mL) cup, jar, or other container. You may use a larger container and add, by weight, 15 grams of the cream base. Use a sanitized utensil to scoop the unscented cream. Stir the essential oil drops into the cream with a sanitized utensil.

Step 3. Add these ingredients to the mixture:

6 drops (0.3 mL) sea buckthorn CO_2 extract (use a pipette to drop this viscous CO_2. Most pipettes have measurements in mL.)

0.5 mL d-alpha-tocopherol or mixed vitamin E. (You may use the contents of one or two vitamin E capsules.)

Mature Skin

Formulation type: 2 percent essential oils in an unscented cream base
Container: 15mL (approx. 1/2 ounce) cup or jar

Application: Used as a facial moisturizer and skin conditioner. Can be used over the whole body to condition dry and damaged skin.

Formula:

Step 1. Pre-blend this recipe into a separate bottle (5 mL to 15 mL) with a dropper (orifice reducer). No carrier oil is added to this bottle.

4 drops geranium EO

2 drops myrrh EO

2 drops frankincense EO

8 drops rosemary verbenone EO

4 drops rose EO

4 drops *Helichrysum italicum* EO

6 drops palmarosa EO

Step 2. Add 5 drops of this formula to an unscented cream base in a small (15 mL) cup, jar, or container. You may use a larger container and add, by weight, 15 grams of the unscented cream base. Use a sanitized utensil to scoop the unscented cream. Stir the essential oil drops into the cream with a sanitized utensil.

Step 3. Add these ingredients to the mixture by stirring completely into the formula. Be sure powdered ingredients are well mixed. The formula may feel grainy, but all ingredients dissolve quickly into the skin.

3 drops (0.15 mL) sea buckthorn CO_2 extract (Use a pipette to drop this viscous CO_2. Most pipettes have measurements in mL.)

0.5 mL d-alpha-tocopherol or mixed vitamin E. (You may use the contents of one or two vitamin E capsules.)

100 mg alpha lipoic acid (R-lipoic acid is preferred). Empty a supplement capsule into the mixture.

1000 mg ascorbyl palmitate (or Ester-C®). Empty a supplement capsule.

Wraps and Masks

Formulations for wraps and masks vary greatly. The essential oil blends can be structured according to skin type, by condition, or to soothe, stimulate, or detoxify. The blends can be applied several ways, such as added to a preexisting mask or wrap or applied to the skin before the mask or wrap formula. Formulation percentages range between 2 and 10 percent, depending on the purpose of the treatment. Your mask/wrap formulation should match the function of your essential oil choices. Several choices would include clay, moor mud, seaweed, and volcanic ash. See Tables 10-2 and 10-3 for specific uses.

Table 10-2 Seaweeds and Their Uses

Main Group	General Group Properties	Subgroups	Properties	Recommended Body Condition and Treatment
Algae (alginates)	Aids in skin firmness, cell renewal, and moisturization			
Clorophyta (green)	Softening, antibacterial, anti-inflammatory	*Lichen moss*		
Cyanophyta (blue-green)	High nutritional group, rich in vitamins A, B, C, E; stimulates cell metabolic rate	*Spirulira*	Rich source of betacarotene, total food source, sugars (moisturizing), antioxidant	Detox, cellulite, softening, and conditioning
Phaeophyta (brown)	Probably the strongest group for blood and metabolic stimulation	*Laminaria digita*	Sugar (moisturizing); vitamins (antioxidants, etc.); provitamins (carotenoids, vitamin D, etc.); minerals (iodine, etc.); antibacterial, metabolic stimulation	More active treatments using heat and stronger stimulation, detox, cellulite, moisturizing and conditioning, revitalizing

Continued

Table 10-2 Seaweeds and Their Uses

Main Group	General Group Properties	Subgroups	Properties	Recommended Body Condition and Treatment
		Fucus Fucus vesibulosus	Similar to *Laminaria digita*	Similar to *Laminaria digita*
Rhodophyta (red)	Contains highly balancing emollient algae	*Chrondrus crispus*	Highly viscous (thick and stabilizing), balancing, emollient (soothing)	Moisturizing and conditioning
		Carageenan	Highly viscous (thick, slippery), emollient (soothing)	Moisturizing and conditioning

Table 10-3 Muds and Clays

Group	Properties	Subgroup	Properties	Use
Kaolinite	Fine powder	China clay		Drawing, tightening, toning
Illite/clorite (sea mud)	High in minerals, magnesium, potassium			
Smectites (volcanic ash)	Rich in minerals. Used to congeal thinner clays; stimulating, vasodilation	Fango mud	High volcanic content; used in Italian hot spring spas	Masks; remineralizing, detoxifying; combine with paraffin for greater benefit. Mud easier to remove when combined with paraffin
Moor (peat) mud	Obtained from bogs rich in decayed plant material, essential oils, minerals			Masks: face, body, hydrotherapy

Hydro-Therapeutic Essential Oil Baths and Salt Glow

Formulation type: 20 to 65 drops of essential oil added to bath or foot soak

Container: Bath, foot basin

Application: Add 20 drops of essential blend to a capful of unscented liquid soap (shampoo), vodka, or whole milk. Swish this mixture into a foot basin and soak feet.

Add 65 drops of essential oil blend to a large capful of unscented liquid soap (shampoo), vodka, or whole milk. Swish mixture into bath.

Foot Formula:

6 drops lemon EO

6 drops bay laurel EO

4 drops MQV EO

4 drops cedarwood EO

Soothing Bath

10 drops neroli EO

15 drops mandarin EO

8 drops ylang-ylang EO

10 drops lavandin EO

5 drops fennel EO

5 drops myrrh EO

6 drops cistus EO

6 drops peru balsam EO

Salts (Dead Sea salt, Great Salt Lake salt, etc.) can be added to the bath or foot water for added benefit.

CHAPTER SUMMARY

The quality of products used in practice and on a daily basis will determine the results. Every ingredient used in a skin formulation has an effect on its overall activity, including contraindications and potential for sensitivity. Because of the interaction of essential oils with product formulation, it is vitally important to be aware of all the ingredients in the formula. Marketing is used to sell ideas and desire and therefore may mislead in identifying the quality or type of ingredients used in various products. A good understanding of the many types of ingredients and of their use in cosmetics, and an ability to identify individual ingredients, will help you in purchasing and using quality ingredients and formulations.

REVIEW QUESTIONS

1. Why does the quality of the ingredients used in skin care matter?
2. Why is it important to know the ingredients used in formulas with essential oils?
3. What is the value of knowing the manufacturing philosophy of a manufactured skin care product?
4. How does marketing affect a natural product?
5. What precautions should you take when using essential oils in pre-made product bases?
6. What is an emulsifier?

CHAPTER REFERENCES

1. Rutledge, M. (2001). *Products of Misinformation*. Irving, TX: Tapestry Press.
2. Carstens, R. (2006, January). "The Dark Side of Beauty." *Alternative Medicine Magazine.*
3. Klimkiewicz, J. (2006, December 6). "Campaigning of Safe Cosmetics, Tougher FDA." *The Hartford Courant.*
4. Rutledge, M. (2001). *Products of Misinformation*. Irving, TX: Tapestry Press.
5. Wikipedia. (2007). *Organic certification*. Retrieved July 30, 2007 from http://www.en.wikipedia.org.
6. Porter, W. P., Jaeger, J. W. & Carlson, I. H. (1999). "Endocrine, immune, and behavioral effects of aldicarb (carbamate), atrazine (triazine), and nitrate (fertilizer) mixtures at groundwater concentrations." *Toxicology and Industrial Health 15* (1–2); 33–150.
7. Answers.com. (2007). Atropine. Retrieved August 6, 2007 from http://www.answers.com.

8. Murray, M. (1996). *Encyclopedia of Nutritional Supplements*. Rocklin, CA: Prima Publishing.
9. Physical & Theoretical Chemistry Laboratory, Oxford University. (2005). "Safety (MSDS) Data for 1,8 Cineole." In *Chemical and Other Safety Information*. Oxford, England.
10. Koh, K. J., Pearce, A. L., Marshman, G., Finlay-Jones, J. J. & Hart, P. H. (2002). "Tea tree reduces histamine-induced skin inflammation." *British Journal of Dermatology 147* (6); 1212–1217.
11. Heinemann, C., Paschold, C., Fluhr, J., Wigger-Alberti, W., Schliemann-Willers, S., Farwanah, H., Raith, K., Neubert, R. & Elsner, P. (2005). "Induction of a hardening phenomenon by repeated application of SLS: Analysis of lipid changes in the stratum corneum." *Acta Dermato-Venereologica 85* (4); 290–295.
12. Rapp, D. (1997). *Is This Your Child's World? How You Can Fix the Schools and Homes That Are making Your Children Sick*. New York, NY: Bantam Books.
13. Lopez, S. (2005, June 8). "Sorry, but we've got really bad chemistry." *Los Angeles Times*. Accessed August 7, 2007 at http://www.breastcancerfund.org/.
14. "Cosmetic Ingredient Review Panel Finds Parabens Safe." (2006, February). *The ICMAD Digest*.
15. Darbre, P. D., Aljarrah, A., Miller, W. R., Coldham, N. G., Sauer, M. J. & Pope G. S. (2004). "Concentrations of parabens in human breast tissue." *Journal of Applied Toxicology 24* (1); 5–13.
16. Cashman, A. L. & Warshaw, E. M. (2005). "Parabens: A review of epidemiology, structure, allergenicity, and hormonal properties." *Dermatitis 16* (2); 57–66.
17. Golden, R., Gandy, J. & Vollmer, G. (2005). "A review of the endocrine activity of parabens and implications for potential risks to human health." *Critical Reviews in Toxicology 35* (5); 435–458.
18. Antczak, S. & Antczak, G. (2001). *Cosmetics Unmasked*. Hammersmith, London: Thorsons.
19. Erikson, K. (2002). *Drop Dead Gorgeous: Protecting Yourself From the Hidden Dangers of Cosmetics*. New York, NY: Contemporary Books.
20. CIR publication: Final Report on the Safety Assessment of Sodium Lauryl Sulfate. *The Journal of the American College of Toxicology*; 1983; 2(7).

21. Rutledge, M. *Products of Misinformation*. Irving, TX: Tapestry Press.
22. Lijinsky, W., Reuber, M.D. & Manning, W. B. (1980). "Potent carcinogenicity of nitrosodiethanolamine in rats." *Nature, 288*(5791); 589–590.
23. National Toxicology Program. (1997, April). "NTP Toxicology and Carcinogenesis Studies of D&C Yellow No. 11" (CAS No. 8003-22-3) in F344/N Rats (Feed Studies). *National Toxicology Program technical report series 463*. Washington, DC.
24. Harrison, J. (2003). *Will the Real Aromatherapy Please Stand Up*. Bellevue, WA: Phytotherapy Institute.
25. US Environmental Protection Agency. (1991).
26. Bridges, B. (2002). "Fragrance: Emerging health and environmental concerns." *Flavour and Fragrance Journal 17* (5); 361–371.
27. Matura, M., Sköld, M., Börje, A., Andersen, K. E., Bruze, M., Frosch, P., Goossens, A., Johansen, J. D., Svedman, C., White, I. R. & Karlberg, A. T. (2005). "Selected oxidized fragrance terpenes are common contact allergens." *Contact Dermatitis 52* (6); 320–328.
28. US Department of Labor Occupational Safety and Health Administration. (2002). *OSHA Fact Sheet: Formaldehyde*. Washington, DC.
29. Erikson, K. (2002). *Drop Dead Gorgeous: Protecting Yourself From the Hidden Dangers of Cosmetics*. New York, NY: Contemporary Books.
30. No author listed. (1997). Final Report on the Safety Assessment of Cetrimonium Chloride, Cetrimonium Bromide, and Steartrimonium Chloride. *International Journal of Toxicology 6*(3); 195–220.
31. Perricone, N. P. (2002). *The Perricone Prescription*. New York, NY: HarperCollins Publishers.
32. Bierhaus, A., Chevion, S., Chevion, M., Hofmann, M., Quehenberger, P., Illmer, T., Luther, T., Berentshtein, E., Tritschler, H., Müller, M., Wahl, P., Ziegler, R. & Nawroth, P.P. (1997). "Advanced glycation end product-induced activation of NF-kappaB is suppressed by alpha-lipoic acid in cultured endothelial cells." *Diabetes 46*(9);1481–1490. Christine Northrup, Inc.
33. English, J. (2005, February). R-Dihydro-Lipoic Acid: The Optimal Form of Lipoic Acid. *Life Extension Magazine*. Accessed August 11, 2007 at http://search.lef.org.

34. Naguib, Y. M. A. (2000). "Antioxidant activities of astaxanthin and related carotenoids." *Journal of Agricultural Food Chemistry 48* (4); 1150–1154.
35. Savouré, N., Briand, G., Amory-Touz, M. C., Combre, A., Maudet, M. & Nicol, M. (1995). "Vitamin A status and metabolism of cutaneous polyamines in the hairless mouse after UV irradiation: Action of beta-carotene and astaxanthin." *International Journal for Vitamin and Nutrition Research 65* (2); 79–86.
36. O'Connor, I. and O'Brien, N. (1998). "Modulation of UVA light-induced oxidative stress by beta-carotene, lutein and astaxanthin in cultured fibroblasts." *J. Dermatol. Sci. 16;* 226–230.
37. Lee, S. J., Bai, S. K., Lee, K. S., Namkoong S., Na H. J., Ha K. S., Han, J. A., Yim, S. V., Chang, K., Kwon, Y. G., Lee, S. K. & Kim, Y. M. (2003). "Astaxanthin inhibits nitric oxide production and inflammatory gene expression by suppressing I(kappa)B kinase-dependent NF-kappaB activation." *Molecules and Cells 16*(1);97–105.
38. Dimpfel, W., Wedekind, W. & Keplinger I. (2003). "Efficacy of dimethylaminoethanol (DMAE) containing vitamin-mineral drug combination on EEG patterns in the presence of different emotional states." *European Journal of Medical Research* 8(5);183–191.
39. Perricone, N. P. (2002). *The Perricone Prescription.* New York, NY: HarperCollins Publishers.
40. Jacob, S., Lawrence, R. & Zucker, M. (1999). *The Miracle of MSM: The Natural Solution to Pain*. New York, NY: G. P. Putnam Press.
41. Jacob, S., Lawrence, R. & Zucker, M. (1999). *The Miracle of MSM: The Natural Solution to Pain*. New York, NY: G. P. Putnam Press.
42. Hoffman, D. (1983, 1990). *The New Holistic Herbal.* Rockport, MA: Element Books.
43. Hoffman, D. (1983, 1990). *The New Holistic Herbal.* Rockport, MA: Element Books.
44. Grieve, M. (1971). *A Modern Herbal*. New York, NY: Dover Publications.
45. Katiyar, S. K. & Elmets, C. A. (2001). "Green tea polyphenolic antioxidants and skin photoprotection." *International Journal of Oncology 18* (6); 1307–1313.
46. Xing, J., Yang, B., Dong, Y., Wang, B., Wang, J. & Kallio, H. P. (2002). "Effects of sea buckthorn (*Hippophae rhamnoides* L.)

seed and pulp oils on experimental models of gastric ulcer in rats." *Fitoterapia 73* (7–8); 644–650.

47. Zeb, A. (2004). "Important therapeutic uses of sea buckthorn: A review." *Journal of Biological Science 4* (5); 687–693.
48. Novell, S. (2003, July 11). "Canada: Sea buckthorn." *Agriculture and Agri-Food Canada Bi-Weekly Bulletin, 16* (13).
49. Ianev, E., Radev, S., Balutsov, M., Klouchek, E. & Popov, A. (1995). "The effect of an extract of sea buckthorn (*Hippophae rhamnoides* L.) on the healing of experimental skin wounds in rats." *Khirurgila* (*Sofiia*) *48* (3); 30–33.
50. Darbre, P. D., Aljarrah, A., Miller, W. R., Coldham, N. G., Sauer, M. J. & Pope G. S. (2004). "Concentrations of parabens in human breast tissue." *Journal of Applied Toxicology 24* (1); 5–13.
51. Lavy, L. & Horton, D. (1995, December). "Arkansas Department of Agronomy." *Arkansas Pesticide News 9.*
52. Friends of the Earth. (2006, September 12). "Use of manufactured nanoparticles in sunscreens, cosmetics and personal care products." Washington, DC.

Essential Oils' Synergistic Relationship with Nutrition, Diet, and Supplements

CHAPTER 11

It's bizarre that the produce manager is more important to my children's health than the pediatrician.

—Meryl Streep

LEARNING OBJECTIVES

1. Discover the holistic and synergistic relationship among essential oils, diet, and a healthy lifestyle.
2. Understand the relationship and effect physical health has on health and vitality of the skin.
3. Learn to work with diet, nutritional and herbal supplements, and lifestyle in conjunction with an aromatherapy practice.

PREVENTION

The purpose of this chapter is to propose methods to prevent systemic imbalance and disease through proper nutrition and a healthy lifestyle. Prevention is the first line of defense against disease and skin disorders. A well-balanced diet, nutritional supplementation, exercise, and relaxation may help to prevent, as well as correct, imbalances in the body and skin. Essential oils can be integrated into a preventative program in conjunction with nutrition and lifestyle.

HEALTHY DIET = HEALTHY BODY

It is an undeniable truth that "You are what you eat." Your cells, and your entire body, are composed of the ingredients that you ingest, including the oxygen you breathe. A healthy diet and lifestyle produces healthy cells and a vital skin condition. A poor diet offers an inadequate source of the building materials and nourishment necessary to keep the body strong and healthy. Nutrient deficiencies are a major cause of imbalance and disease. A proper diet that provides an adequate source of nutrients will result in a well-nourished and smoothly functioning healthy body. This is the simple and obvious reality that we have been taught since childhood.

DIET, ILLNESS, AND ESSENTIAL OILS

The following topics are basic elements of nutritional knowledge pertinent to the use of essential oils. There are links between essential oils and diet, beginning with the obvious limits to the results that can be achieved with essential oils if the body is deprived of the nutrients necessary for it to function properly. If a symptom is directly caused by a nutrient deficiency, it will not go away with an aromatherapy treatment. The outcome will not be positive if essential oils are used to treat symptoms that are directly related to a diet that consists of nutritionally vacant foods or toxic elements.

A high-calorie and processed-food diet challenges the therapeutic activity of essential oils. For a therapist to prescribe essential oils to reduce inflammation while the client is eating an inflammation-producing diet is similar to trying to reduce moisture in a small room while running a dehumidifier *and* a humidifier at the same time. As an aromatherapist, you need to recognize the effects of dietary intake. Basic nutritional knowledge assists you in understanding how food, nutrient deficiency, and eating habits factor into symptoms and disease. A true working knowledge of diet and nutrition information is beyond the scope of this book. This knowledge must be gained through continuing education classes and by using expert sources. Internet search engines, such as Google and Yahoo, are especially useful tools for finding current research on specific nutritional topics.

How You Eat What You Eat

Although the nutritional value of food is important, the way and setting in which it is consumed will also influence nutritional outcome. Eating a meal at lightning speed or under stressful conditions is detrimental to digestion and slows absorption of nutrients.[1] Stress prevents the parasympathetic nervous system (PSNS) from functioning properly. The PSNS slows down certain body systems so that digestion and other functions can take place. The way a person eats should be considered, and adjusted if necessary, for essential oil therapy to be fully effective.

LIFESTYLE AND ESSENTIAL OILS

The influence lifestyle has on overall health is also important and should not be underestimated. A destructive lifestyle becomes a negative force for physical, emotional, and spiritual health. The most relevant lifestyle issues are work, living environment, rest habits, and activity level. Both dietary and lifestyle issues must be addressed before a treatment with essential oils can be successful in addressing the related symptoms. Though essential oils may have little to no effect on the conditions that result from a continuing harsh lifestyle, they can be used to influence a change in behavior patterns that drive lifestyles. This is also true when diet is a lifestyle issue. If diet is the result of negative behavior patterns, it can also be treated with aromatherapy as an emotionally driven lifestyle issue.

PHYSICAL HEALTH AND SKIN HEALTH

Beauty and health are synonymous, and the skin is a barometer of internal health. Nutrients bring health to the skin through their direct influence on other systems or functions of the body, which in turn brings vibrancy and balance to the skin. In terms of holism, two nutritional paths can be taken to promote healthy skin. The direct approach is one in which attention is paid to those nutrients used to treat or maintain skin health; the indirect path focuses on body systems and overall health. Certain skin conditions expose obvious internal disorders, such as the yellow hue of the skin with jaundice. Although the skin is affected, jaundice is not a disease of the skin. It is caused either by obstruction of bile passageways or by disturbance in the functioning of liver cells.[2] The system that needs treatment is the liver or bile ducts, not the skin. Acneic skin is an imbalance of body systems, including the skin. This disruption could be caused by imbalance of the endocrine, nervous, or digestive systems or by some combination of all three systems. Once the imbalance is exposed and treated, the skin will find its natural balance and health, clearing the acneic condition. Acne can be treated directly. But if acne is a symptom of systemic imbalance that is not addressed, the result of treatment will be less than satisfactory.

HOMEOSTASIS

Homeostasis is a feedback mechanism that enables the body to adapt to change. It is the dynamic equilibrium needed to protect the internal environment of the body.[3] Homeostasis is our body's way of maintaining stability in an ever-changing external environment. The body adapts through feedback mechanisms, some of which are maintained by the skin (Table 11-1). Homeostasis allows the body to go through temperature and environmental changes yet maintain a steady state.

SKIN HOMEOSTASIS AND THE HEALTH OF THE BODY

The skin's homeostasis mechanisms communicate with other body systems, including the hypothalamus. This feedback loop can be disrupted, either by external or internal causes.

Table 11-1 Functions of the Skin Involved in Homeostasis[4]

- Protection
  The skin protects us from microorganism and parasitic infection and resists the entry of toxins and harmful chemicals.
- Regulation of body temperature
  Body temperature is regulated by the skin's control of blood flow at the surface and through the evaporation of sweat at its surface.
- Water balance
  The skin assists in homeostatic fluid balance, providing output through the sudoriferous (sweat) glands and controlling evaporation with a healthy lipid barrier.
- Sensory reception
  Millions of nerve endings receive and transmit to keep the body informed of environmental changes.
- Synthesis of vitamin D
  The fat-soluble vitamin D_3 (cholecalciferol) is synthesized in human skin when it is exposed to ultraviolet (UV) B radiation from the sun. It is biologically activated in the liver and is then used to maintain calcium levels in the bones and support normal function of the nervous system.
- Synthesis of hormones
  Hormones produce insulin-like growth factors, steroid and other hormones from diet derived retinoids, and eicosanoids from fatty acids. Hormones also exert biological effects on the skin.

The internal causes can be related to disease, stress, or improper diet and lifestyle. If the body is in a healthy state and adequately supplied with vital nutrients, it generally quickly recovers from imbalances or injuries. Homeostasis of individual skin cells, as with all cells, must be maintained for complete holistic health. A solid nutritional and lifestyle program for health and well being will assist the homeostatic functions of the skin and the cells.

NUTRITIONAL BASICS FOR HEALTH AND VITALITY

Some basic dietary rules are helpful to develop a holistic balance among the body, mind, spirit, and skin. An array of philosophies, scientific theories, and opinions are propounded about diet and nutrition. A review of these perspectives is beyond the scope of this book. The following sections include basic holistic health information and recommendations. Keep in mind that quality is a key qualifier in selecting food, water, and nutritional supplements.

Water (Filtered)

Water is the most important ingredient for a properly functioning body. The amount of water required is determined by many factors that include body size, living environment, and lifestyle. The standard rule is to drink at least eight 8-ounce glasses of water daily (pure water; not tea, soda, etc.). Water is the moisturizer of the skin and the carrier of all soluble nutrients within the body. It also carries toxins and waste products from the tissues. Water is an important daily nutrient. There are holistic practitioners who use water as a medicinal tool with great success.

Making a water choice may seem challenging. Water supplies are a cause of increasing concern. Community tap water is filtered but, in many areas, may still contain impurities, toxins, metals, and microorganisms. Chlorine is often mentioned as a hazardous ingredient of tap water. Chlorine, though it protects against harmful microorganisms, may be a danger to human health, especially to skin health. Chlorine in the water is also thought to disrupt the beneficial flora in the intestines, which are necessary for health. Check your local health department or the EPA website, http://www.epa.gov, to determine the quality of your water supply.

Bottled water may pose risks as well, so consumers must note both the source of water and the bottling practices. Plastics may leach compounds, such as vinyl chloride or phthalates, that are hazardous to health. Filters are another system of achieving and drinking pure, clean water. The effectiveness and quality of the many filters on the market are important issues that need to be carefully considered. Useful Internet resources include consumerresearch.com and consumerreports.com. Highly efficient water filters are available that eliminate some, if not most, of the hazardous elements from water.

Whole, Organic, and Fresh High Quality Foods

An enormous amount of information is available on the subject of a well balanced diet and proper nutrition. The diet philosophy is not as important as the quality of the food that is eaten. Many factors must be considered in determining food quality. We will take some of the basics from leading holistic nutritionists.

- Eat only whole, unprocessed foods. Processed foods are depleted of much of their nutritional value and are not necessarily good for proper digestion and absorption.
- Eat organically grown foods when attainable. Eating organically produced foods is a good way to avoid pesticides or other chemical residues. Organic farming is also the safest and most sensible method of farming for the environment. It prevents soil erosion, protects water supplies, and saves energy.[5] This text's support of organic food is based on the same reasoning that requires the use of pure and authentic essential oils described in Chapter 4. Supporting organic foods includes avoiding GMOs (genetically modified organisms). These are foods grown from seeds that have been genetically modified; for instance, a tomato combined with a gene from a fish. Industrialized chemical farming and the use of GMOs do not have a place in holistic practice.
- Foods should be fresh. Buy fruits, vegetables, meats, and grains as fresh as possible. Some nutrients in fruits and vegetables are diminished as the food is exposed to air. Check the expiration dates on all packaging and throw away any foods that have expired.
- Use sensible cooking procedures. Overcooking foods depletes their nutrient value, and some foods like spinach and dark greens lose their vital enzyme content when heated.

Become knowledgeable and aware of as many factors as possible about food choices and preparation. Good quality, organic, and healthy foods are becoming widely available. Be aware that stores known to sell "health foods" may still carry foods that are not of the best quality for a healthy lifestyle. These foods may contain hydrogenated fats, refined sugars or corn syrup, and nitrate preservatives. Carefully read all ingredient lists on packaged foods and look for information regarding produce, meats, and bulk foods.

Vegetables and Fruits

The nutrients derived from fresh fruits and vegetables are continually praised for numerous health benefits. Variety allows you to take advantage of as many of these nutrients as possible. What you get from vegetables and fruits are antioxidants, chlorophyll, vitamins, minerals, and enzymes, and the benefits derived from these nutrients. You needn't read about the nutritional content and benefit of every vegetable and fruit. Just eat a wide variety, with variations in color that include red, orange, yellow, and dark green vegetables. This strategy will ensure the greatest assortment of beneficial, health giving, and healing nutrients.

Protein

Protein is an important source of building material for the entire body. Your body can manufacture twelve of the twenty amino acids required to grow and function. Whether you are a vegetarian or carnivore, the remaining eight amino acids must come from the diet. The U.S. government sets the Recommended Daily Allowance (RDA) of protein at 0.8 grams per kilogram (2.2 pounds) of body weight.[6] Protein foods can be measured for their biological value, with eggs at 94 percent, fish at 75 to 90 percent, rice at 86 percent, legumes at 70 to 80 percent, and poultry and meat at 75 to 80 percent.[7] Animal products contain complete proteins. It was formerly believed that a completely vegetarian diet was missing amino acids; therefore, it was necessary to combine foods, such as rice with nuts, aduki beans, and soy or other combinations of nuts, seeds, grains, and legumes.[8] Research now demonstrates that this belief is founded on misinformation. A vegetarian diet based on any single one of these unprocessed starches (e.g., rice, corn, potatoes, beans), with the addition of vegetables and fruits, supplies all the protein, amino acids, essential acids, minerals, and vitamins (with the exception of B_{12}) necessary for excellent health.[9]

Protein deficiency leads to various breakdowns and malfunctions of the body. Skin and hair are especially lifeless from a protein-deficient diet. On the other hand, some evidence shows that high levels of protein, mainly animal derived, can lead to detrimental effects caused by a greater demand on the liver and kidneys.[10]

AUTHOR'S **NOTE**

DIET AND HAIR LOSS

I had a client whose hair was brittle and thinning. Her skin was also looking more haggard than should be expected of a 28-year-old woman. Diet is a reasonable first suspect in this condition. She had been a vegetarian for about 12 years. Her diet, from her description, seemed reasonable, though she did ingest some processed carbohydrates and soda. Other factors to consider are stress levels, hormone balance, and bad habits normally attributed to a rock star. She was not stressed, did not have a particularly wild lifestyle and practiced yoga a few times a month.

Six months later, I was noticing that her hair was looking thicker and healthier, and her skin had a youthful vitality fitting her age. I asked what changes she had made. She told me that about four months previously she had had a ravenous craving for a steak. She obliged her desire and had since had meat three to four times per week. Protein deficiency may be related to hair loss,[11] and it is common, though not true, to think that a vegetarian diet lacks sufficient protein. A deficiency of vitamin B_{12} is more likely in a vegetarian diet,[12] but it is not usually related to weakness of the hair or skin.

Obviously, something was missing from my client's diet that meat provided, whether it was protein, B_{12}, or something else. She has blood type O, the meat eater of the *Eat Right for Your Type*,[13] philosophy. Dr. Peter D'Adamo introduced the idea that blood type is an evolutionary marker of what foods are best for you. I've known many fervent type O meat eaters and a few type O vegetarians. Many of the type O vegetarians didn't eat meat for philosophical reasons. I have noticed that some, but not all, still craved meat, and

Continued

a few reverted back to a carnivorous diet. I'm a type O and have no craving or taste for animal proteins beyond salmon and halibut, and these need to be wild caught from the Alaskan waters. There's a certain quality to these fish that suits my fish eating, or pescatarian, ways. The blood type theory doesn't absolutely explain why the change in diet brought my client's skin and hair back to life. It does explain the importance of a healthy and complete diet that includes the needs of the individual.

You'll be limited as a therapist to what you can do with topical treatments if the body requires an element that only diet can provide. I used the best of what I had to offer in skin and hair care, including essential oils, but these external remedies didn't fully satisfy the condition of my client's hair loss and haggard skin. My familiarity with nutrition, diet, and lifestyle gave me the wisdom to know that what I had to offer was not the answer. I let my client know this, and our professional relationship was never compromised. As a beauty therapist, I was not expected to resolve a suspected nutrient deficient condition.

FOOD ALLERGIES

Food allergies may cause imbalances within the body. Food allergies may be detected by an unhealthy appearance of the skin, nails, hair, or eyes. Essential oils may provide some relief from food allergies. They can be effective in two ways: (1) to strengthen the immune system so that sensitivities are decreased and the body is better able to handle allergy-producing foods, or (2) to decrease the symptoms of a food allergy, such as inflammation. It is better to determine which foods are causing reactions and eliminate them from the diet. There are relatively simple tests that determine food allergies. See a naturopath or other health professional knowledgeable in detecting food sensitivity.

NUTRITIONAL SUPPLEMENTATION

Although eating a healthy amount and variety of whole organic foods may provide an adequate diet, it is still reasonable to supplement with nutrients, herbs, and essential fatty acids. Nutrients are in their most usable form when they come from food, so a healthy diet is by far the most effective source of nutrition. In our modern society, getting the necessary and complete amount of nutrients from food isn't always possible. Supplementation is a way to ensure that your body gets everything it needs. In a perfect world, it would not be necessary to supplement the diet. Today's living conditions place increased demands on the body as it is exposed to environmental pollutants and excessive stressors. This added demand justifies the added protection the body receives from supplementation. Nutritional supplements are also used for therapeutic and medicinal purposes.

Nutrient Knowledge for Proper Supplementation

Be sensible, cautious, and knowledgeable in the use of supplements. Realize that all nutrients work together in the body in a holistic manner and that particular combinations are required for certain functions and results. For instance, calcium is a necessary mineral for bone density. But calcium cannot do its job if the necessary cofactors, such as magnesium and vitamin D, are not present.[14] All nutrients work together. For this reason, a whole-food diet that emphasizes variety is the foundation of a healthy body. Supplementing should mimic food as closely as possible to achieve the best results. This is accomplished through vitamins and supplements that combine nutrients in ways that they would appear in foods or as you would receive in a whole food diet. Because of the many variables that occur in nature there is much controversy surrounding the use of supplements as a way to receive nutrients in their proper food-state form and combination.

Absorbing Nutrients

An important issue regarding nutrients is the ability to absorb them. Nutrients from food are in a form the body can assimilate, or absorb. Supplements must also be in an assimilable form to be of value. Much controversy exists over supplements' ability to be absorbed in a usable manner. Assuming that the nutrients are assimilable, there may still be congestion in the digestive tract or other digestive issues that hinder the individual from reaping the benefits of healthy food choices or nutrient supplementation. Digestive support from essential oils, such as peppermint to stimulate digestive processes, can be beneficial in this situation.

HIGH QUALITY MULTIPLE VITAMINS AND MINERALS

Each person has individual nutritional requirements. Nutritional needs vary among male, female, young, old, active, and the stressed. Many vitamin manufacturers are creating products designed for the individual. Whether you can find an individually tailored multiple vitamin and mineral supplement, learn about individual requirements before selecting a brand or product. You may find vitamin and nutrient deficiencies through a hair or blood analysis available through your health practitioner or through the Life Extension Foundation, http://www.lef.org. Your individual needs may be more difficult to determine and may require a long term professional analysis, or period of adding and/or subtracting nutrients and vitamins under professional guidance. When choosing your own supplements pay attention to how many tablets (or capsules) the manufacturer says it takes to get the nutrient amounts printed on the label.

Quality is, as always, of ultimate concern. Many vitamins are prepared using binders or other ingredients that do not break down in the digestive system. High-quality brand vitamins are prepared using ingredients that the body can absorb, break down, and use.

Using a holistic perspective is valuable in selecting multivitamin and mineral supplements. A few companies are now producing supplements made from whole foods or, as in the probiotic method,[15] developed in a manner similar to that in which the nutrients occur naturally in whole foods. Again, food is the best way to ensure proper absorption and use of nutrients. A vitamin that can mimic and provide nutrients close to their natural state in foods is a good choice for supplementation.

NUTRIENT RECOMMENDATIONS

Consulting a qualified "whole food" nutritionist is often a wise step to take to determine optimal nutrient consumption. The following list provides an overview of some important nutrients that are especially supportive of healthy skin. The study of nutrition is constantly growing and shifting as science adds to our understanding of this body of knowledge. This list serves only as a basic guideline and does not include recommended daily amounts. Consult with a professional regarding your daily needs or follow the manufacturer's instructions.

Vitamin A (Retinol, Retinal, Retinoic Acid)

Vitamin A has many functions in the human body. It is well known for its antioxidant action and especially valued for the functions it performs for eyesight. It promotes tissue growth and healing, and it supports the cellular structure of the skin. It is especially helpful for aging skin and for preventing wrinkles, psoriasis,[16] and other skin disorders. Vitamin A supports immune function, including the enhancement of white blood cells. Foods that contain vitamin A are butter, milk, fatty fish like mackerel and salmon, eggs, and foods containing carotenoid compounds, which are described in the next section.

Vitamin A is a fat-soluble vitamin and is stored in the body. Therefore, be cautious when supplementing with a preformed vitamin A, which includes any of the retinoid compounds retinol, retinal, and retinoic acid. Toxicity can occur with high dosages (in excess of 50,000 IU daily over several years) and when vitamin A is taken during pregnancy.[17] These safety issues are nonexistent when vitamin A is taken in the form of carotenoids.

Carotenoids

The carotenoid complexes are a number of individual compounds, each of which has its unique individual properties. All carotenoids share an important function as valuable and powerful antioxidants, making them an important nutrient for healthy aging and protection of the body and skin. Some carotenoids, including beta-carotene and beta-cryptoxanthin,[18] are converted into vitamin A by the body. Foods that are high in carotenoids are colored fruits and vegetables such as carrots (beta carotene), tomatoes (lycopene), and corn (zeaxanthin).

The carotenoid's antioxidant properties function especially well on the skin, protecting the skin against cancer,[19]

UV radiation,[20] and other free radical damage. Astaxanthin, the carotenoid compound found in the Hawaiian algae, was discussed for its UV protection in Chapter 10. Food sources of astaxanthin include wild salmon, shrimp, and lobster, which explains the red color found in these seafoods.[21]

Zeaxanthin and lutein have recently been well documented for their ability to prevent and reverse macular degeneration.[22] The carotenoids in general are extremely useful for preventing many age-related issues and promoting healthier skin.

Vitamin C (L-Ascorbic Acid and Ascorbyl Palmitate)

The antioxidant and immune stimulating effects of vitamin C are very powerful and beneficial for the entire body. Vitamin C fulfills several functions in the body, many of which are important to the skin. Vitamin C assists in collagen production, fortifying the tissues of the body and skin,[23] and works as an important antioxidant, preventing premature aging.[24] Good nutritional sources of vitamin C are vegetables , like broccoli and red peppers, and fruits, such as oranges, kiwis, and strawberries.

Vitamin E

Vitamin E is an antioxidant that protects fatty acids in cell membranes.[25] It also helps regenerate skin cells after injuries or other damaging factors. Topically, it is used to stimulate healthy cell growth and prevent bad scarring.[26] Vitamin E is a must in any anti-aging program. Use vitamin E to revitalize the skin or as protection from a toxic or polluted environment.

The major food sources of vitamin E are nuts, seeds, whole grains, and some fruits and vegetables. Many cosmetic formulas now contain vitamin E. This ingredient has the dual role of therapeutic agent and preservative (because it prevents oxidation). Both natural and synthetic vitamin E formulations are available. Discerning the difference is important, because natural vitamin E is more effective in the human body.[27] Naturally occurring vitamin E is called d-alpha-tocopherol or sometimes just d-tocopherol. The synthetic version is dl-alpha-tocopherol or tocopherol acetate. There are four forms of tocopherol that exist, alpha-, beta-, delta-, and gamma. A good supplement would contain a complex of all four forms of vitamin E, d-alpha-tocopherol, d-beta-tocopherol, d-delta-tocopherol, and d-gamma-tocopherol.

To complete the vitamin E picture, there is another group of vitamin compounds identified as tocotrienols. These compounds are even stronger antioxidants than the tocopherols and have their own specific functions. Tocotrienols also occur as alpha-, beta-, delta-, and gamma. D-alpha-tocotrienol possesses 40–60 times more antioxidant protection than d-alpha-tocopherol.[28] The most complete vitamin E supplement would include all eight tocopherol and tocotrienol compounds.

Essential Fatty Acids (EFAs)

Essential fatty acids are fats that are required for their many health- and skin-nourishing benefits. These fatty acids are called *essential* because they are not manufactured by the body and therefore must be included in the diet. Two major groups of essential fatty acids exist: omega-3 and omega-6. Omega-3 fatty acids, like eicosapentaenoic acid (EPA) and docosahexaenoic acid (DHA), are found in seaweed and fatty fish like salmon, herring, and mackerel. Their main properties include supporting cellular membrane function protecting the cardiovascular system;[29] they also act as anti-inflammatory agents.[30] EFAs are an especially important nutrient to support the myelin sheath, the cellular membrane of the central nervous system and the parasympathetic nervous system.[31,32] Research has demonstrated that a diet rich in EFAs is essential for brain function and development.[33]

Omega-6 fatty acids, specifically gamma-linoleic acid (GLA), is found in cold-pressed vegetable oils such as borage, evening primrose, and sunflower seed oils. Omega-6 fatty acids have a special role in skin care. GLA has a calming effect on skin cells. It is an anti-inflammatory and prevents redness and dryness of the skin.[34] A diet rich in essential fatty acids works synergistically with topical use of oils that contain fatty acids. Refer to Chapter 9 for more information on those carrier oils that contain essential fatty acids.

MSM (Methylsulfonylmethane)

MSM is a sulfur-containing compound essential to many functions of the body. MSM is a supplement that helps correct inflammation and pain.[35] MSM is important in collagen health and helps normalize cross-linking, and over time diminishes scarring.[36] MSM-containing food sources include eggs, broccoli, cabbages, onions, garlic, and fish.

Probiotics

Probiotics are supplements that contain beneficial bacteria that normally live in our body. These bacteria (*Lactobacillus acidophilus, Bifidobacterium bifidum,* and others) reside in places of the body that come into contact with the outer world, e.g., on the skin and in the digestive tract. The main function of these "good" bacteria is to create a barrier to protect the body from harmful influences from the outside, especially infectious microorganisms. Yeast infections or candidiasis commonly result from a lack of these protective bacteria.

The friendly bacteria residing in the digestive tract are called *intestinal flora*. Other functions of the intestinal flora include aiding the process of digestion and synthesis of vitamin K. The bacteria of the colon also manufacture vitamin B_{12}, though there may not be enough of this vitamin produced by the bacteria for useful absorption, a concern for vegetarians who have a limited source of this nutrient and may be depending on probiotic production.[37] Use of antibiotics[38] or other medicines, stress, poor diet, and lack of exercise put a strain on the friendly flora, which weakens this immune barrier of the body. A deficiency of intestinal flora can easily result in health problems, such as gastro-intestinal (GI) trouble and skin diseases such as acne and atopic dermatitis.[39] Use a probiotic product regularly, particularly if diarrhea or constipation is a problem. Probiotics are highly recommended after using antibiotics, when general health is poor, when the diet is high in sugar or refined carbohydrates, and where water sources contain chlorine. Fiber content in foods provides a healthy environment for friendly bacteria.

Avoid using antibacterial soaps on the skin. The layer of bacteria on the skin provides protection against infections.[40] Antibacterial soaps destroy these beneficial bacteria and increase pathogenic bacteria's resistance to antimicrobial agents.[41] Essential oils may be used topically to prevent and eliminate pathogenic infection. Tea tree oil has demonstrated safe and effective results in topical elimination of harmful bacteria and fungus.[42,43] The action of essential oils does not harm beneficial bacteria.

ANTIOXIDANTS

Antioxidants are used to prevent free radical damage. Free radicals have been popularly associated with disease and aging. Free radicals may play an important role in healing injuries[44] and occur as a natural phenomenon of metabolism. The trouble begins when too many free radicals are present or when free radicals are in the wrong place. They are related to many illnesses, such as cancer and cardiovascular disease.[45] Free radicals can cause intracellular functional disorders related to the aging of the body.[46] As mentioned in Chapter 3, the body produces enzymes as free radical scavengers. The production of these enzymes depends on many nutrients, especially iron, manganese, copper, and zinc.

Valid studies on antioxidants such as beta-carotene,[47] vitamin E, and alpha-lipoic acid[48] document their effectiveness when they are used topically. Results show that these compounds prevent excessive aging of the skin and sun damage.

Supplemental Antioxidants

Supplemental antioxidants prevent an excess of free radicals and protect skin and body from age-related damage.[49] Vitamins A, C, and E provide supplemental antioxidant protection. Other supplements valued for their antioxidant properties are alpha-lipoic acid, co-enzyme Q10, and proanthocyanidins.

- Alpha-lipoic acid
  This is a very powerful antioxidant and anti-inflammatory[50] nutrient. Alpha-lipoic acid is part of an enzyme complex within the cell and is responsible for energy production. It is both water and fat soluble and so protects both the aqueous cell compartment and the lipid membrane. Supplementation with alpha lipoic acid is extremely beneficial for preventing premature aging and age-related systemic damage[51] and is used to prevent and reverse diabetic neuropathy.[52,53]

  An important feature of alpha lipoic acid is in its ability to protect from glycation,[54] a process in which sugars break down proteins within the body. Glycation is generally caused by high-glycemic carbohydrate diets and large amounts of sugar (glucose or fructose) in the bloodstream. Glycation causes aging damage to all protein body systems, including cross-linking of collagen and wrinkles of the skin.[55] Skin aging is slowed and damage reversed by the combination of anti-glycation, antioxidant, and anti-inflammatory activities of alpha lipoic acid. Alpha lipoic acid is effectively absorbed and used by the cells, both when used internally[56] and with topical application.[57]

- Coenzyme Q10
  Coenzyme Q10 (CoQ10) is made naturally in the body and supports energy production. It acts as an antioxidant and anti-inflammatory[58] and has the ability to stimulate the immune system. Coenzyme Q10 is a cancer preventive and protects the body from cardiovascular disease and diabetes. It is suggested for use as a supplement to prevent age related damage.[59]
- Proanthocyanidins (PCO; proanthocyanidin oligomers)
  This group of compounds is found in many foods, such as blueberries, pomegranates, and green tea and provides a rich source of antioxidants. Their action includes cancer prevention and reducing cardiovascular disease. Studies have shown that PCO compounds increase longevity[60] and provide anti-aging capabilities.[61] Topical use in cosmetics is supplied by ingredients such as grape skins, cocoa, green tea, and many fruits.

HERBAL SUPPLEMENTS

Many herbs can be taken as supplements for specific conditions that may affect health and beauty. Some herbs act as tonics, strengthening the entire body or specific organs. The following herbs are a few that are recommended for overall health. The common application methods for herbal supplementation are teas, capsules, and tinctures, usually as an alcohol or glycerine extract. Follow the manufacture's dosage instructions when taking herbs unless otherwise directed by an herbal nutritional practitioner.

Echinacea (Echinacea angustifolia)

Echinacea is a common remedy for colds, flu, and allergies because of its strong antimicrobial actions. It is an often overused herb and for our purpose is recommended for use only when protection from bacterial or viral infection is necessary, such as seasonal susceptibility to colds and flu, or to strengthen a weakened immunity. It combines well with many other herbs[62] and essential oils for overall protection and healing of the body and skin.

Ginseng (*Panax ginseng*)

Ginseng is a well-known herbal tonic and is recommended to increase strength and vitality.[63] Ginseng has been used in China for centuries. The Chinese believe ginseng is the herb of eternal youth.

Milk Thistle (*Silybum marianum*)

Milk thistle herb is used to support the function of the liver.[64] It assists in the formation of new liver cells and helps the liver eliminate toxins that pass through that organ. When the liver is overworked, the skin can lose its vitality and will look sickly and pallid. Milk thistle can play an important role in overcoming health problems and some skin diseases[65] such as psoriasis, which may benefit by liver support.

EMOTIONAL, SPIRITUAL, AND PHILOSOPHICAL HEALTH

Emotional, philosophical, and spiritual balances are important factors in overall health.[66] Poor emotional health has a detrimental effect on the nervous, cardiovascular, and digestive systems and on the skin. These effects in turn have synergistic damaging effects on the entire body. Stress is an established marker of compromised health and disease.[67] Skin sensitivities, blotchiness, psoriasis, hair loss, and similar conditions are all symptoms of stress and other forms of poor emotional health.[68] Stress is known to elevate blood levels of **cortisol**, a hormone responsible for maintaining stability during the "fight or flight" response of the body. Cortisol is believed to create inflammation and is attributed to causing fat storage, hypertension, and accelerated aging.[69]

Emotional balance is influenced by spiritual and philosophical health, which is much harder to define and describe in relation to the health of the body. According to many spiritual teachers and philosophers, a positive philosophy and spiritual outlook help to overcome emotional instability and a victim consciousness. Victim consciousness develops from a mindset that attributes to others, or to society, all the bad or negative things that happen to the individual. Self-empowerment was introduced in Chapter 1 as a way to overcome victim consciousness. Fear is factored into victim consciousness and, in relation to health, is especially apparent in Western society's fear-based approach to aging, disease, and death.[70] The fear, or victimization, of disease and death are said by many mind-body philosophers to create these very things. The result of a victim consciousness is poor health and compromised beauty.

LIFESTYLE

Negative lifestyle factors generally create an emotional, spiritual, or physical imbalance. Some lifestyle issues that affect health and beauty are work, rest, play, environment, and exercise.

Work

A stressful work environment relates to the issues of emotional health. Negative feelings about a job may translate into negative feelings about the self and may compromise health. Could this possibly be the reason why most heart attacks occur on Monday mornings?[71,72] Work habits affect and influence health also. Even if a person loves his or her job, overwork creates a situation that often leads to physical and emotional stress.

Environmental conditions are also a consideration of work-related health. This category includes chemical toxins used at work and office environments that may be engorged with microorganisms and airborne toxins because of poor ventilation.

Rest

Rest or downtime is necessary to give the body and mind time to heal, to cleanse and relax from life's high demands. Adequate sleep has many healthful influences on the body and mind and is important to achieve health, well-being, and beauty.

Play

Play is also a lifestyle factor that has an indirect influence on health and beauty. Play is activity that helps release tension and stress from the body and mind. Play should be fun and also emotionally and spiritually fulfilling.

Environment

The environment that a person lives within has varied effects on health. Where you live can be an unknown cause of imbalance. Be aware of as many environmental factors as possible. Toxins, molds, pollens, and many other environmental considerations should be observed for their effect on health and beauty. The harmony between you and the area in which you live is also of importance. It is healthful to understand and accept who you are in relation to the area in which you live. For instance, if you are a politically liberal person who lives in a highly conservative area, you may experience stress even if the situation is not fully apparent to you. Stress may also be related to the geographical environment. Some people find the clamor and congestion of city life comfortable, while others are stressed from the constant noise and pace of the city.

Exercise

Exercise improves cardiovascular function, respiration, digestion, muscle tone, bone strength, and lymphatic drainage. A fit body is a healthy and beautiful body. Exercise has an effect on spiritual and emotional balance that should not be underestimated. This effect is apparent in the dual spiritual and physical strengthening role of yoga and tai chi.

Exercise does not have to be strenuous. Walking is considered one of the better forms of exercise. Strenuous exercise may in fact be a detriment to health. With a "work hard, play hard" mentality, stress may result from both work and exercise. Over-doing exercise could result in systemic inflammation.[73] When weight training, it is also important to focus on flexibility, using either yoga or stretching exercises.

CHAPTER SUMMARY

A holistic and synergistic relationship exists among essential oils, diet, and a healthy lifestyle. Acquiring knowledge about a healthy diet and supplementation will bring increased value to the use of essential oils in aromatherapy. This chapter reviews many of the factors that contribute to a healthy diet and body. Nutritional supplements, including vitamins, antioxidants, and herbs can be used to bring balance to body systems and prevent damage caused by aging and, in turn, bring vibrancy and health to the skin. The direct link that emotions, lifestyle, and exercise have to overall health is included as part of a holistic health model.

REVIEW QUESTIONS

1. What are some of the benefits of a healthy diet?
2. What is the first line of defense against disease and skin disorders?
3. What is homeostasis?
4. What should you consider when choosing foods for a healthy diet?
5. What benefits are achieved by supplementing the diet with carotenoids? Essential fatty acids? Alpha-lipoic acid?
6. How does emotional health affect the health of the body and the skin?

CHAPTER REFERENCES

1. Haas, E. (1992). *Staying Healthy With Nutrition.* Berkeley, CA: Celestial Arts.
2. Venes, D. (Ed.) (1997). *Tabor's Cyclopedic Medical Dictionary* (18th edition). Philadelphia, PA: F. A. Davis Company.
3. Murray, M. (1996). *Encyclopedia of Nutritional Supplements.* Rocklin, CA: Prima Publishing.
4. Farabee, M. J. (2001). *The Integumentary System.* Accessed on August 11, 2007 at http://www.emc.maricopa.edu.
5. 11 Reasons Why You Should Eat Organic Food. (2005). The Organic Grocer Int. Pty. Ltd. Accessed on August 11, 2007 at http://www.theorganicgrocer.com.au.

6. U.S. Department of Agriculture, Agricultural Research Service. (2005). *USDA Nutrient Database for Standard Reference, Release 18.* Nutrient Data Laboratory Home Page. Accessed on August 11, 2007 at http://www.nal.usda.gov.
7. Haas, E. (1992). *Staying Healthy With Nutrition.* Berkeley, CA: Celestial Arts.
8. Haas, E. (1992). *Staying Healthy With Nutrition.* Berkeley, CA: Celestial Arts.
9. McDougall, J. (2002). "Plant foods have a complete amino acid composition." *Journal American Heart Association, 105* (25); 197.
10. Strychar, I. (2006). "Diet in the management of weight loss." *Canadian Medical Association Journal 174* (1); 56–63.
11. Pitchford, P. (2002). *Healing with Whole Foods: Asian Traditions and Modern Nutrition.* Berkeley, CA: North Atlantic Books.
12. Pitchford, P. (2002). *Healing with Whole Foods: Asian Traditions and Modern Nutrition.* Berkeley, CA: North Atlantic Books.
13. D'Adamo, P. J. & Whitney, C. (1993). *Eat Right for Your Type.* New York, NY: Putnam.
14. Haas, E. (1992). *Staying Healthy With Nutrition.* Berkeley, CA: Celestial Arts.
15. Saranat, R., Schulick, P. & Newmark, T. (2002). *The Life Bridge: The Way to Longevity With Probiotic Nutrients.* Brattleboro, VT: Herbal Free Press.
16. Brzezinska-Wcislo, L., Pierzchala, E., Kaminska-Budzinska, G., Bergler-Czop, B. & Trzmiel, D. (2004). "The use of retinoids in dermatology." *Wiadomosci Lekarskie 57* (1–2); 63–69.
17. Murray, M. (1996). *Encyclopedia of Nutritional Supplements.* Rocklin, CA: Prima Publishing.
18. Nidus Information Services, Inc. (2001). *Vitamins, Carotenoids, and Phytochemicals.* Accessed on August 11, 2007 at http://www.well-connected.com.
19. Mindell, E. (2002). *Natural Remedies for 101 Ailments.* North Bergen, NJ: Basic Health Publications.
20. Darwin, M., Schanzer, S., Teichmann, A., Blume-Peytavi, U., Sterry, W. & Lademann, J. (2006). "Functional food and bioavailability in target organ skin." *Der Hautarzt 57* (4); 288–290.
21. Astaxanthin: Biochemical Properties. (2002). *Mera Pharmaceuticals, Inc.* Accessed on August 11, 2007 at http://www.astaxanthin.org.

22. Torrey, G. (2006). *Zeaxanthin may decrease your risk of macular degeneration.* American Macular Degeneration Foundation. Accessed on August 11, 2007 at http://www.macular.org.
23. Murray, M. (1996). *Encyclopedia of Nutritional Supplements.* Rocklin, CA: Prima Publishing.
24. Perricone, N. P. (2002). *The Perricone Prescription.* New York, NY: HarperCollins Publishers.
25. Null, G. (1999). *Gary Null's Ultimate Anti-Aging Program.* New York, NY: Broadway Books.
26. Milchak, L. M. & Douglas, Bricker J. (2002). "The effects of glutathione and vitamin E on iron toxicity in isolated rat hepatocytes." *Toxicology Letters 126* (3):169–177.
27. Murray, M. (1996). *Encyclopedia of Nutritional Supplements.* Rocklin, CA: Prima Publishing.
28. Sen, C. K., Khanna, S. & Roy, S. (2006). "Tocotrienols: Vitamin E beyond tocopherols." *Life Sciences 78* (18): 2088.
29. Life Extension Foundation. (2006, January 21). *Life Extension Update.* "Fish and Omega 3's: Sometimes More is More." Life Extension Foundation. Accessed on August 11, 2007 at http://www.lef.org.
30. Davis, B. (2002). *Essential fatty acids in vegetarian nutrition.* Andrews University Nutrition Department. Accessed on August 11, 2007 at http://www.andrews.edu.
31. Venes, D. (ed.) (1997). *Tabor's Cyclopedic Medical Dictionary* (18th edition). Philadelphia, PA: F. A. Davis Company.
32. Salvati, S., Attorri, L., Avellino, C., Di Biase, A. & Sanchez, M. (2000). "Diet, lipids and brain development." *Developmental Neuroscience 22* (5–6); 481–487.
33. Yehuda, S., Rabinovitz, S. & Mostofsky, D. I. (2005). "Essential fatty acids and the brain: From infancy to aging." *Neurobiology of Aging 26* (Suppl 1); 98–102.
34. Klimaszewski, A. (1999). *Ditch the Itch! Borage Oil, Containing GLA, Relieves the Symptoms of Eczema, Including Itching, Redness, and Oozing.* Bioriginal Publishing. Accessed on August 11, 2007 at http://www.fatsforhealth.com.
35. Jacob, S. & Appleton, J. (2003). *MSM: The Definitive Guide.* Topanga, CA: Freedom Press.
36. Jacob, S., Lawrence, R. & Zucker, M. (1999). *The Miracle of MSM: The Natural Solution for Pain.* New York, NY: Penguin Putnam Inc.

37. Pitchford, P. (2002). *Healing with Whole Foods: Asian Traditions and Modern Nutrition.* Berkeley, CA: North Atlantic Books.
38. Schmidt, M., Smith, L. & Sehnert, K. (1994). *Beyond Antibiotics: 50 (or so) Ways to Boost Immunity and Avoid Antibiotics.* Berkeley, CA: North Atlantic Books.
39. Meletis, C. & Barker, J. (2003, May). "Skin health, eczema, and prevention strategies." *The Townsend Letter for Doctors and Patients 238.* 56–58.
40. Todar, K. (2002). *The Bacterial Flora of Humans.* University of Wisconsin-Madison Department of Biology. Accessed on August 11, 2007 at http://www.textbookofbacteriology.net.
41. Doolitte, M. (2000). *Antibacterial Soap: Common Cold Killer or Dangerous Fad?* Accessed on August 11, 2007 at http://www.colorado.edu.
42. Wilkinson, J. M. & Cavanaugh, H. M. (2005). "Antibacterial activity of essential oils from Australian native plants." *Phytotherapy Research 19* (7); 643–646.
43. Halcon, L. & Milkus, K. (2004). "*Staphylococcus aureus* and wounds: A review of tea tree oil as a promising antimicrobial." *American Journal of Infection Control 32* (7); 402–408.
44. Venes, D. (ed.) (1997). *Tabor's Cyclopedic Medical Dictionary* (18th edition). Philadelphia, PA: F. A. Davis Company.
45. Floyd, R. A. (1990). "Role of oxygen free radicals in carcinogenesis and brain ischemia." *FASEB J 4 9*; 2587–2597.
46. Zs-Nagy, I. (2002). "Pharmacological interventions against aging through the cell plasma membrane: A review of the experimental results obtained in animals and humans." *Annals of the New York Academy of Sciences 959*; 308–320.
47. Idson, B. (1993). "Vitamins and The Skin (Vitamins in Cosmetics)." *Cosmetics and Toiletries 108* (12); 179.
48. Perricone, N. P. (2002). *The Perricone Prescription.* New York, NY: HarperCollins Publishers.
49. Miquel, J. (2002). "Can antioxidant diet supplementation protect against age related mitochondrial damage?" *Annals of New York Academy of Sciences 959*; 508–516.
50. Ha, H., Lee, J. H., Kim, H. N., Kim, H. M., Kwak, H. B., Le, S., Kim, H. H. & Lee, Z. H. (2006). "Alpha lipoic acid inhibits inflammatory bone resorption by suppressing prostaglandin E2 synthethis." *Journal of Immunology 176* (1); 111–117.

51. Savitha, S. Tamilselvan, J., Anusuyadevi, M. & Panneerselvam, C. (2005). "Oxidative stress on mitochondrial antioxidant defense system in the aging process: Role of DL-alpha-lipoic acid and L-carnitine." *Clinica Chimica Acta: International Journal of Clinical Chemistry 355* (1–2); 173–180.
52. Ziegler, D. (2004). "Thiotic acid for patients with symptomatic diabetic polyneuropathy: A critical review." *Treatments in Endocrinology 3* (3); 173–189.
53. Malinska, D. & Winiarska, K. (2005). "Lipoic acid: Characteristics and therapeutic application." *Postepy Higieny I Medycyny Doswiadczalnej (Online) 59;* 535–543.
54. Thirunavukkarasu, V., Anitha Nandhini, A. T. & Anuradha, C. V. (2005). "Lipoic acid improves utilisation and prevents protein glycation and AGE formation." *Die Pharmazie 60* (10); 772–775.
55. Perricone, N. P. (2002). *The Perricone Prescription.* New York, NY: HarperCollins Publishers.
56. Malinska, D. & Winiarska, K. (2005). "Lipoic acid: Characteristics and therapeutic application." *Postepy Higieny I Medycyny Doswiadczalnej (Online) 59*; 535–543.
57. Podda, M., Rallis, M., Traber, M. G., Packer, L. & Mailbach, H. I. (1996). "Kinetic study of cutaneous and subcutaneous distribution following topical application of [7,8–14C]rac-alpha-lipoic acid onto hairless mice." *Biochemical Pharmacology 52* (4); 627–633.
58. Bauerova, K., Kucharska, L., Mihalova, D., Navarova, J., Gvozdjakova, A. & Sumbalova, Z. (2005). "Effect of coenzyme Q(10) supplementation in the rat model of adjuvant arthritis." *Biomedical papers of the Medical Faculty of the University Palacky, Olomouc, Czechoslovakia 149* (2); 501–503.
59. Dhanasekaran, M. & Ren, J. (2005). "The emerging role of coenzyme Q-10 in aging, neurodegeneration, cardiovascular disease, cancer, and diabetes mellitus." *Current Neurovascular Research 2* (5); 447–459.
60. Wilson, M. A., Shukitt-Hale, B., Kalt, W., Ingram, D. K., Joseph, J. A. & Wolkow, C. A. (2006). "Blueberry polyphenols increase lifespan and thermotolerance in *Caenorhabditis elegans.*" *Aging Cell 5* (10); 59–68.

61. Sangeetha, P., Balu, M., Haripriya, D. & Panneerselvam, C. (2005). "Age related changes in erythrocyte membrane surface charge: Modulatory role of grape seed proanthocyanidins." *Experimental Gerontology 40* (10); 820–828.
62. Hoffman, D. (1990). *The New Holistic Herbal.* Rockport, MA: Element Books.
63. Hoffman, D. (1990). *The New Holistic Herbal.* Rockport, MA: Element Books.
64. Green, J. (2000). *The Herbal Medicine-Makers Handbook: A Home Manual.* Berkeley, CA: The Crossing Press.
65. Jacknin, J. (2001). *Smart Medicine for Your Skin.* New York, NY: Penguin Putnam Inc.
66. Weil, A. (1995). *Spontaneous Healing.* New York, NY: Alfred A. Knopf.
67. Pert, C. (1999). *Molecules of Emotion.* New York, NY: Touchstone.
68. Choi, E. H., Brown, B. E., Crumrine, D., Chang, S., Man, M. Q., Elias, P. M. & Feingold, K. R. (2005). "Mechanisms by which psychologic stress alters cutaneous permeability barrier homeostasis and stratum corneum integrity." *Journal of Investigative Dermatology 124* (3); 587–595.
69. Miller, G. E., Ritchey, A. K. & Cohen, S. (2002). "Chronic psychological stress and the reduction of pro-inflammatory cytokines: A glucocorticoid-resistance model." *Health Psychology 21* (6); 531–541.
70. Harrison, J. (2001). *The Essentials for Beauty and Skin: A Practice and Philosophy in Pursuit of Inner and Outer Beauty.* Bellevue, WA: Phytotherapy Institute.
71. Murakami, S., Otsuka, K., Kubo, Y., Shinagawa, M., Yamanaka, T., Ohkawa, S. & Kitaura, Y. (2004). "Repeated ambulatory monitoring reveals a Monday morning surge in blood pressure in a community-dwelling population." *American Journal of Hypertension 17* (12 Pt); 1179–1183.
72. Friedman, E. H. (1994). "Morning and Monday critical period for the onset of AMI." *European Heart Journal 15* (12); 1727.
73. Mastorakos, G., Pavlatou, M., Diamanti-Kandarakis, M. & Chrousos, G. P. (2005). "Exercise and the stress system." *Hormones (Athens) 4* (2); 73–89.

The Holistic Consultation and Aromatherapy Treatment

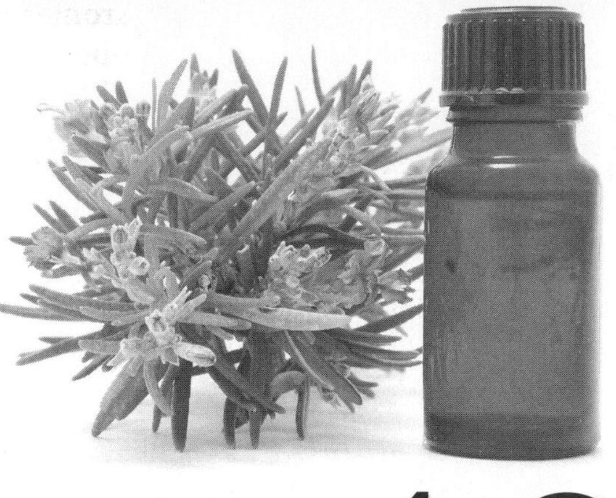

CHAPTER 12

It is more important to know what sort of person has a disease than to know what sort of disease a person has.

–Hippocrates

LEARNING OBJECTIVES

1. Create a thorough and in-depth consultation form.
2. Learn unique and powerful analysis of consultation data.
3. Organize your essential oil knowledge base into a holistic client consultation and treatment plan.
4. Carry conclusions of analysis into an essential oil treatment.

HOLISTIC CLIENT EVALUATIONS

Each chapter of this book offers a distinct feature of aromatherapy. Reading and understanding the information provides a solid foundation of essential oil knowledge and a starting point for developing a therapeutic practice using essential oils. This chapter covers evaluating the client to determine the therapeutic focus of your aromatherapy formulation and application. This is where you put all of the information you have learned so far into practical use.

If you are a practitioner or clinician, you have already learned or developed from experience a suitable method for consultation and analysis. Specific areas of concern that relate to your profession must be covered in a consultation. For example, an esthetician is interested in the features of the skin and therefore asks questions about skin type and sensitivities. Body therapists extract information about pain and physical discomfort in their consultations. The more holistic your practice, the more the boundaries between specific professional consultations dissolve. A massage therapist will want to know about skin condition, and the esthetician will ask questions regarding pain. Naturopaths, by the nature of their practice, are already attuned to the diversity of holistic consultation procedures. These dissolving boundaries do not mean that therapists will consult or perform services beyond their professional expertise. The holistic consultation accepts all information as a tool to better understand conditions that may influence symptoms or conditions that are the focus of the practice.

CONSULTATION IS AN ADDED SERVICE

A thorough, holistic client consultation takes time. This is an added service to your practice and should be viewed accordingly. You can approach a consultation in several ways. For a first visit, the client may fill out a form, which you briefly review and discuss, along with the reason for the visit. You then go on to perform expected services. This type of consultation may be a 15-minute block of time already included in the fee for your service. From this starting point, a more detailed consultation is conducted during the service. When appropriate, note further information regarding the client and potential influential factors. In any clinician-client relationship, consultation is ongoing and may be accomplished casually. No matter what the consultation procedure, all pertinent facts are recorded in the client's file.

If a formal and lengthy consultation is performed during the first or succeeding visits, you and the client need to be clear about compensation for the visit. An hour of consultation time is adequate in most cases. Your client should be educated about the benefits derived from the consultation and informed that an additional hourly charge is charged for a consultation that exceeds the time limit that may already be included in the fee for the requested services. An in-depth and holistic consultation is an important element of a successful clinical service and should be regarded as such. As a professional, you must consider your consultation skills as valuable as your treatment skills.

THE CONSULTATION FORM

The consultation form is a starting point for most therapists and clinicians. A generic, yet very detailed, example is used in this chapter to demonstrate one method that accommodates a thorough and holistic aromatherapy consultation. Your consultation form may be longer or shorter. A consultation also includes visual observations, such as body posture, eye contact, and general appearance (clothing, hair, etc.). There is no right way to perform a consultation. The results achieved from your practice are what matter. Some practitioners are intuitively intense and are able to diagnose or recommend procedures without any conversation or consultation at all. If it works, then it is an appropriate method.

AUTHOR'S **NOTE**

THE EVOLUTION OF A CONSULTATION

I gradually cultivated my method of consultation through years of beauty practice and teaching in esthetic and massage schools. Like everyone, I began with the common protocol, extracting the most basic information. This basic consultation is chiefly designed to keep you out of trouble. You need to

Continued

know about any allergies, sensitivities, medications, disease history, and a few other things that help to avoid application or treatment contraindications. This protocol is a good idea and is information that's included on my form. A typical consultation will also include pertinent facts related to the service and will determine what is expected of the service by asking questions that guide you to the client's anticipated outcome.

I have created a form much larger in scope, possibly too extensive for some practitioners. I arrived at this form following years of studying skin, hair, physiology, biology, essential oils, herbs, massage, nutrition, and an assortment of alternative health and healing practices. The goal of beauty is a goal of health. The consultation form must reflect this. No matter what your knowledge base or practice, the information included on a thorough consultation form can be used. I have repeated this point in so many ways throughout this book. It's a holistic methodology.

It would appear that the information extracted cannot be used by non-medical practitioners. What would you, as an esthetician, have done if your client came to you knowing she had a gum infection that was causing a rash, like the woman described in Chapter 1, who had a leg rash? The rash is on the skin, your area of expertise. The cause is a gum disease, which is not in your treatment jurisdiction.

My intent is to connect with what I can't treat as much as it is to know what I can. It is not my place to treat a gum infection. I did the best for this woman by relieving, temporarily, the symptom of the gum infection: her rash. Had the client informed me that she had a gum related disease, I may have asked, "Have you seen a dentist?"

ANALYZING A CLIENT CONSULTATION FORM

The following sample questionnaire provides a thorough and in-depth analysis.[1] A brief explanation follows many of the questions included on this form. These explanations are included to assist you in finding a deeper awareness from the client's answers. Essential oil recommendations are included to help you incorporate an aromatherapy association to the consultation.

The questions are generic and not specific to the service you are providing. The questions are designed to stimulate communication that will contribute to an accurate holistic consultation and treatment. The most important results from this questionnaire may not be in the written answers but in the dialogue that follows. The data you acquire will assist you in developing essential oil formulations.

Part One: Personal Information

The consultation form generally begins with basic personal information. As basic as it may appear, it contains facts that may provide direction for therapeutic focus or treatment.

1. Date
2. Name

   A person's name does not generally trigger any value in treatment focus. A name may say a lot about a person, however. Does a "common" name produce a common person? Does an unusual name develop a creative or quirky personality?[2] A numerologist, one who studies the esoteric effects of numbers, would extract more than just letters from the name to develop a personality overview similar to astrology. Names also affect how others perceive a person.[3]

3. Street Address
4. City/State/ZIP

   An address has the potential to be a hidden source of physical, emotional, or psychological stress.[4] Certain locations are associated with environmental concerns, such as living near industry known to emit pollutants, living near power lines, and other living situations that may trigger disease or imbalance in the body. These same conditions can also create emotional problems that may manifest physically.[5]

   An issue concerning address that may be overlooked is the effect of social environment. Neighborhoods, communities, cities, states, and countries have personalities; they have conditions that all are expected to live by. Neighborhoods may also reflect social values. If a person lives in an area that does not harmonize with her beliefs, living style, or social attitudes, the situation could provoke stress, anxiety, self-esteem issues, or other emotionally challenging matters.[6] A conservative person living in a liberal area may feel isolated. If the person is aware of conflicts that involve social, political, or spiritual beliefs, acknowledging and accepting the contrasts may lead to healthy acceptance of the situation. If the person is not aware of how conflict may affect mental and physical health, the situation may result in a stress-related disease.

Another area of distress may be that the locale does not fit the person's personality, as with a "city girl" who is living on a country farm. The personal questions portion of this consultation form includes a question asking how the client "feels" about where she lives. The answer to this question may lead you to ask other questions about how the living environment affects the client.

Essential oil choices may be made based on your analysis. If the environment is physically toxic or challenging to the immune system, an essential oil such as MQV may be selected to support the immune system, or bay laurel to support lymphatic drainage and detoxification. If social issues are involved, you need more information to formulate or recommend essential oils precisely. Jasmine is often recommended for self-esteem problems. Ester oils, such as lavender and clary sage, are appropriate when stress or anxiety is present.

5. Phone, Mobile Phone, Work Phone
6. E-Mail

   Every once in a while, a client will have an e-mail address that may say something about their personality, self-image, or interests, almost like a vanity license plate. This information may not carry much weight in an evaluation, but it could trigger further conversation or be a door that opens on areas of greater interest.

7. Birth Date, Birth Place/Time

   Birth date, place, and time are only of value as an effective consultation tool if you are versed in astrology.

8. Marriage Status

   There are obvious issues surrounding marriage and being single or divorced. Relationships, or lack thereof, have a powerful influence on health and the body. This question can lead to a conversation and inquiries that may be too personal and should be entered within the limits of a professional relationship.

9. Number of Children

    This is another relationship question and also has direct influence on the health of body and emotions.

10. Occupation

    Work is an obviously important piece of data. You want to know as much as possible about the client's job. Is it a high-pressure job? Does the client work in a contaminated environment? Is it a job that requires an abundance of overtime? Are any possible allergens present? Self-esteem issues may also be addressed under this category, especially related to hierarchies in the workplace.

    The answers to these questions will have a strong influence on your essential oil choices. Oils such as peppermint and basil may be necessary for mental fatigue. Tea tree or lavender may be required for anti-infectious properties and immune support. Workplace stress is addressed on an individual basis and oils are selected according to the stress involved, such as esters for emotional stress, pine for fatigue or MQV for detoxification and support of immune function during exposure to potentially toxic environments.

11. Referred By

    Knowing who referred the client may provide further information. Did the client come in for treatment of similar symptoms? If so, do they live in the same neighborhood? Work in the same place? Are there any other comparisons that may be derived from the referral?

Part Two: Medical Profile

The next section in our example consultation form is used to extract medical information. Information regarding health will support diagnostic accuracy and contribute to your therapeutic direction. A medical profile will also direct you to avoid any oils or procedures that may be contraindicated.

These questions are pretty straightforward and do not require further explanation. The amount of information asked here may seem like medical information overload and unnecessary to some practitioners. Edit this list as needed to keep it in line with your practice. Remember, no matter what your specialty, in a holistic practice, all conditions past and present give clues to the overall health of the body. The more information you have to develop an assessment of the client's conditions, the better your selection of oils.

12. Have you had any major illnesses, accidents, or surgery? If so, please explain.
13. Are you under a doctor's care now? Explain.
14. List any prescription medications or prescription cosmetics you are currently using.
15. List any known allergies you have.
16. What is your current weight?
17. What is your ideal (or desired weight)?
    You may use this question to diagnose self-image. If a client seems thin, but writes in their ideal weight as lower, or much lower, than the current weight, this information will alert you to possible self-esteem issues or anorexia. If this is not your area of expertise, you will be limited in your options for dealing with it. Essential oils may be effective for some emotional or psychological situations, but it will not replace professional support.
18. What is your height?
19. Please circle Y if you currently have any of the listed conditions. Please circle P if you have had the condition in the past but are no longer experiencing it.

Abdominal Pains	Y	P
Attention Deficit Disorder (Hyperactivity)	Y	P
Alcoholism	Y	P
Anemia	Y	P
Arthritis or Joint Pain	Y	P
Asthma	Y	P
Back Pain	Y	P
High Blood Pressure	Y	P
Low Blood Pressure	Y	P
Cancer (Explain)	Y	P
High Cholesterol	Y	P
Colitis	Y	P
Constipation	Y	P
Diabetes Type I	Y	(under control)
Diabetes Type II	Y	(under control)
Eczema/Atopic Dermatitis	Y	P
Fatigue	Y	P
Gout	Y	P
Heart Attack	Y	P
Heart Disease	Y	P
Headache (not migraine)	Y	P
HIV	Y	

Irritable Bowel Syndrome		Y	P	
Lupus		Y	P	
Migraine		Y	P	
Menopause	Post	Peri	Pre	Not Sure
Menstrual Cramps		Y	P	
Menstrual Cycle Imbalance (no bleeding, excessive bleeding, etc.)		Y	P	
Mental Illness (Explain)		Y	P	
PMS		Y	P	
Psoriasis		Y	P	
Rosacea		Y	P	
Stroke		Y	P	
Teeth/Gum Disease		Y	P	
Telangiectasias/Couperose (dilated superficial blood vessels)		Y	P	
Ulcer		Y	P	
Varicose Veins		Y	P	

20. Please list and describe other conditions that are not listed above.

Part Three: Diet

The following questions investigate diet by providing a checklist of foods the client consumes daily (D), moderately (M), hardly at all (H), or not at all (N). This is not a complete list, and you may need to ask other questions. For example, for a client who eats fish, does he look for fish that is not farmed or avoid fish known to contain heavy metals or PCB contaminants? You will gain a clearer view of the client's nutritional awareness from this information. Suspected food allergies may also be unveiled by these questions. Some obvious food-to-disease relationships may appear, such as the consumption of large amounts of sugar and processed foods with inflammatory conditions. Again, this information may be outside of your area of expertise. Use this data as best you can for successful treatment within your modality.

21. Circle the appropriate letter after each item listed.
    D: Consume food or substance daily to three times per week.
    M: Consume food less than three times per week.
    H: Consume food less than twice a month.
    N: Never consume a particular food or substance.

Artificial Sweetener	D	M	H	N
Beer	D	M	H	N
Black Tea	D	M	H	N
Coffee	D	M	H	N
Chocolate (over 70 percent cocoa)	D	M	H	N
Dairy (eggs, butter, milk; not yogurt)	D	M	H	N
Fast Food or Chain Restaurant Food (McDonalds, Red Lobster, Denny's, etc.)	D	M	H	N
Fish	D	M	H	N
Fried Food	D	M	H	N
Grains (quinoa, amaranth, wheat)	D	M	H	N
Green Tea	D	M	H	N
Herbal Tea	D	M	H	N
Hydrogenated Vegetable Oils (margarine, shortening, packaged foods)	D	M	H	N
Junk Food (include chocolate under 70 percent cocoa)	D	M	H	N
Liquor	D	M	H	N
Meat (beef, pork, lamb, buffalo)	D	M	H	N
Nicotine	D	M	H	N
Nuts	D	M	H	N
Poultry	D	M	H	N
Processed Packaged Foods	D	M	H	N
White Rice	D	M	H	N
Brown Rice	D	M	H	N
Salt	D	M	H	N
Soda	D	M	H	N
Sugar	D	M	H	N
Sweet Desserts	D	M	H	N
Colored Vegetables (dark green, red, yellow)	D	M	H	N
Raw Vegetables	D	M	H	N
Cooked to Soft Vegetables	D	M	H	N

Vegetable Oils (cold pressed, not hydrogenated)	D	M	H	N
Water (filtered)	D	M	H	N
Water (tap)	D	M	H	N
Wine	D	M	H	N
Yogurt	D	M	H	N

22. Do you eat organic foods? If so, what percentage of your diet is organic?
23. Are you a vegetarian?
24. Describe three common meals.
25. How many meals do you eat each day?
26. How long do you take to eat lunch?
27. How long do you take to eat your average dinner?
28. What time do you generally eat dinner?
29. Do you have any known food allergies?
30. Do you take vitamin, herbal, green (wheat grass, spirulina, powdered green) food drinks, or nutritional supplements? If yes, list them.
31. Are you dieting? Explain.

Part Four: Habits, Feelings, and Relationships

Questions about the client's personal feelings, habits, relationships, and opinions make up this next section. You are limited by your profession as to how you use this information. Tell your client to skip any questions that they believe are too personal or irrelevant to the treatment requested. Though each of these questions is valid in diagnosing health and skin related conditions, they are exceedingly personal and, depending on your practice, may not be appropriate and can be left off the consultation form.

Confidentiality pledge statement: **We pledge to protect the confidentiality of all your personal information**.

32. Are you moody and emotional?
33. Do you easily become angry or irritated?
34. Explain any experience you feel is relevant to the condition for which you are seeking treatment. If appropriate, include family history and relationships.
35. Is your job satisfactory?
36. Describe your home life.
37. Briefly describe your place of residence, town, neighborhood, etc.

38. Do you have a partner? On a scale of 1–10, how would you rate this relationship? (1 = least and 10 = most satisfying.)
39. How do you feel about your personal relationships (friends, co-workers)?
40. Are you concerned about political issues?
41. Are you concerned about environmental issues?
42. Are you concerned about living conditions and lifestyles around the world?
43. Do you feel that you make a positive contribution to the world?
44. Do you have a spiritual practice or philosophy? Include meditation, prayer, religion, tai chi, yoga, or anything you feel inspires a non-physical existence.

Part Five: Exercise and Physical Activity

The next set of questions assesses the client's quality of activity. Your personal knowledge of exercise and physical activity will determine your use of these questions and answers. Physical activity is a well-known factor in positively enhancing mental and physical health.

Activity and exercise can cause physical pain and inflammation. Essential oils are often recommended and applied for inflammation, bruising, and other similar physical conditions. *Helichrysum italicum*, applied directly on a bruised area, sports injury, or swelling from over-exercise, will help relieve pain and inflammation almost immediately.

45. Describe your daily physical activity, such as sitting at a desk eight hours, standing all day, driving all day, gardening three hours a day, etc.
46. Do you exercise (include walking, yoga, tai chi, martial arts, etc.)?
    If yes, how often do you exercise?
47. Describe your exercise routine.

Part Six: Alternative and Natural Therapies

In a consultation for any alternative or natural therapy, it is helpful to know how familiar the client is with the service being provided and with alternative and natural healing in general. This knowledge will help you to be clear with the language you use, because some words are exclusive to, or have different meaning, when used in reference to alternative and natural therapy. You want to be sure the client understands the words you are using, so be aware if more or less detail is necessary in your explanations. This topic relates to the issue of communication and perception, discussed in Chapter 1. Ask your client to describe what she knows about natural healing, especially aromatherapy, as the answer will enable you to determine whether their expectations are realistic and if their expectations match your anticipated outcome. In general, it is wise to discuss expected results and to elicit the client's perception of any treatment you provide.

The last two questions are directly related to a client who asks for an aromatherapy treatment.

48. Have you ever had or used alternative treatments?
    If so, please explain and describe the treatment(s), the reason for the treatment, the results you expected, and the results you achieved.
49. What is your overall impression of natural therapies?
50. Why did you choose an aromatherapy treatment?
51. What results would you like to achieve from aromatherapy?

Part Seven: The Skin

The next set of questions will pertain to the condition of the skin. This section is useful for any holistic treatment, though it may seem applicable to esthetic treatments only. The skin is a barometer, and it shows signs of systemic imbalance or disease. "Reading" the skin is a valuable diagnostic technique.

The way a client may answer these questions could provide clues to self-esteem, self-awareness, and other emotional or psychological factors. Knowing what skin care or cosmetic products the client is using is beneficial to alert you to potential toxicity or allergies. An esthetician, or any therapist, keeps a client record card. On this card, the clinician's evaluations and analysis are documented, separately, from the client questionnaire. The client record is used to evaluate the success of treatments by documenting changes in the skin over time.

52. What is your skin type? (oily, normal, or dry)
53. Do you have a specific skin condition or conditions that are of special concern?
54. Does your skin type, or condition, change from morning to evening? In winter? In summer? In fall? In spring?

55. How do you "feel" about your skin?
56. How has your skin changed over the past 10 years?
57. Does your skin react to stress? In what way?
58. Do you notice any changes in the skin, such as heat, rash, blotchiness, oiliness, or dryness, after eating particular foods?
59. Does your skin change after exercise?
60. Are you satisfied with your skin type?
61. Describe your skin care regimen, including the names of the products you use daily.
62. Describe and name specific cosmetic products you use occasionally?
63. Do you wear makeup? Name all products.
64. Do you use sunscreen? Name all products and when you use it.
65. How often are you exposed to direct sunlight?
66. How often are you exposed to fluorescent lights?
67. How much time do you spend on caring for your skin in the morning? In the evening?

ARE YOU QUALIFIED TO RECOMMEND ESSENTIAL OILS FOR . . . ?

In the explanations provided on the client consultation form, the suggested analysis contains elements that would be considered under the jurisdiction of medicine, psychology, or psychiatry. Note that a diagnosis and prescription based on your evaluations should be guided by your licensing or legitimate qualifications. Your selection of essential oils will be based on your professional or personal abilities as well as your experience with the oils.

That said, aromatherapy as well as other plant based therapies, has not traditionally abided by the rules of professional qualifications. Dr. Schnaubelt, in *Aromatherapy Lifestyle*, Part 3 of his PIA Masters Series, has introduced five laws of aromatherapy. Law four states: "Aromatherapy benefits its users without the need for conventional expertism."[7] Law four does not dismiss legal qualifications; rather, it makes a broad statement that essential oils are commonly used by those who *do not* have conventional degrees or licensing in psychiatry, psychology, medicine, or other related health fields. Because of the current qualifying standards of aromatherapy (see Chapter 13), a gap exists when it comes to defining an essential oil "expert." At this time, we are stranded in search of qualifying factors and licensing that allow aromatherapists, as independent professionals, to work with essential oils for emotional and medical conditions that are associated with the oil's properties and uses. By the very nature of essential oil use you are, or will be, treating psychological and medical conditions.

The consultation example form includes suggestions for psychological and medical conditions, with an understanding that, in your own consultations, you will proceed in an appropriate manner. The following evaluations are presented as a guide to integrating previously described properties and actions of essential oils based on scientific and experiential evidence.

Common Sense Evaluation

This text is not intended to create or define the qualifications of an aromatherapy expert. Remember to use common sense and obey all legal standards that limit professional use of essential oils. This message is conveyed several times in this text. The best advice I can give to help you understand how to employ the information presented in this text is to use common sense. Common sense is, like many of the stipulations of aromatherapy, an elusive term that is open to interpretation and definition.

EVALUATION AS A NON-LINEAR PROCESS

Understand that a consultation is not a linear process. While evaluating section one, you may jump to consider information from section three or five. In this example, however, I will attempt to proceed in a linear manner, following the form from section one to section seven.

SELECTION OF ESSENTIAL OILS

The process of a holistic consultation is your best guide to determine specific essential oils you will use for treatment.

This text provides you with more than enough aromatherapy knowledge to begin. To demonstrate a process for selecting essential oils, this section presents a sample client consultation with recommendations for aromatherapy formulation. An annotated approach to the consultation form is used to clarify the essential oil choices.

DEMONSTRATION CONSULTATION: AN ESTHETICS CONSULTATION

Following is an annotated and generalized example of an esthetic consultation. If you are not an esthetician you should be able to adapt this example to any practice or therapeutic modality.

Treatment Goal

A treatment goal is not included on the sample consultation form of this chapter but may be placed there at your discretion.

AUTHOR'S **NOTE**

MY CONSULTATIONS

This consultation demonstration is extracted from my work with real clients. It's an example of how I take the information expressed in this book and put it into practice. You'll see how I can address non-skin care conditions, such as sinus inflammation caused by allergies, through a skin care application. I do not, in any way, claim to be treating the sinus condition. My knowledge and experience of essential oils informs me that the selected oil, German chamomile, is known to reduce inflammation from seasonal allergies. It's a great oil selection for this client's skin, so it doesn't matter if it helps the sinus condition or not. I wasn't asked to treat that condition and I'm not including it in my treatment presentation to the client.

I may feel obliged to inform the client if I have selected treatment oils that address conditions that are not related to their skin condition. This, again, becomes an area of licensing and professionalism. Don't address conditions out of your realm. But as a contradiction to this statement, you do need to be concerned about those health conditions that affect the skin. You'll find that the oils selected for an area out of your professional jurisdiction will likely be correct for the skin condition. That's why there's so much information in this book that is not specifically about essential oils. The more you know, the more you can address. Essential oils are a holistic modality. You are, whether you are conscious of it or not, treating the overall health of your client with essential oils. The esthetician accomplishes this feat with a simple skin-focused application.

AUTHOR'S **NOTE**

RECOMMENDED BY YOUR ESTHETICIAN

In Chapter 1, I state that estheticians are in the best place for professional essential oil use. I would like to explain and begin by saying estheticians are not better aromatherapists. Aromatherapy is a holistic and healing treatment within any modality, whether that modality is massage, naturopathy, or reflexology. The difference is in the professional products recommended or prescribed by the practitioner. Clients are more likely to use an aromatherapy product that you blend or recommend if it is part of their normal daily regimen. People use skin-care products on a daily basis, so when essential oils are incorporated into these products, nothing is added to their daily routine.

The human factor should always be taken into account with any recommendation. How often have you gone back to a health practitioner expressing your forgetfulness in taking the required treatment? It's normal. How easy is it for the person to use your product or treatment, and how much of a challenge is it for them to remember to use it? The reason I say the esthetician is in a unique position is because they are treating with, and suggesting, take-home products that already exist in a person's daily routine. When it comes to skin care, who do you think will have the overriding influence over products used by a client? I haven't taken an official poll, but my guess is that the client will use the esthetician-suggested product A over the health professional's product B. I've talked to clients who have sidelined a dermatologist-prescribed product to use the spa product sold by an esthetician. Working as an esthetician in a holistic setting, in conjunction with naturopaths and other whole body professionals, to me is the ideal situation.

Chapter 1 notes the importance of stating the treatment goal. This text's demonstration and explanation of a holistic consultation assumes that the goal is included in a verbal interview before each service. The goal is recorded on the client's record card.
Example Goal: Reduce fine lines and wrinkles for a more youthful appearance.

PERSONAL INFORMATION

The client is a 45-year-old female of mixed Asian and European descent, married, with no children. She lives and works in Cambridge, Massachusetts, a city bordering Boston. The client is an executive in marketing management at a bio-tech company. Based on this personal information, an essential oil list is created to address potential factors that may cause aging or damage to the skin.
Sample Evaluation and Oil Selection Based on Personal Information: Essential oils are selected to provide protection from, and detoxification of, city living that may cause free radical damage and skin congestion created by exhaust and other environmental factors. The stress of a high-pressure job is also addressed. Stress may create hormonal imbalance, a concern because of pre-menopausal conditions (determined by a non-linear jump to the medical evaluation in section two). Environmental and work-related stress may cause premature aging of the skin that will influence the essential oil selection. Essential oils can then be selected by using the Structure-Effect Diagram and knowledge of individual oils.
Structure-Effect Diagram: Ester compounds are selected for stress reduction and soothing qualities to the skin.

Sesquiterpene alcohols protect and regenerate skin, so oil choices include carrot seed, cedarwood, frankincense, vetiver, and Australian sandalwood.

Monoterpene hydrocarbon content, oxides, or both are possibly included for detoxification of environmental impurities that may accumulate in the tissues.

Oil	Properties
Rose (*Rosa damascena*)	Selected for diversity of action; regeneration of cells to reduce and prevent fine lines and wrinkles;

	protection from environmental pollutants; calming to relieve tension.
Geranium (*Pelargonium asperum*)	Adaptogen. Best choice for women. Excellent for skin rejuvenation.
Neroli (*Citrus aurantium*)	Very soothing for stress-related issues. Relaxing.
Clary Sage (*Salvia sclarea*)	Relaxing and stress-reducing ester. Use as a skin conditioner and to mimic estrogen for hormonal balance. A recommendation is made to combine clary sage with *Vitex agnus castus* to address menopausal imbalances.
Frankincense *(Boswellia carterii)*	Cell regenerative and great for mature skin. Spiritual support.
MQV (*Melaleuca quinquenervia viri*)	Immune support and detoxification of skin tissue.
Eucalyptus radiata	Antiseptic; detoxification.

Medical Information and Evaluation

The client has no specific medical conditions that require special attention. She has been relatively healthy with no major illnesses. She has noticed some symptoms that could be related to pre-menopause. She has had migraines sporadically for many years; when asked more specific questions, identified that they occur in spring and fall. This pattern may be related to seasonal allergies, because the pain occurs with tension in the neck and occipital area as well as behind the eyes, a problem that is often caused by swollen sinuses. It appears that other pains and problems are caused by overwork and stress.

Sample Evaluation and Oil Selection Based on Medical Information: The same essential oils chosen for personal evaluation would be suitable for this medical evaluation. Eucalyptus and MQV address possible seasonal allergies and sinus congestion. Clary sage, rose, geranium, and MQV all address hormonal and menopausal issues.

Additions may include:
Structure-Effect Diagram: Sesquiterpene hydrocarbons to reduce allergic inflammation caused by seasonal allergies.

Oils	Properties
German chamomile *(Matricaria recutita)*	Reduce sinus inflammation caused by seasonal allergies.
Lavender *(Lavandula angustifolia)*	Headache and stress relief; balancing.

Diet Information and Evaluation

The client's diet is fair to good. It is lacking in organic foods but does have variety. She drinks moderate amounts of coffee (one to two cups daily) and does not consume sweets or junk foods very often, so this is not a major concern. Alcohol consumption is moderate, and there is no nicotine. The client mentioned that her diet falters while she is traveling; she tends to feel fatigued and bloated, and her skin breaks out during those occasions.

You will find that you rarely select essential oils because of diet. Eating habits and diet are evaluated to detect possible food-related causes of the symptoms being addressed in treatment. Oil choices may help to relieve emotional attachment or addiction to foods. This is an advanced aspect of aromatherapy, however, and comes with skills developed from experience. Evidence of essential oils having this kind of effect is based purely on empirical anecdotes presented within the aromatherapy community.

Structure-Effect Diagram: Ether compounds, primarily anethole, may be recommended as a result of the client's expression of often having rushed meals. Anethole, in anise and fennel, is useful after the meal to help autonomic function and support proper digestion.

(Indian restaurants supply fennel seeds to chew following a meal for this purpose.)

Oil	Properties
Peppermint (*Mentha piperita*)	Used to help digestion and liver function following an "impure" meal. This oil is useful when traveling and when unable to fully control the quality of meals. Peppermint is used independently, rather than in a

	formulation. The oil is useful following a meal, especially after a junk meal or consuming too much alcohol. This function is demonstrated by the custom of eating mint following a meal. (A real mint, not the toxic waste pellets commonly offered by restaurants.)
Anise seed (*Pimpinella anisum*)	A drop of this oil following a rushed meal, or any meal, aids in proper digestion by providing equilibrium to the autonomic nervous system. It can be combined with the peppermint to aid digestion and liver function. Anise also relieves the symptoms of stress, such as quickened breathing and heart rate.

Habits, Feelings, and Relationships Information and Evaluation

The answers in this section may alert you to emotional conditions that can influence symptoms and skin condition. Even if you are not licensed or knowledgeable in psychological evaluation, you may find information here that could guide the direction of your essential oil choices. Situations that cause stress are sometimes very obvious.

Our example client does not reveal detail to any questions answered. She appears self confident and self-satisfied with the direction of her life, job, and relationships. Her desire to reduce and prevent signs of aging does not appear to be emotionally driven or arising from issues of low self esteem. In conversation, the reason (the "why") she is seeking treatment is based upon her desire to compete in a competitive work environment, as well as her wish to maintain a healthy and vibrant appearance.

The client's answers do not call for any added oil recommendations. This client did not disclose or does not have a spiritual practice. The already recommended frankincense is a suitable oil to help lift this client out of a physical awareness and to help her connect with a more energetic, alternate, or spiritual reality. This is a difficult area to define. In the context and design of this holistic consultation there is scientific reasoning that merits questioning how consciousness or thought molds our physical existence. This is an advanced study of aromatherapy; this text will merely suggest, without further explanation, that using spiritual type oils, such as frankincense and myrrh, may be recommended when a client needs mental "downtime" and spiritual expansion.

Oils	Properties
Frankincense	Spiritual expansion and quieting of mental "chatter."

Exercise Information and Evaluation

Client is active at work, seldom sitting for more than two hours. She does not practice a regular exercise routine but does walk once or twice a week and is active at home. This information does not suggest any apparent imbalances that may be caused by exercise routines, or lack thereof, and thus does not warrant an essential oil recommendation. Yoga may be suggested for a valued combination of exercise, stress reduction, and spiritual expansion. Each of these practices is beneficial for reducing fine lines and preventing wrinkles, the client's stated goal.

Alternative and Natural Therapies Information and Evaluation

The client had acupuncture treatment in the past, seeking this remedy for a temporary experience of shoulder and neck pain. She reports that the treatment was moderately successful. She is aware of natural therapies through magazine articles, television reports, and conversations with friends. This client needs explanations of specific language related to alternative treatment. This need is not uncommon in any practice if you want the client to fully understand procedures.

This questioning did uncover a pain that the client did not mention in the medical section. Neck pain is so common that unless clients seek treatment for that reason, they often do not see it as a concern. Neck tension and pain are often related to stress. The ester-containing essential oils already selected will be adequate for stress related neck pain. Additional oils may be suggested for spasm or muscle inflammation.

Oils	Properties
Helichrysum italicum	Reduces muscle pain and inflammation.

Skin Information and Evaluation

Our sample client has medium pigmented skin, a Fitzpatrick IV on the **Fitzpatrick Scale** used to measure a skin type's tolerance to the sun's burning rays.[8] She has slight folds beginning to form at the mouth and some loss of elasticity apparent around chin and neck. Some puffiness and darkness is present under the eyes. Fine expression lines, or crow's feet, have formed around the eye and is apparent only when smiling or squinting. Dehydration is detected, though the client's skin is a "normal" skin type. She has apparent loss of the lipid barrier function, but not to a degree at which the skin looks or feels dry. Some comedones (blackheads) have formed in the jaw line and around the nose.

The client is, on the whole, satisfied with her skin. She has noticed undesirable changes over the past three years that relate to her interest in creating more vitality and youthfulness to her skin tone and texture. The client's answers in Part Seven: The Skin, are consistent with the issues noted in the preceding questions. She is exposed to pollutants, fluorescent lights, and other conditions that may contribute to the loss of skin tone and firmness. Stress is known to contribute to all the signs of aging mentioned by the client.

Rose, clary sage, frankincense, lavender, geranium, and neroli essential oils may be suggested here for stress relief of the skin and cellular rejuvenation. Sesquiterpene alcohols, ketones, and esters are useful to counteract aging skin conditions.

Many more oils could be added to this list. We added a few more to give an ample essential oil collection from which to select the final formulation.

Oils	Properties
Palmarosa (*Cymbopogon martini*)	Cell regenerative, calming.
Cistus (*Cistus ladaniferus*)	Cell regenerative, wrinkle reduction.
Australian sandalwood (*Santalum spicatum*)	Relieves tension and stress; promotes skin elasticity.
Eucalyptus dives	Contains ketones; promotes regeneration of skin cells.

HOLISTIC TREATMENT

This consultation practice is primarily an exercise in selecting essential oils, based on the data gathered from a client consultation. Some elements of the holistic consultation introduced in Chapter 1 were not used. Here is a review and final analysis of the client consultation:

Aromatherapy treatment will address several causes of aging skin that include stress, inflammation, and free radical damage (oxidation).

Treatment with essential oils includes these properties: cell regenerative, antioxidant, anti-inflammatory, tissue and skin strengthening, and stress reduction. Botanical oils (rose hip seed, olive, and others) may be used to reduce inflammation, regenerate cells, and prevent free radical damage.

An anti-inflammatory diet and antioxidant supplementation is recommended. This recommendation could be expressed as a suggestion to visit a holistic nutritionist or read books related to diet and skin health.

Alert the client to the detrimental effects (fine lines and wrinkles) that overwork and lack of rest have on the skin. Yoga is a good recommendation for a combination exercise and relaxation practice.

CREATING A FORMULA AND CHOOSING A METHOD OF APPLICATION

More than enough essential oils have been selected for the example client. Many of these oils have similar properties and activity. This similarity does not mean that it doesn't matter which oil you use. Each essential oil is distinctive, and one may be more effective than another, even though they possess similar composition and properties. We will now go through an exercise of choosing the final oils for a blend, along with the application method that will be used.

Choosing the Final Oils

No precise methodology is used to choose the essential oils for the final blend. Every aromatherapist has his or her way of accomplishing this selection. As with so many other aspects of aromatherapy, there is not a wrong or right way to select oils.

Selection and Fragrance Aversion or Attraction

Some aromatherapists believe that allowing the client to smell the oils is a proper method for formulating blends. The reasoning underlying this practice is that people may be attracted to what they need. This text supports the idea that we are biologically and emotionally tuned into our needs through fragrance. The attraction concept has been taught through many schools of aromatherapy and may have demonstrated enough validity to warrant passing this method on to students. Alternatively, some clinicians believe the opposite and choose oils for which the client has an aversion. This is not as common a practice, but by no means is it wrong. There is a third group, clinicians who don't lean either way and generally do not present oils to the client for approval or disapproval.

If a client doesn't like the oil's odor, some aromatherapists may find a way to slip it into the blend if they believe that adding it will provide therapeutic value. Be aware of the lessons taught in Chapter 3 about emotional connection to fragrance. If a client has a negative memory association stored along with the oil's odor, it is best to leave it out of a blend to avoid a possible allergic or emotional reaction from associated memories. With so many oils available, it is not necessary to make the client uncomfortable.

Inevitably, some questions arise from the attraction or aversion method of oil selection. Does this system work for people with anosmia, the inability to detect smell (introduced in Chapter 3)? Schizophrenics may have smell disorders, as may people who detect all odors as foul. How does letting the client smell oils affect the choice with these people? These are not questions to be answered, but ones that need to be considered when selecting a method to choose essential oils.

NO RIGHT WAY, NO WRONG WAY

We have already developed an instructive method of creating a list of oils that depends on the client consultation and therapeutic focus. The final word on selecting oils used in the formulation is rooted in individual preference. The ongoing challenge, or blessing, of aromatherapy remains. There are no definite rules, no right way and no wrong way. There are only common sense ways. You are again left to make decisions from an intuitive sense, a random decision, a pseudo-scientific methodology, or any other method that suits your needs at the time.

Fragrance Considerations The overall fragrance of the blend usually is considered to some extent. This consideration is not a rule, but after all, this practice is called "aroma" therapy. This step is where you may incorporate the concepts of top, middle, and base fragrance notes (Chapter 8). Look at your list and determine the notes you have available.

Making the Final Selection In this example, five oils are selected for the final blend. They are listed in this section with an explanation of why they were chosen. Some explanations are based on science, some on empirical study, and some on an esoteric basis or according to the "common" use of the oil. Remember, the reasoning is always driven by individual preference.

Oil	Reason
Rose	Chosen for its feminine character, creating balance for this client, who plays a strong role in a masculine field of work. Hormonally balancing. Relaxing. Rose is known to be good for the emotional heart and is selected based on an intuitive sense that the client will benefit from rose's ability to energetically satisfy the need to be loved. Cell regenerative and skin strengthening. Reduces wrinkles and fine lines.
Clary sage	Adds a potent stress-reducing quality; phyto-hormone properties are chosen to help balance stress-related and menopausal hormonal issues. Cell strengthening.

Frankincense	Spiritual emphasis. Cell regeneration. Wrinkle and fine line reduction.
Palmarosa	Cell regeneration. Antiseptic.
Australian sandalwood	Cell regeneration. Emotional balance.

This selection of essential oils addresses the therapeutic focus and goals expressed by both the client and the clinician in an esthetic practice. The oils were chosen based on the experience of how these oils blend together to create a therapeutic synergy as well as a fragrance synergy. The selected oils also offer therapeutic diversity based on the client's needs.

METHOD OF APPLICATION

Which method of application you choose may be determined by the clinical situation. In our example, an esthetic clinic, the facial treatment entails adding the essential oil blend to selected products. In a massage practice, the essential oils would be added to a carrier blend for body massage, reflexology treatment, or both. Choose the method of application that fits your clinical practice. You may also want to include energy work using a spray mist or diffuser carrying the blend. A perfume oil or personal massage formula may also be created for the client's daily use.

Creating and Applying the Essential Oil Blend

Our example, using an esthetic treatment, contains several treatment opportunities. The facial includes products for cleansing, exfoliating, toning, and a mask, as well as a treatment complex and moisturizing. Review Chapter 10 for products and ingredients. If all the products are unscented, a blend could be incorporated into them. In our example, we formulate a treatment blend in a one-ounce container and give it to the client to take home for daily use. We begin by formulating the oil blend, using the directions taught in Chapter 8 for a 2.5 percent dilution of the selected oils, resulting in 15 drops total of essential oil.

4 drops - Rose
4 drops - Palmarosa
2 drops - Clary sage
2 drops - Frankincense
3 drops - Australian sandalwood

Added Fees for Expensive Oils

In this blend, rose oil is used at a high percentage. The client should be charged a reasonable added fee for the expense of the rose oil. This additional cost should be discussed in advance with the client, and if she or he does not agree, a lower percentage of rose could be used, or the rose could be replaced by geranium or other suitable oil.

Formulating the Base Oil Blend The selected method of application is a treatment complex made with 2.5 percent essential oil in a mixture of base oils. The base oil blend is formulated to address the treatment focus and includes essential fatty acids and other components for treating inflammation, antioxidant activity, and cell regeneration (see Chapter 9). The formulation is written in percentages and liquid milliliter measurement for a one-ounce, 30-mL container. The blend will consist of:

25 percent (7.5 mL) - Olive oil
15 percent (4.5 mL) - Rose hip seed oil
52.5 percent (16.5 mL) - Hazelnut oil
5 percent (1.5 mL) - Raspberry seed oil

The base oil blend and the essential oils used in this treatment complex will provide a holistic remedy formulated according to the results of the consultation. In an esthetic facial, this treatment is applied after the mask and before moisturizing. One treatment in a spa setting will not do much for the conditions being addressed. The client may take the remaining formula home and use it daily after cleansing and toning and before moisturizing. This formula can also be used for full body massage.

ANALYZING TREATMENT PROGRESS AND EFFICACY

The effectiveness of the treatment is determined by whether it achieves the expected results. In follow-up appointments with the client, visual, or alternate, determining factors should make it obvious whether the aromatherapy protocol is working. Results may be divided into stages: Immediate, Short Term, and Long Term. Individual and professional standards apply to defining the time allotted to these stages.

You may have a protocol in place to observe and record results from treatment. This same protocol may be used for essential oil therapy. Unanticipated or surprising benefits are always appreciated and often are expected with the use of essential oils. A massage therapist, using neroli in treatment for anxiety and stress, may observe improvement in skin condition, and an esthetician working on adult acne may hear from the client that an ongoing neck pain has diminished. Pay attention to unexpected results, because they offer clues to further treatment and oil selection. If results are not adequate, you may need to revise the formulation and select different essential oils. Trial and error is used in essential oil therapy, as it is in most healing and clinical work.

CHAPTER SUMMARY

The consultation is an important part of a successful holistic aromatherapy treatment. This chapter includes a detailed consultation form and explains how to analyze the information collected, including clues embedded in such items as the name and address. The consultation form is used to create a sample client, identify a treatment goal for that client, and develop the rationale behind the selection of essential oils and application method.

REVIEW QUESTIONS

1. The holistic consultation is used as a tool to achieve what goal?
2. How is a person's name analyzed in a holistic consultation? Address?
3. What value can you derive from the medical checklist to help you select essential oils?
4. Why would you want to discuss a client's familiarity with alternative therapies?
5. How do you choose essential oils based on information gathered during consultation?
6. How are aromatherapy results determined?

CHAPTER REFERENCES

1. Harrison, J. (2000). *Global Healthy Aging Consultation and Analysis.* Bellevue, WA: Phytotherapy Institute.
2. Flora, C. (2004, March/April). "Hello, My Name is Unique." *Psychology Today.* Accessed on August 16, 2007 at http://www.psychologytoday.com.
3. Erwin, P. G. (1993). "First names and perceptions of physical attractiveness." *Journal of Psychology 127* (6); 625–631.
4. Harrison, J. (2000). *Global Healthy Aging Consultation and Analysis.* Bellevue, WA: Phytotherapy Institute.
5. *Environment Can Affect Your Health.* (2006). Texas Medical Association. Accessed on August 16, 2007 at http://www.texmed.org.
6. Harrison, J. (2001). *The Essentials for Beauty and Skin.* Bellevue, WA: Phytotherapy Institute.
7. Schnaubelt, K. (2004). *Aromatherapy Lifestyles: Science Based Self-Medication with Essential Oils.* San Rafael, CA: Terra Linda Scent and Image.
8. Milady/Thompson Delmar Learning. (2003). *Milady's Standard Comprehensive for Training Estheticians.* Clifton Park, NY: Thomson Delmar Learning.

Aromatherapy Licensing and Regulations

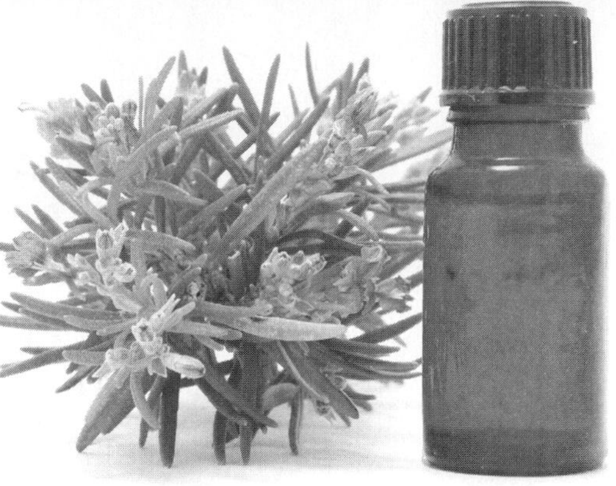

CHAPTER 13

Most aromatherapy courses on the market are intended for the lay person[.] While these courses are interesting, they are not relevant to clinical practice.

–Jane Buckle, PhD

LEARNING OBJECTIVES

1. Understand which government agencies and standards regulate the practice of aromatherapy and the use of essential oils.
2. Learn the guidelines for proper use of essential oils under your professional licensing in the clinical setting.
3. Become knowledgeable in the language that is used for essential oil claims and the labeling requirements for aromatherapy products.
4. Understand the laws, regulations, and standards that have been established for aromatherapy education and essential oil classes or certification.

AROMATHERAPY AND CAM THERAPISTS

Many of the uses and applications of essential oils presented in this book lean toward medical interpretation. Essential oils have pharmaceutical-like activity and are "prescribed" by aromatherapists in ways that mimic traditional medicine. The practice of aromatherapy and the use of essential oils must stay within the guidelines of licensing and legal practice. Regulations, codes and standards that are specific to essential oils are reviewed in this chapter.

Aromatherapy is primarily practiced by therapists who function outside the mainstream medical community. Clinical use of essential oils is practiced by **CAM** (Complimentary Alternative Medicine) therapists, which include naturopaths (ND), traditional Chinese medical practitioners, Ayurvedic doctors and medical massage therapists. Essential oil therapy, classified as an herbal therapy, is considered a CAM therapy (see Table 13-1).

Table 13-1 CAM Therapies Listed by The White House Commission of Complimentary Alternative Medicine Policy: CAM Systems of Health Care, Therapies, or Products[1]

Major Domains of CAM	Domain Examples
Alternative health care systems	Ayurvedic medicine
	Chiropractic
	Homeopathic medicine
	Native American medicine (e.g., sweat lodge, medicine wheel)
	Naturopathic medicine
	Traditional Chinese medicine (e.g., acupuncture, Chinese herbal medicine)
Mind-body interventions	Meditation
	Hypnosis

Table 13-1 (continued)

Major Domains of CAM	Domain Examples
	Guided imagery
	Dance therapy
	Music therapy
	Art therapy
	Prayer and mental healing
Biological based therapies	Herbal therapies
	Special diets (e.g., macrobiotics, extremely low-fat or high carbohydrate diets)
	Orthomolecular medicine (e.g., megavitamin therapy)
	Individual biological therapies (e.g., shark cartilage, bee pollen)
Therapeutic massage, body work, and somatic movement therapies	Massage
	Feldenkrais
	Alexander method
Energy therapies	Qigong
	Reiki
	Therapeutic touch
Bioelectromagnetics	Magnet therapy

Nurses and Aromatherapy

Registered Nurses are in a unique position in the mainstream medical setting for the use of essential oils and other CAM therapies. They are allowed to use CAM therapy within the scope appropriate to their educational level, knowledge, skills, and abilities.[2] This is a useful guideline for all practitioners who use essential oils. At this time, the practice is rarely found, or understood, in hospitals or doctors offices. There remains a lack of valid and consistent information and knowledge regarding essential oils for use in medical practice. Jane Buckle and her company, RJ Buckle Associates, have done much to overcome this lack by providing essential oil education in 45 Planetree Medical Centers and Facilities across the United States.[3]

In the traditional Western medical setting, introducing essential oils for something other than "relaxation" may be more challenging. It would depend strongly on the head of the medical staff and his or her awareness and acceptance of essential oil therapy. Government licensing and insurance regulate the medical field in ways that may make it a "risk" to incorporate essential oils topically, internally or for claims other than vague references to calming, soothing, and energizing. The American Medical Association (AMA) oversees ethical behavior among their members and does not impose regulations for essential oil use.

Aromatherapy and the Spa

The FDA does not allow any drug claims to be made for essential oils, which eliminates statements of specific therapeutic results for medical conditions (see Standards and Laws Governing Essential Oil Use, in this chapter). This rule creates a special place for essential oils in the spa industry. Essential oils can be incorporated into a formula and applied to the skin for acne or to release muscle tension in massage and will have potential healing activity in other areas. The clinician can formulate with purposeful focus on a medical issue without expressing a medical claim. The "claim" may be left out of the therapeutic consultation, but the effect will remain in the application. If estheticians or therapists wish to work medicinally, they may approach healing without making drug claims, so long as their manner is appropriate for their profession and they follow all safety guidelines. "Appropriate" is a generalized term that is defined by the practice, job title, and position within the clinic and attitudes and approval of co-workers and management.

The esthetician, massage therapist, and other spa professionals have essential oils already in place as an accepted therapeutic tool. Reading and understanding this text provides a knowledge base for proper use of essential oils. The next step is practice and experience to furnish the skills required for expert use. The opportunity in the spa setting is distinctive, in that it offers the therapeutic benefit of essential oils veiled beneath a beauty treatment. It is permissible to formulate according to medical data extracted from a consultation, even though your primary goal is a specific treatment for beauty or massage. Doing so is simply a way of adopting holistic use of the therapeutic qualities of essential oils that have been repeatedly emphasized in this text.

Essential Oils in the Medical Spa The medical esthetic and medi-spa environments offer a wide range of opportunity for the aromatherapy trained esthetician and therapist. Many procedures conducted within the medical spa can benefit from the use of essential oils. Incorporating the use of essential oils for pre- and post-surgery may promote a positive healing process and assist in scar prevention. Medical spa procedures may produce anxiety and essential oils become a valuable adjunct as relaxing agents. Essential oils are quite successful in reducing stress and anxiety in hospitals.[4,5]

Doctors in the medical spa setting may restrict the use of essential oils as part or follow-up to a medical procedure. It is imperative to follow the guidelines expressed by doctors and others who create the regulations in a place of employment. Any use of essential oils in a medical spa may have to be approved by the head medical supervisor or by management. An appropriate manner to discuss the value and safety of aromatherapy is to present solid academic studies from published sources, especially peer-reviewed journals that document the effects of essential oils.

Standards and Laws Governing Essential Oil Use

In the United States, no laws govern the use of essential oils or aromatherapy. None of the 50 states currently issue a license for an "Aromatherapist." When using essential oils in a professional practice, you are governed by any guidelines or regulations stated for the licensing of your profession. If you practice as an aromatherapist and do not hold any other licensing, you must be aware of the laws that govern practicing medicine without a license. All 50 states have laws that prohibit the practice of medicine, which means treating or diagnosing disease, by individuals without a proper license.

FDA Regulations

The FDA regulates claims made by manufacturers. They have established rules for all products and advertising claims. Essential oils are regulated by the FDA, and claims that have not been approved by the FDA may not be written on the label of packaged essential oils. Essential oils are listed as GRAS (generally regarded as safe) by the FDA. They are not regulated as therapeutic agents or for medical use, however.

When labeling any aromatherapy product, you are permitted to say what the product is used for, such as "for psoriasis, atopic dermatitis, and inflamed skin," but you may not say "will heal," "cures," or "stops" the specific condition. Language becomes the tool to direct the use of essential oils on a label. The language may suggest use for a condition but must not explicitly state that the product will make any physiological changes to the body or skin. Refer to the FDA web site for laws and conditions regarding labeling.

TRAINING AND CERTIFICATION

Education in the field of aromatherapy is not regulated by state or government agencies. No standards or qualifications are in place regarding the educational requirements for essential oil use or for certification as an aromatherapist. Some private groups that have made attempts to self-regulate aromatherapy as an industry and have set core curriculum guidelines for aromatherapy training. Certification in aromatherapy is only as valid as the quality of the education and educators from which it is received.

Aromatherapy schools or others specializing in essential oil education may be registered or licensed within a state. This licensing means only that the state recognizes them as a school operating in the state's jurisdiction. A school can be licensed by a state, even though the curriculum does not qualify for professional license.

Aromatherapy training can be accomplished through correspondence or through the Internet. Private technical schools, such as massage, esthetic, and cosmetology schools, may offer aromatherapy certification as a part of their curriculum or as continuing education. The quality of essential oil education and curriculum varies from school to school. The best method of determining the qualification of a particular school is through diligent research and consideration.

CHAPTER SUMMARY

Aromatherapy is often practiced outside of the medical profession. It is included under herbal therapies in the White House Commission on Complementary and Alternative Medicine (CAM) Policy. Currently, as a profession, aromatherapy and the use of essential oils does not offer any state or federal standards or licensing. The FDA lists essential oils as GRAS (generally regarded as safe) and does not consider them to be drugs. Essential oil actions considered as drug claims cannot legally be listed on a label. No essential oil or aromatherapy education standards exist. Anyone can claim to be an aromatherapist or an aromatherapy educator. To seek training, it is up to the individual to fully research the quality of the educator and training curriculum.

REVIEW QUESTIONS

1. What is CAM? Name at least 3 health care systems listed by the White House Commission on CAM Policy.
2. What qualifications does a Registered Nurse need to practice aromatherapy?
3. How may a spa therapist or esthetician address a medical issue responsibly?
4. What are the standards and laws governing essential oil use?
5. What kind of claims cannot be made on the bottle label containing essential oils?
6. What standards exist to qualify or license aromatherapy education, and what is the best way to choose a school for certification?

CHAPTER REFERENCES

1. The White House Commission of Complimentary Alternative Medicine Policy. "Chapter 2: Overview of CAM in the United States: Recent History, Current Status, And Prospects for the Future." March 2002; pp 9–10.
2. Buckle, J. (2003). *Clinical Aromatherapy: Essential Oils in Practice.* Philadelphia, PA: Churchill Livingston.
3. Planetree. Derby, CT. Accessed on August 16, 2007 at http://www.planetree.org.
4. Dunn, C., Sleep, J. & Collett, D. (1995). "Sensing an improvement: An experimental study to evaluate the use of aromatherapy, massage, and periods of rest in an intensive care unit." *Journal of Advanced Nursing 21* (1); 34–40.
5. Hudson, R. (1995). "Use of lavender in a long term elderly ward." *Nursing Times 91*; 12.

Appendix A

THERAPEUTIC FORMULAS

The following essential oil formulas are written in drop amounts and can be added to any one-ounce carrier or base blend. There are more essential oils listed than are used in the formulas. These may be swapped and used as alternate choices to those used in the formulas.

COLDS/FLU

Essential oils – Bay laurel, *Eucalyptus radiata*, *Euc. globulus*, green myrtle, lavender, lemon myrtle (*Backhousia citriodora*), MQV, pine, ravensare, spruce, tea tree

Formula:	**Chest Rub**	**Inhalation (in bowl of hot water)**
	4 Euc. radiata	2 Euc. globulus
	4 MQV	2 Pine
	2 Cedarwood	2 Lavender
	3 Lavender	
	2 Lemon myrtle	

MUSCLE ACHE, SPASM, AND CRAMPS/JOINT PAIN

Essential oils - Birch, black pepper, German chamomile, Roman chamomile, *Eucalyptus globulus* (or *radiata*), ginger, *Helichrysum italicum*, juniper, *Kunzea ambigua* (spring flower), lavender, lemon, peppermint, rosemary, vetiver, wintergreen (use extreme caution, small amounts)

Formula:	**Pain Remedy**	**Muscle Soothing**
	4 Birch (or wintergreen)	2 *Kunzea ambigua*
	3 Black pepper	2 Ginger
	4 German chamomile	5 Juniper
	8 *Helichrysum italicum*	3 Lavender
	4 Lavender	3 Lemon
	4 Peppermint (or spearmint)	
	3 Vetiver	

FEMALE REPRODUCTIVE BALANCE

Essential oils - Angelica, carrot seed, Roman chamomile, clary sage, cypress, fennel, geranium, lavender, marjoram, nutmeg, rose, sage *(Salvia lavandulaefolia)*, vitex

Formula:	**PMS**	**Cramps**	**Menopause**
	2 R. chamomile	3 R. chamomile	2 Cypress
	5 Clary sage	5 Clary sage	5 Geranium
	4 Lavender	2 Cypress	3 Rose
	2 Ylang-ylang	1 Marjoram	2 Sage
	2 Vetiver	2 Nutmeg	2 Aus. sandalwood
			2 Vitex

SCARS/STRETCH MARKS

Essential oils: Cistus, *Eucalyptus dives,* frankincense, *Helichrysum italicum,* lavender, rose, rosemary verbenone

Formula:	**Scars**	**Stretch Mark Prevention**
	7 *Helichrysum italicum*	4 Rose
	7 Rosemary verbenone	4 Lavender
	4.5 mL rose hip seed oil	4.5 mL Rose hip seed oil

CELLULITE/DIURETIC/LYMPHATIC

Essential Oils - Angelica, bay laurel, carrot seed, cedarwood, cypress, *Eucalyptus citriodora*, fennel, fir, grapefruit, lemon, MQV, orange, pine, spruce

Formula:	**Cellulite**	**Circulation**	**Glandular Secretions**
	4 Cedarwood	5 Cedarwood	2 Angelica
	4 Cypress	5 Cypress	4 Carrot seed
	4 Grapefruit	3 Lemon	4 Cedarwood
	4 Lemon	3 Fir	4 Fennel

ANXIETY/TENSION/STRESS/ NERVOUSNESS/DEPRESSION

Essential Oils - Bergamot, cedarwood, Roman chamomile, clary sage, geranium, jasmine, lavender, lemon verbena, mandarin, mandarin petitgrain, marjoram, melissa, neroli, orange, rose, ylang-ylang

Formula:	**Anxiety**	**Stress**	**Depression**
	2 Cedarwood	4 Bergamot	2 Cedarwood
	2 R. chamomile	2 Cedarwood	3 Geranium
	2 Clary sage	3 Lavender	4 Lavender
	4 Mandarin	2 Mandarin petitgrain	2 Melissa
	3 Neroli	3 Marjoram	3 Rose

Appendix B

SUGGESTED ESSENTIAL OIL KITS

The following sets are suggestions for essential oil starter sets.

Basic Three

Lavender
Peppermint
MQV (Alternate choices are *Eucalyptus globulus, Eucalyptus radiata,* or tea tree)

Versatile Five

Lavender
Peppermint
MQV (same choices as above)
Cedarwood
Geranium (or other floral oils like ylang-ylang, neroli, or rose)

Skin Care Complete

Carrot seed
All skin types and conditions, regenerative

Cistus
All skin types, regenerative, wrinkles and mature skin

Cape chamomile
All skin types and conditions, anti-inflammatory, soothing

Geranium

All skin types and conditions

Lavender

All skin types and conditions

Palmarosa

General skin care, anti-infectious, regenerative

Patchouli

All skin types and conditions, regenerative, fungicidal, decongestant

Rose

All skin types and conditions, regenerative, aging and wrinkled skin

Rosemary verbenone

General skin care, regenerative, vitalizing, mucolytic

Ylang-ylang

All skin types

Appendix C

EMOTIONS AND MIND

	Anger	Anxiety	Aphrodisiac	Ego/Insecurity	Depression	Grief	Irritability	Insomnia	Mental Stimulant/ Memory	Relaxation	Sedative	Sensitivity	Shock	Stress	Tension
Essential Oils															
Anise seed (*Pimpinella anisum*)	X	X	X		X		X					X	X	X	X
Basil (*Ocymum basilicum*)		X		X	X				X					X	X
Bay laurel (*Laurus nobilis*)	X	X						X				X		X	X
Bergamot (*Citrus bergamia*)	X	X				X	X	X				X		X	X
Birch (*Betula lenta*)															
Cardamon (*Elettaria cardamomum*)	X	X	X											X	X
Carrot seed (*Daucus carota*)										X					
Cedarwood (*Cedrus atlantica*)	X	X			X	X	X	X		X		X		X	X
Chamomile, Cape (*Eriocephalus punctulatus*)	X	X			X		X	X		X		X	X	X	X
Chamomile, German (*Matricaria recutita*)												X		X	

	Anger	Anxiety	Aphrodisiac	Ego/Insecurity	Depression	Grief	Irritability	Insomnia	Mental Stimulant/ Memory	Relaxation	Sedative	Sensitivity	Shock	Stress	Tension
Chamomile, Roman (*Anthemis nobilis*)	X	X			X	X	X	X		X	X	X	X	X	X
Cinnamon, bark (*Cinnamomum zeylanicum*)			X						X						
Cistus (*Cistus ladaniferus*)		X		X								X		X	X
Clary sage (*Salvia sclarea*)	X	X			X		X	X		X	X	X		X	X
Citronella (*Cymbopogon nardus*)					X										
Clove bud (*Eugenia caryophyllata*)			X						X						
Coriander (*Coriandrum sativum*)					X		X		X					X	X
Cypress (*Cupressus sempervirens*)						X								X	
Eucalyptus citriodora	X														
Eucalyptus dives										X					
Eucalyptus globulus	X														X
Eucalyptus radiata	X														
Eucalyptus staigeriana		X													
Everlasting (see Helichrysum)														X	X
Fennel (*Foeniculum vulgare*)				X	X		X						X	X	X
Fir (*Abies alba*)															
Frankincense (*Boswellia carterii*)		X	X	X	X	X	X					X		X	X
Galbanum (*Ferula galbaniflua*)		X	X	X			X					X		X	X
Geranium (*Pelargonium graveolens*)	X	X			X	X	X	X				X		X	X

Ginger (*Zinziber officinale*)														X	
Grapefruit (*Citrus paradisi*)							X					X		X	X
Helichrysum (*Helichrysum italicum*)					X		X	X				X		X	X
Inula graveolens		X												X	
Hyssop (*Hyssopus officinalis*)		X					X		X	X				X	X
Jasmine (*Jasminum grandiflorum*)		X	X	X	X	X	X			X		X		X	X
Juniper (*Juniperus communis*)														X	
Kunzea ambigua								X		X				X	X
Lavandin (*Lavandula hybrida*)		X					X	X		X		X		X	X
Lavender (*Lavandula angustifolia*)	X	X			X	X	X	X		X	X	X	X	X	X
Lemon (*Citrus limon*)		X			X		X							X	X
Lemongrass (*Cymbopogon citratus*)	X														X
Lemon verbena (*Lippia citriodora*)		X					X			X	X				
Lime (*Citrus limetta*)		X			X		X	X				X		X	X
Litsea cubeba							X					X		X	
Manadrin (*Citrus reticulata*) peel	X	X			X	X	X			X	X	X		X	X
Mandarin petitgrain (*Citrus reticulata*) leaves	X	X			X	X	X	X		X	X	X		X	X
Marjoram (*Origanum hortensis*)		X			X		X	X		X	X	X		X	X
Melissa (*Melissa officinalis*)	X	X					X	X		X		X		X	X
MQV (*Melaleuca quinquenervia viridiflora*)	X														X

Continued

	Anger	Anxiety	Aphrodisiac	Ego/Insecurity	Depression	Grief	Irritability	Insomnia	Mental Stimulant/ Memory	Relaxation	Sedative	Sensitivity	Shock	Stress	Tension
Myrrh (*Commiphora myrrha*)				X			X							X	X
Myrtle (*Myrtus communis*)														X	
Neroli (*Citrus aurantium*) blossom	X	X	X		X	X	X	X		X		X		X	X
Nutmeg (*Myristica fragrans*) seed		X	X						X					X	X
Orange, bitter (*Citrus aurantium*) peel		X			X		X					X		X	X
Orange, sweet (*Citrus sinensis*)		X			X		X					X		X	X
Oregano (*Origanum vulgaris*)															X
Palmarosa (*Cymbopogon martini*)							X							X	X
Patchouli (*Pogostemon cablin*)		X	X		X		X					X		X	X
Pepper (*Piper nigrum*)									X					X	X
Peppermint (*Mentha piperita*)					X				X						
Peru balsam (*Myroxylon pereira*)							X	X				X		X	X
Petitgrain (*Citrus aurantium*) leaves					X		X							X	X
Pine (*Pinus sylvestris*)									X						
Ravensare (*Ravensara aromatica*)															X
Rose (*Rosa damascena* or *centifolia*)	X	X	X	X	X	X	X	X		X	X	X		X	X

Rosemary, cineol type (*Rosmarinus officinalis*)	X					X			X						
Rosemary, supercritcal CO_2 extract (*Rosmarinus officinalis*)**									X						
Rosemary, verbenone type (*Rosmarinus officinalis*)										X					
Sage (*Salvia officinalis*)						X								X	
Saint John's wort (*Hypericum perforatum*)	X	X			X		X	X		X	X	X		X	X
Sandalwood, Australian (*Santalum spicatum*)		X	X		X	X	X					X		X	X
Savory (*Satureja hortensis*)									X						
Spearmint (*Mentha spicata*)									X						
Spike lavender (*Lavandula latifolia*)										X					X
Spikenard (*Nardostachys jatamansi*)				X		X				X	X	X	X	X	X
Spruce (*Picea mariana*)		X							X						
Tanacetum annuum												X		X	
Tarragon (*Artemisia dracunculus*)		X					X		X			X	X	X	X
Tea tree (*Melaleuca alternifolia*)															X
Thyme, geraniol type (*Thymus vulgaris*)												X			
Thyme, linalol type (*Thymus vulgaris*)		X					X					X			

Continued

	Anger	Anxiety	Aphrodisiac	Ego/Insecurity	Depression	Grief	Irritability	Insomnia	Mental Stimulant/ Memory	Relaxation	Sedative	Sensitivity	Shock	Stress	Tension
Thyme, thymol type (*Thymus vulgaris*)					X				X						
Thymus satureioides									X						
Tuberose (*Polianthes tuberosa*)		X	X	X		X	X					X		X	X
Vanilla (*Vanilla planifolia*)		X	X		X		X					X		X	X
Vetiver (*Vetiveria zizanoides*)					X		X					X		X	X
Vitex (*Vitex agnus castus*)					X		X					X			X
Wintergreen (*Gaultheria fragrantissima*)									X						
Yarrow (*Achillea millefolium*)		X					X					X			X
Ylang-ylang (*Cananga odorata*)		X	X		X	X	X	X		X	X	X		X	X
****Supercritical CO_2 extracts contain important components not found in the essential oil or described on the Structure-Effect Diagram.**															

PHYSICAL PROPERTIES

	Allergies	Cramping - Digestive	Cramping - Muscular	Constipation	Aids Circulation	Digestive Aid	Expectorant/Decongestant	Fever	Headaches	Indigestion	Inflammation	Pain Relief/Analgesic	Liver Tonic	Lymphatic	Menstrual Cramps	Menopause Imbalance	Spasm
Essential Oils																	
Anise seed (*Pimpinella anisum)*		X		X		X				X					X	X	X
Basil (*Ocymum basilicum*)						X		X		X						X	X
Bay laurel (*Laurus nobilis*)	X		X				X			X	X			X	X		X
Bergamot (*Citrus bergamia*)															X		X
Birch (*Betula lenta*)			X						X		X	X					X
Cardamon (*Elettaria cardamomum*)		X		X		X											X
Carrot seed (*Daucus carota*)						X				X						X	X
Cedarwood (*Cedrus atlantica*)	X	X			X		X				X			X	X	X	X
Chamomile, Cape (*Eriocephalus punctulatus*)	X		X					X			X	X			X	X	X
Chamomile, German (*Matricaria recutita*)	X		X					X			X				X		
Chamomile, Roman (*Anthemis nobilis*)			X	X					X		X				X	X	X
Cinnamon, bark (*Cinnamomum zeylanicum*)				X	X							X					
Cistus (*Cistus ladaniferus*)	X										X						
Citronella (*Cymbopogon nardus*)											X						X

Continued

	Allergies	Cramping - Digestive	Cramping - Muscular	Constipation	Aids Circulation	Digestive Aid	Expectorant/Decongestant	Fever	Headaches	Indigestion	Inflammation	Pain Relief/Analgesic	Liver Tonic	Lymphatic	Menstrual Cramps	Menopause Imbalance	Spasm
Clary sage (*Salvia sclarea*)			X												X		X
Clove bud (*Eugenia caryophyllata*)												X					
Coriander (*Coriandrum sativum*)		X		X		X				X							
Cypress (*Cupressus sempervirens*)							X				X		X	X	X		
Eucalyptus citriodora																	
Eucalyptus dives							X										
Eucalyptus globulus							X				X			X		X	
Eucalyptus radiata							X				X			X			
Eucalyptus staigeriana							X							X			
Everlasting (see Helichrysum)																	
Fennel (*Foeniculum vulgare*)		X		X		X				X				X	X	X	X
Fir (*Abies alba*)							X										
Frankincense (*Boswellia carterii*)	X		X					X	X		X					X	X
Galbanum (*Ferula galbaniflua*)	X		X								X					X	
Geranium (*Pelargonium graveolens*)	X		X			X			X		X		X		X	X	X
Ginger (*Zinziber officinale*)			X			X			X		X	X			X	X	
Grapefruit (*Citrus paradisi*)														X			
Helichrysum (*Helichrysum italicum*)	X		X					X	X		X				X	X	X
Inula graveolens							X										
Hyssop (*Hyssopus officinalis*)					X					X	X						

Jasmine (*Jasminum grandiflorum*)															X	X	
Juniper (*Juniperus communis*)											X						
Kunzea ambigua	X		X								X				X	X	
Lavandin (*Lavandula hybrida*)											X						X
Lavender (*Lavandula angustifolia*)	X		X		X			X	X	X	X	X			X	X	X
Lemon (*Citrus limon*)							X	X		X	X			X			
Lemongrass (*Cymbopogon citratus*)							X										
Lemon verbena (*Lippia citriodora*)		X									X	X					X
Lime (*Citrus limetta*)														X			
Litsea cubeba																	
Manadrin (*Citrus reticulata*) peel			X	X		X											X
Mandarin petitgrain (*Citrus reticulata*) leaves			X						X				X		X		X
Marjoram (*Origanum hortensis*)				X											X	X	X
Melissa (*Melissa officinalis*)			X						X		X				X	X	X
MQV (*Melaleuca quinquenervia viridiflora*)	X		X				X				X				X		
Myrrh (*Commiphora myrrha*)	X										X						
Myrtle (*Myrtus communis*)							X										
Neroli (*Citrus aurantium*) blossom			X												X		X
Nutmeg (*Myristica fragrans*) seed											X						
Orange, bitter (*Citrus aurantium*) peel						X				X				X			
Orange, sweet (*Citrus sinensis*)						X				X				X			

Continued

	Allergies	Cramping - Digestive	Cramping - Muscular	Constipation	Aids Circulation	Digestive Aid	Expectorant/Decongestant	Fever	Headaches	Indigestion	Inflammation	Pain Relief/Analgesic	Liver Tonic	Lymphatic	Menstrual Cramps	Menopause Imbalance	Spasm
Oregano (*Origanum vulgaris*)					X						X	X					
Palmarosa (*Cymbopogon martini*)																	
Patchouli (*Pogostemon cablin*)	X				X						X	X					
Pepper (*Piper nigrum*)				X				X			X	X			X		
Peppermint (*Mentha piperita*)		X	X	X	X	X		X	X	X	X		X				
Peru balsam (*Myroxylon pereira*)	X										X						
Petitgrain (*Citrus aurantium*) leaves																	X
Pine (*Pinus sylvestris*)							X							X			
Ravensare (*Ravensara aromatica*)	X						X										
Rose (*Rosa damascena* or *centifolia*)	X		X	X			X		X		X		X		X	X	X
Rosemary, cineol type (*Rosmarinus officinalis*)					X	X	X			X	X	X	X				
Rosemary, supercritcal CO_2 extract (*Rosmarinus officinalis*)**													X				
Rosemary, verbenone type (*Rosmarinus officinalis*)						X					X		X				
Sage (*Salvia officinalis*)										X	X				X		X
Saint John's wort (*Hypericum perforatum*)								X	X								
Sandalwood, Australian (*Santalum spicatum*)										X	X				X		
Savory (*Satureja hortensis*)												X					

Spearmint (*Mentha spicata*)						X					X	X	X				
Spike lavender (*Lavandula latifolia*)			X									X					X
Spikenard (*Nardostachys jatamansi*)	X		X					X		X	X				X	X	X
Spruce (*Picea mariana*)							X										
Tanacetum annuum	X		X								X	X			X		
Tarragon (*Artemisia dracunculus*)		X		X		X				X					X		X
Tea tree (*Melaleuca alternifolia*)							X										
Thyme, geraniol type (*Thymus vulgaris*)			X						X								
Thyme, linalol type (*Thymus vulgaris*)			X						X								
Thyme, thymol type (*Thymus vulgaris*)					X							X					
Thymus satureioides					X												
Tuberose (*Polianthes tuberosa*)																	
Vanilla (*Vanilla planifolia*)																	
Vetiver (*Vetiveria zizanoides*)											X						
Vitex (*Vitex agnus castus*)															X	X	
Wintergreen (*Gaultheria fragrantissima*)			X								X	X					X
Yarrow (*Achillea millefolium*)	X							X			X				X	X	
Ylang-ylang (*Cananga odorata*)			X												X	X	X
****Supercritical CO_2 extracts contain important components not found in the essential oil or described on the Structure-Effect Diagram.**																	

SKIN CARE

	Acne	Allergies	Astringent	Boils	Bug Bites	Burns	Chapped/Cracked	Congestion/Water Retention	Dandruff	Dermatitis/Eczema	Detoxify/Purify	Dry Skin	Mature Skin	Oily Skin	Psoriasis	Regenerative	Rosacea	Scars/Stretch Marks	Sensitive Skin	Varicose Veins	Warts	Wrinkles	Wounds
Essential Oils																							
Anise seed (*Pimpinella anisum*)																							
Basil (*Ocymum basilicum*)									X														
Bay laurel (*Laurus nobilis*)	X	X			X			X		X	X			X		X				X			X
Bergamot (*Citrus bergamia*)				X				X			X			X									
Birch (*Betula lenta*)																							
Cardamon (*Elettaria cardamomum*)																							
Carrot seed (*Daucus carota*)	X				X	X	X	X		X	X	X	X		X	X	X	X	X	X		X	X
Cedarwood (*Cedrus atlantica*)	X	X	X		X	X	X	X	X	X	X	X	X	X	X	X	X	X	X	X		X	X
Chamomile, Cape (*Eriocephalus punctulatus*)	X	X		X	X	X	X		X	X			X	X	X		X	X	X			X	X
Chamomile, German (*Matricaria recutita*)	X	X		X	X	X				X					X		X		X				
Chamomile, Roman (*Anthemis nobilis*)	X	X			X	X				X					X				X				

Cinnamon, bark (*Cinnamomum zeylanicum*)																							
Cistus (*Cistus ladaniferus*)		X		X	X	X	X			X		X	X	X	X	X	X	X	X	X		X	X
Citronella (*Cymbopogon nardus*)	X		X		X						X												
Clary sage (*Salvia sclarea*)	X								X					X									
Clove bud (*Eugenia caryophyllata*)																							
Coriander (*Coriandrum sativum*)																							
Cypress (*Cupressus sempervirens*)	X		X					X	X		X			X						X			
Eucalyptus citriodora	X							X			X			X									
Eucalyptus dives	X				X					X	X	X	X	X	X	X	X	X	X			X	X
Eucalyptus globulus	X	X		X	X			X			X			X						X			X
Eucalyptus radiata	X	X		X	X			X			X			X						X			
Eucalyptus staigeriana	X				X			X			X			X						X			
Everlasting (see *Helichrysum*)																							
Fennel (*Foeniculum vulgare*)	X							X						X						X			
Fir (*Abies alba*)																							
Frankincense (*Boswellia carterii*)		X	X	X	X	X	X		X	X		X	X		X	X	X	X	X	X		X	X
Galbanum (*Ferula galbaniflua*)		X				X	X		X	X		X	X						X			X	

Continued

	Acne	Allergies	Astringent	Boils	Bug Bites	Burns	Chapped/Cracked	Congestion/Water Retention	Dandruff	Dermatitis/Eczema	Detoxify/Purify	Dry Skin	Mature Skin	Oily Skin	Psoriasis	Regenerative	Rosacea	Scars/Stretch Marks	Sensitive Skin	Varicose Veins	Warts	Wrinkles	Wounds
Geranium (*Pelargonium graveolens*)	X	X	X	X	X	X	X	X	X	X	X	X	X	X	X	X	X	X	X	X	X	X	X
Ginger (*Zinziber officinale*)		X								X													
Grapefruit (*Citrus paradisi*)	X							X			X			X						X			
Helichrysum (*Helichrysum italicum*)	X	X		X	X	X	X		X	X		X	X	X	X	X	X	X	X	X		X	X
Inula graveolens	X	X		X				X			X			X									
Hyssop (*Hyssopus officinalis*)										X		X				X							
Jasmine (*Jasminum grandiflorum*)							X					X	X						X			X	
Juniper (*Juniperus communis*)	X		X					X	X		X			X									
Kunzea ambigua		X		X	X					X					X		X		X				
Lavandin (*Lavandula hybrida*)	X	X		X	X	X	X					X	X	X	X				X		X		X
Lavender (*Lavandula angustifolia*)	X	X		X	X	X	X		X	X	X	X	X	X	X	X	X	X	X	X	X	X	X
Lemon (*Citrus limon*)	X			X				X	X		X			X						X	X		
Lemongrass (*Cymbopogon citratus*)	X			X				X	X		X			X									
Lemon verbena (*Lippia citriodora*)			X						X		X												

Lime (*Citrus limetta*)	X			X				X	X		X			X									
Litsea cubeba	X			X				X			X			X									
Manadrin (*Citrus reticulata*) peel	X		X											X									
Mandarin petitgrain (*Citrus reticulata*) leaves	X											X		X				X				X	
Marjoram (*Origanum hortensis*)		X			X																		
Melissa (*Melissa officinalis*)	X													X									
MQV (*Melaleuca quinquenervia viridiflora*)	X	X		X	X	X		X	X	X	X		X	X	X	X				X			X
Myrrh (*Commiphora myrrha*)	X	X	X	X	X	X	X		X	X		X	X		X		X	X	X	X	X	X	X
Myrtle (*Myrtus communis*)	X																						
Neroli (*Citrus aurantium*) blossom				X			X												X				
Nutmeg (*Myristica fragrans*) seed																							
Orange, bitter (*Citrus aurantium*) peel	X			X				X			X			X						X			
Orange, sweet (*Citrus sinensis*)	X			X				X			X			X						X			
Oregano (*Origanum vulgaris*)	X																						
Palmarosa (*Cymbopogon martini*)	X	X		X	X	X	X			X		X	X	X	X	X	X		X	X	X	X	X
Patchouli (*Pogostemon cablin*)		X	X	X	X	X	X		X	X	X	X	X	X	X	X	X	X	X	X	X	X	X

Continued

	Acne	Allergies	Astringent	Boils	Bug Bites	Burns	Chapped/Cracked	Congestion/Water Retention	Dandruff	Dermatitis/Eczema	Detoxify/Purify	Dry Skin	Mature Skin	Oily Skin	Psoriasis	Regenerative	Rosacea	Scars/Stretch Marks	Sensitive Skin	Varicose Veins	Warts	Wrinkles	Wounds
Pepper (*Piper nigrum*)													X										
Peppermint (*Mentha piperita*)	X		X					X	X		X			X									
Peru balsam (*Myroxylon pereira*)							X		X	X		X	X		X		X	X			X	X	
Petitgrain (*Citrus aurantium*) leaves	X				X																		
Pine (*Pinus sylvestris*)								X			X												
Ravensare (*Ravensara aromatica*)	X			X	X			X	X		X			X						X			
Rose (*Rosa damascena* or *centifolia*)	X	X	X	X	X	X	X	X	X	X	X	X	X	X	X	X	X	X	X	X	X	X	X
Rosemary, cineol type (*Rosmarinus officinalis*)	X		X	X				X	X		X			X						X			
Rosemary+A88, supercritcal CO_2 extract (*Rosmarinus officinalis*)**	X			X	X		X		X	X			X	X	X	X	X	X	X	X		X	X
Rosemary, verbenone type (*Rosmarinus officinalis*)	X			X	X		X		X	X		X	X	X	X	X	X	X	X	X		X	X
Sage (*Salvia officinalis*)							X		X	X					X	X	X	X	X			X	X
Saint John's wort (*Hypericum perforatum*)		X					X								X				X				X

Sandalwood, Australian (*Santalum spicatum*)	X	X	X	X	X	X	X		X	X		X	X	X	X		X	X	X			X	X
Savory (*Satureja hortensis*)																							
Spearmint (*Mentha spicata*)	X								X					X									
Spike lavender (*Lavandula latifolia*)	X	X		X		X	X			X		X	X		X	X	X	X	X		X	X	X
Spikenard (*Nardostachys jatamansi*)		X		X		X	X			X		X	X		X	X	X				X	X	
Spruce (*Picea mariana*)																							
Tanacetum annuum	X	X		X	X	X				X					X		X		X				
Tarragon (*Artemisia dracunculus*)																							
Tea tree (*Melaleuca alternifolia*)	X			X	X	X	X	X	X	X	X			X	X					X	X		X
Thyme, geraniol type (*Thymus vulgaris*)	X			X	X	X	X		X			X	X		X						X		X
Thyme, linalol type (*Thymus vulgaris*)	X			X	X	X	X			X					X		X				X		X
Thyme, thymol type (*Thymus vulgaris*)																							
Thymus satureioides	X																				X		
Tuberose (*Polianthes tuberosa*)							X																
Vanilla (*Vanilla planifolia*)							X					X											
Vetiver (*Vetiveria zizanoides*)				X	X	X	X			X		X	X		X		X		X		X	X	
Vitex (*Vitex agnus castus*)													X										

Continued

	Acne	Allergies	Astringent	Boils	Bug Bites	Burns	Chapped/Cracked	Congestion/Water Retention	Dandruff	Dermatitis/Eczema	Detoxify/Purify	Dry Skin	Mature Skin	Oily Skin	Psoriasis	Regenerative	Rosacea	Scars/Stretch Marks	Sensitive Skin	Varicose Veins	Warts	Wrinkles	Wounds
Wintergreen (*Gaultheria fragrantissima*)																							
Yarrow (*Achillea millefolium*)		X		X	X	X											X		X				
Ylang-ylang (*Cananga odorata*)	X			X					X					X					X				
****Supercritical CO_2 extracts contain important components not found in the essential oil or described on the Structure-Effect Diagram.**																							

CHEMICAL FAMILY

X = Predominant chemical class. Main or important influence comes from the compounds in the chemical family.

* = Contains compounds from the chemical family in lesser amounts or is not as influential in overall effects of the oil.

	Monoterpene Hydrocarbons	Sesquiterpene Hydrocarbons	Monoterpene Alcohols	Sesquiterpene Alcohols	Diterpene Alcohols	Monoterpene Aldehydes	Monoterpene Ketones	Sesquiterpene Ketones	Diketones	Monoterpene Esters	Monoterpene Oxides	Phenols	Phenylpropanes	Ethers	Sesquiterpene Lactones
Essential Oils															
Anise seed (*Pimpinella anisum*)		*	*			*	*							X	
Basil (*Ocymum basilicum*)	*	*	X							*	X		*	X	

Bay laurel (*Laurus nobilis*)	*	X	X				*			X	X		X		
Bergamot (*Citrus bergamia*)	X		X							X					
Birch (*Betula lenta*)										X					
Cardamon (*Elettaria cardamomum*)	X		X							X	X				
Carrot seed (*Daucus carota*)	X	X	X	X						*	*			*	
Cedarwood (*Cedrus atlantica*)		X		X				X							
Chamomile, Cape (*Eriocephalus punctulatus*)	X	X	*					*		X	*				
Chamomile, German (*Matricaria recutita*)		X		X							*				
Chamomile, Roman (*Anthemis nobilis*)			*				*			X					
Cinnamon, bark (*Cinnamomum zeylanicum*)	*	*	*							*			X		
Cistus (*Cistus ladaniferus*)	X		X		X	*	*			*					
Citronella (*Cymbopogon nardus*)	X		X			X				*					
Clary sage (*Salvia sclarea*)	*	X	X	X	X	*	*			X	*			*	
Clove bud (*Eugenia caryophyllata*)		X								X	*		X		
Coriander (*Coriandrum sativum*)			X			X	*							*	
Cypress (*Cupressus sempervirens*)	X	X	*	X	*					*					
Eucalyptus citriodora			X			X				*					
Eucalyptus dives	X	*	X				X								
Eucalyptus globulus	X	X	X			*	X			X	X				
Eucalyptus radiata	*		X			X					X				
***Eucalyptus polybractea* - cineole type**	*		*								X				
***Eucalyptus polybractea* – cryptone type**	X		X			*	X				X				
Eucalyptus staigeriana	X		*			X				*	X				

Continued

	Monoterpene Hydrocarbons	Sesquiterpene Hydrocarbons	Monoterpene Alcohols	Sesquiterpene Alcohols	Diterpene Alcohols	Monoterpene Aldehydes	Monoterpene Ketones	Sesquiterpene Ketones	Diketones	Monoterpene Esters	Monoterpene Oxides	Phenols	Phenylpropanes	Ethers	Sesquiterpene Lactones
Everlasting (*see* Helichrysum)	*		*			*				X					
Fennel (*Foeniculum vulgare*)	*						X							X	
Fir (*Abies alba*)	X									X					
Frankincense (*Boswellia carterii*)	X	X	*	X											
Galbanum (*Ferula galbaniflua*)	X	X		X						*					
Geranium (*Pelargonium graveolens*)	*	*	X			X	*			X	*				
Ginger (*Zinziber officinale*)	*	X	X	X		X	*				*				
Grapefruit (*Citrus paradisi*)	X	X						X	X						
Helichrysum (*Helichrysum italicum*)	*	X	*						X	X					
Inula graveolens										X					X
Hyssop (*Hyssopus officinalis*)	*	X	X				X				*				
Jasmine (*Jasminum grandiflorum*)			X				X			X					
Juniper (*Juniperus communis*)	X	X	*							*					
Kunzea ambigua	X		X	X							X				
Lavandin (*Lavandula hybrida*)	*		X							X					
Lavender (*Lavandula angustifolia*)	*	*	X			*	*			X	X				
Lemon (*Citrus limon*)	X	*	*			X									
Lemongrass (*Cymbopogon citratus*)	X		*			X				*					

Lemon verbena (*Lippia citriodora*)	*	X	X			X					*				
Lime (*Citrus limetta*)	X		X							X					
Litsea cubeba	X	*	X			X				*					
Manadrin (*Citrus reticulata*) peel	X		X			*				X					
Mandarin petitgrain (*Citrus reticulata*) leaves			X							X					
Marjoram (*Origanum hortensis*)	X	*	X							X					
Melissa (*Melissa officinalis*)	*	X	*			X				*	*				
MQV (*Melaleuca quinquenervia viridiflora*)	X	X	X	X		*				*	X				
Myrrh (*Commiphora myrrha*)	X	X	*			*						*			
Myrtle, red (*Myrtus communis*)	X	X	X			*				X	X				
Neroli (*Citrus aurantium*) blossom	X		X	*		X	*			X					
Nutmeg (*Myristica fragrans*) seed	X		X								*	*		X	
Orange, bitter (*Citrus aurantium*) peel	X		X			*				X					
Orange, sweet (*Citrus sinensis*)	X					X	*								
Oregano (*Origanum vulgaris*)	*	*	*							*		X			
Palmarosa (*Cymbopogon martini*)			X	*						X					
Patchouli (*Pogostemon cablin*)	*	X	X	X		*	*								
Pepper (*Piper nigrum*)	*	X	*			*	X								
Peppermint (*Mentha piperita*)	*	X	X	*			X			*	*				
Peru balsam (*Myroxylon pereira*)			X			X				X					
Petitgrain (*Citrus aurantium*) leaves	X	*	X							X					
Pine (*Pinus sylvestris*)	X	X	*							*					
Ravensare (*Ravensara aromatica*)	*	X	X							*	X	*		*	

Continued

	Monoterpene Hydrocarbons	Sesquiterpene Hydrocarbons	Monoterpene Alcohols	Sesquiterpene Alcohols	Diterpene Alcohols	Monoterpene Aldehydes	Monoterpene Ketones	Sesquiterpene Ketones	Diketones	Monoterpene Esters	Monoterpene Oxides	Phenols	Phenylpropanes	Ethers	Sesquiterpene Lactones
Rose (*Rosa damascena* or *centifolia*)	X		X				X			*	*	*			
Rosemary, cineol type (*Rosmarinus officinalis*)	*	*	X				*			*	X				
Rosemary, supercritcal CO_2 extract (*Rosmarinus officinalis*)**	X	X	X				X			*	X				
Rosemary, verbenone type (*Rosmarinus officinalis*)	X	*	X				X			*	X				
Sage (*Salvia officinalis*)	X	X	X	X	*		X			*	*	*			
Saint John's wort (*Hypericum perforatum*)	*	X	*				*				*				
Sandalwood, Australian (*Santalum spicatum*)	*	X		X											
Savory (*Satureja hortensis*)	X	*	*									X			
Spearmint (*Mentha spicata*)	X	X	X				X			*	*				
Spike lavender (*Lavandula latifolia*)	X		*				X			*	X				
Spikenard (*Nardostachys jatamansi*)		X		X		*	*	X							
Spruce (*Picea mariana*)	X	*	*	*						X					
Tanacetum annuum	*	X					*								
Tarragon (*Artemisia dracunculus*)														X	

Tea tree (*Melaleuca alternifolia*)	*	*	X								X				
Thyme, geraniol type (*Thymus vulgaris*)	*		X							X					
Thyme, linalol type (*Thymus vulgaris*)	*	*	X							X		*			
Thyme, thymol type (*Thymus vulgaris*)	X	X	X				*			*	*	X		*	
Thymus satureioides	X			X								X			
Tuberose (*Polianthes tuberosa*)			X	X						X					
Vanilla (*Vanilla planifolia*)			*			X				*				X	
Vetiver (*Vetiveria zizanoides*)		X		X			*			*					
Vitex (*Vitex agnus castus*)	X	X	*	X	X										
Wintergreen (*Gaultheria fragrantissima*)			*			*				X		*		*	
Yarrow (*Achillea millefolium*)	*	X	*				X				*				*
Ylang-ylang (*Cananga odorata*)	*	X	X							X		*			
****Supercritical CO_2 extracts contain important components not found in the essential oil or described on the Structure-Effect Diagram.**															

Appendix D

FRAGONIA

There's a story to be told about this essential oil, recently introduced to the aromatherapy market. For the complete tale, you'll have to read Volume 36 (August 2006) of the journal *Aromatherapy Today*. The edited version is as follows. The oil, from southwestern Australia, is called Fragonia™. The plant from which the oil is extracted was originally identified only as *Agonis sp.* and received its completed nomenclature, *Agonis fragrans*, in 2001. The story involves a botanist, Chris Robinson, and the husband–wife team of John and Peta Day. Robinson's curiosity about the plant and the Days' willingness to cultivate it have provided the aromatherapy community with an oil that Dr. Daniel Pénoël has called the "oil for the new millennium."

What is strikingly unique about Fragonia is its chemical structure. The ratio in which the chemical structure is formed is very similar to what is called the "Golden Ratio." The Golden Ratio is introduced in Chapter 1 as the formula that Dr. Marquardt used to design his beauty mask and is believed to be the most esthetically pleasing geometric ratio in art and nature. The golden proportion seen in this oil is thought to be a marker of its potential ability to create balance in the body and mind. According to the few aromatherapists who have written about the oil, its balancing properties are remarkable. The proportions at successive levels of the molecular structure — from the golden proportions of the molecular groupings to the proportions of the compounds within the groupings — mimic fractal geometry. Fractals are objects in which the parts are a reduced-sized copy of the whole. Look at a fern. Each leaf is shaped like the whole branch, and each section of the leaf has a similar shape. In Fragonia, the pattern is similar; for instance, the monoterpene group makes up approximately 30 to 39 percent; the main compound in the monoterpene group, alpha-pinene, is 21 to 27 percent; and the lesser monoterpenes are in close-to-equal proportions at 1.4 to 2.9 percent. Dr. Pénoël links the fractal and golden proportions of Fragonia to its actions on the human organism from "cell to psyche."

Fragonia is the first essential oil to have a trademarked name. This fact offers a unique buying situation in aromatherapy. When you purchase a trademarked oil, you are guaranteed a specific quality with a well-defined chemical structure. At the time of this writing, the oil is not commercially available in large quantities.

FRAGONIA[1, 2, 3, 4]

Botanical name	*Agonis fragrans*
Botanical family	Myrtaceae
Derived from	Branches, leaves
Origin	Australia
Cost	—
Fragrance character	Middle note. It is very pleasant with an obvious cineole (tea tree) fragrance and a prevailing linalool (rosewood, lavender) note, along with citrus, woods and spice.
Blends well with	Experimental at this point. Likely to blend well with most oils.
Application	Any
Main components	1:1:1 ratio of monterpenes, oxides, and C-10 alcohols

THERAPEUTIC USES

Properties	Experimental, with preliminary testing demonstrating antimicrobial, anti-inflammatory, emotional balance, expectorant, and immune support
Medicinal use	Preliminary testing has seen results for: antibacterial, candidiasis (yeast infection), congestion, inflammation (tissue injury)
Skin, hair & body	Experimental
Mind/emotions	Preliminary results for: anxiety, balancing, disturbed sleep, stress, tension
Spiritual	Experimental
Contraindications	From chemical analysis, no toxicity is anticipated.

REFERENCES

1. Pénoël, D. "Fragonia™: The Latest Promising Aromatic Gift from Australia." *Aromatherapy Today*. August, 2006; Vol. 3.
2. Day, P., Day, J. "Fragonia™: The Oil for the New Millennium." *Aromatherapy Today*. August, 2006; Vol. 3.
3. Guba, R. "The Chemistry of Fragonia™." *Aromatherapy Today*. August, 2006; Vol. 3.
4. Wallwork, K. "Fragonia™ Essential Oil." *Aromatherapy Today*. August, 2006; Vol. 3.

Glossary

A

Absolute an essence produced by solvent extraction, the method most commonly used to extract the more delicate essences, such as jasmine and tuberose

Adulteration the practice of adding synthetics, isolated compounds common to the specific oil, or cheaper natural oils to the pure essential oil

Aldehyde a functional group defined by a carbonyl group attached to a hydrocarbon group and a hydrogen atom

Allopathic Medicine A system of treating a disease by producing a reaction that is antagonistic to the disease. This is the system used by most Western educated physicians.

Amygdala an area of the limbic system related to memory and emotions

Anosmia the inability to detect odor

Antioxidants compounds that neutralize free radicals by donating an electron to the free radical's electron pair

Aromacology a scientific study of smell, primarily investigating the emotional and behavioral effects of odors

Aromatherapy the art and science of using essential oils derived from plants, flowers, fruits, seeds, and woods for the health and wellness of the body, mind, and spirit

Aromatic Compound a stable class of compounds because of the equal distribution of the electrons

Aromatic Ring a 6 carbon cyclic structure containing three double bonds

Aromatogram test method used by Paul Belaiche to examine the ability of the whole oil, or individual compounds, to inhibit or kill specific microorganisms

Ascorbyl Palmitate a vitamin C ester formed by combining, or reacting, L-ascorbic acid with fatty acids from vitamin C

Atomic Number The number of protons in the nucleus. This number determines the position on the Periodic Table.

Atomic Weight on the Periodic Table, this number is below the element's symbol and represents the sum of the neutrons and protons contained within the atom

Atoms the smallest particle of an element that still retains its character

Autonomic Nervous System the system of the body that controls involuntary bodily functions: heart rate, breathing, and digestion

B

Base a term used to describe a carrier for essential oils, most commonly referring to a therapeutic fixed oil formula, creams or lotions

Beauty the quality of objects, sounds, ideas, etc., that pleases and gratifies as by their harmony, pattern, excellence or truth

Biologically Familiar a term used by the author to describe a quality of ingredients used in skin care that exist in nature as plants, animals, and minerals, or the compounds extracted from those

Biosynthesis the process used by living organisms to produce, change, restructure and eliminate the chemical structures used by the organism

Biosynthetic Pathway The chain of events that occurs in the formation of chemical compounds in a living organism. The chemicals used by mammals and all living organisms are produced, changed, restructured, and eliminated using enzymes, water, atoms, and other compounds in a process called biosynthesis.

C

Candidiasis an infection of the *Candida albicans* yeast

Carbonyl Group a functional group composed of an oxygen atom double bonded to a carbon atom

Carrier Oil A vegetable, nut, or fruit oil in which essential oils are diluted. Carrier oils are often selected for their individual therapeutic and healing properties.

Centrifugation a force created by spinning at high speeds and used to extract essential oil from the citrus peel

Chemical Bonds the bond formed when atoms combine to create a balance in their outer energy levels by sharing electrons with other atoms

Chemical Polymorphism when a plant from one specified botanical origin produces differing composition

Chemotaxis the first sense mechanism of single celled organisms; the ability of cells to sense and move (taxis) toward or away from chemicals (chemo) in the environment

Chemotype an identifying name, usually following the botanical name, that identifies the main component contained in essential oils coming from a plant of a specified botanical origin that prouces differing composition, or chemical polymorphism

Chiral objects that cannot be superimposed on their mirror image, like hands

Chromatogram the record that results from of gas chromatography analysis, showing peaks proportional to the quantity of the corresponding compounds in the essential oil

Civilization Diseases diseases that result from lifestyle or from a poor relationship with the environment, such as cancers, asthma, and autoimmune diseases

Cold Expression the process used to extract the essential oil from citrus peels; also called cold pressing or scarification

Cold Pressed The process used to extract the essential oil from citrus peels. Also called cold expression or scarification.

Compounds the combination of two or more elements created by the sharing of electrons, ionic bonds or hydrogen bonding

Concréte the salve-like substance created by treating plant material with the solvent hexane during the production of absolutes

Cosmeceuticals The term used to define nutrients and vitamins that are added to a cosmetic formula with pharmaceutical like activity. Also called nutraceuticals.

Cortisol a corticosteroid produced by the adrenal cortex and released during times of stress

Coumarin a trace element found in many essential oils, such as lavender and khella (Ammi visnaga)

Covalent Bond nonmetal elements form covalent bonds by sharing electrons

D

Degummed a process that removes phosphorous-containing lipids from fixed oils

Dilution reducing the concentration of essential oil in the entire product or blend

Dipole a molecule with an equal, but opposite charge, or the separation of negative and positive charge, in a polar covalent bond

Distillation the process that uses steam, water, or both to extract the essence from plant materials

Diterpene Alcohol a compound defined by a free hydroxy group (-OH) attached to a diterpene (C-20) hydrocarbon

Double Bond occurs when two atoms bond by sharing two electrons

E

Eczema an acute or chronic skin inflammation

Electron a subatomic particle with a negative charge orbiting the nucleus of the atom

Electron Arrangement the arrangement of electrons orbiting the nucleus

Electron Pair two electrons that join to spin and orbit in opposite directions around a nucleus

Electronegativity the tendency of an element to attract electrons in a bond

Electropositivity the tendency of an element to lose an electron in a bond

Elements The primary substances that build all other objects and things. Elements include oxygen, carbon, hydrogen, silver, and zinc.

Emerging Properties the special quality that arises from the hierarchical order at each stage of development

Empirical Evidence scientific documentation derived from direct experience or observation

Emulsified when ingredients, or substances that normally do not stay together, such as oil and water, have an ability to combine with the help of an ingredient that acts as an emulsifier

Emulsifier a substance or compound used to combine ingredients together, such as oil and water, that do not mix

Enantiomers Molecules with almost identical formula and arrangement, their only difference being its symmetry. They are two non-superimposable mirror images of each other. Enantiomers are two chiral molecules.

Endocrine System a network of glands that secrete hormones into blood or lymph that have a specific action or effect on organs, tissue, or the entire body

Endorphins neurotransmitters known to reduce pain and stimulate sexual arousal

Enfleurage an ancient method of extracting the essence from plants and flowers, using animal fat or a vegetable oil

Energy Levels the term used to describe the arrangement levels of electrons around the nucleus of the atom

Epithelium a mucous layered area at the top of the nostrils containing millions of olfactory nerve endings

Essential Fatty Acids polyunsaturated fatty acids that are vital for many functions of the body in addition to the strength and structure of cells

Essential Oil a volatile oil extracted from plants by distillation with either water or steam or by mechanical process of citrus rinds

Essence An oily, fragrant substance contained within pockets or cells of plants. When the essence is extracted using distillation or by mechanical process of citrus rinds, it is called an essential oil.

Ester a compound that is produced by a reaction of carboxylic acid and an alcohol

Ethers a family of compounds with an oxygen atom connected to two hydrocarbon groups

F

Fatty Acid a hydrocarbon chain with one of the hydrogen atoms replaced by a carboxyl group (COOH)

Fitzpatrick Scale a classification of skin developed by Thomas Fitzpatrick, MD, PhD that classifies skin in a I–VI scale based on its tolerance to the sun's burning rays

Fixative the essential oil(s) that holds together the fragrance aspect of a blend by slowing down the rate of evaporation of the more volatile components in the blend

Fixed Oil a botanically derived and non-volatile oil usually extracted from nuts or the seeds of vegetables and fruits

Folk Medicine intuitive and traditional knowledge of the healing and medicinal use of plants and aromatics that has been passed down from generations of use

Free Radical An atom or molecule with an unpaired electron. In order to regain the stability of an electron pair, the free radical steals electrons from other molecules.

Functional Groups An atom or group of atoms that attaches to a hydrocarbon, usually containing oxygen. The functional group gives a unique characteristic and function to the compound and is organized in chemical families or groups. The functional groups form some of the most versatile and useful properties in aromatherapy.

G

Gas Chromatography/Mass Spectrometry (GC/MS) a method used to analyze the composition of essential oils and uncover falsifications and adulterations

Glycation the breakdown of protein caused by sugar binding

H

Herbal Tincture an herbal remedy using alcohol or glycerin to extract the medicinal properties from the plant material

Hippocampus an area of the limbic system related to memory and emotions

Holism viewing an organism as a unified whole, in which the parts are no longer viewed as individual units but are analyzed in relationship with the whole organism

Holistic Beauty viewing beauty as a dimension of holistic health and health maintenance throughout the aging process

Holistic Health a method of health and healing that cares for the whole person—the physical, mental, and social conditions—not just the physical symptoms, in treating illness

Homeostasis physiological equilibrium or the ability of an organism to maintain internal balance in an ever changing environment

Hormones chemicals produced and released from an organ or part of the body that regulates or initiates an activity in another organ or body part

Humectant an agent that promotes moisture retention

Hydration The chemical combination of a substance with water. The saturation of tissue in the body is also called hydration.

Hydrocarbon compound composed of carbon and hydrogen

Hydrodiffusion Plant material is placed in a still completely immersed in water that is heated causing the evaporation of the oils without the use of steam. Also called water distillation.

Hydrogen Bonds weak bonds or forces between water molecules and other interesting and important molecular arrangements that play an important role in the chemistry of life

Hydrolate The therapeutic water by-product of essential oil distillation. Also called hydrosol.

Hydrosol The therapeutic water by-product of essential oil distillation. Also called hydrolate.

Hypothalamus an area of the brain that plays a predominant role in the production and release of hormone-like substances that control hunger, thirst, body temperature, and other body functions related to homeostasis

I

Inert inactive or substances that have limited chemical interaction with the body or other ingredients in a formula

Ionic Bonds Chemical bonds formed when the electrons of metals are attracted to the nuclei of nonmetals. In this formation the metal loses an electron, or is oxidized, and the nonmetal gains an electron, or is reduced.

Ions atoms with an electrical charge created when the atom loses or gains an electron

Isolate an active compound, such as a vitamin or nutrient, extracted or isolated from a plant, food or other source

Isomers molecules having the same summary formula but of a different structural arrangement of the atoms in the molecule

Isoprene Units hydrocarbon compounds made up of 5 carbon atoms

Isoprenoids the main chemical structure of essential oil compounds

K

Keratolytic an agent that promotes the softening and shedding of the horny outer layer of skin cells, or exfoliation

L

Lactone an ester group integrated into a carbon ring system

Limbic System The most primitive parts of the brain and includes the hypothalamus, the amygdala, and the hippocampus. It influences the endocrine and the autonomic nervous systems.

Lipids fats or fat-like substances

M

Metabolism the sum of all physical and chemical changes that take place in an organism and all the material changes that occur within living cells

Monoterpene Alcohols A compound defined by a hydroxy functional group (-OH) bonded to a monoterpene (C-10) hydrocarbon. These are considered the most beneficial and safest of the essential oil compounds.

Monoterpene Hydrocarbon The most basic essential oil molecule. This is a terpene hydrocarbon containing 10 carbon atoms (C-10).

Mucolytic agents that are able to liquefy or dissolve hardened mucous

N

Nanoparticles manufactured particles that are less than 100 nanometers in size

Neuropeptides peptides released from neurons using chemical signals to communicate with and influence the body and also affect behavior

Neurotransmitters messenger molecules that excite or inhibit a specific activity of its target cell

Neutron a subatomic particle with neutral, or no charge, within the nucleus of the atom

Nutratceutical The term used for vitamins and nutrients when used as pharmaceutical agent or therapeutically. These are called cosmeceuticals when added to cosmetics.

O

Occlusive Layer a barrier, usually produced by an ingredient, that is used to prevent water loss from the skin

Octet Rule the tendency for atoms to adjust to eight valence electrons

Odor Receptor Neurons (ORN) the olfactory nerves, which regenerate and replace dead neurons every 60 days

Oleoresins oils that are extracted from plant resins and gums using an alcohol extraction method

Organic Chemistry the study of carbon based compounds

Organic Compounds compounds containing carbon

Orifice Reducers a fitting inside the neck of a bottle that allows drops of essential oils to be extracted

Oxidation the word used to describe the loss of an electron by an atom, ion or molecule

Oxide A single oxygen with other elements. In the case of essential oils, the oxygen is bound to a terpene ring compound.

Oxidized a molecule that has lost an electron

P

Periodic Table the arrangement of the elements according to their atomic weight and atomic number

Peroxidize a chemical change in the essential oil caused by an oxygen reaction

Petrochemical substances created or processed using petroleum products

Phenol a compound composed of a hydroxy group (-OH) bonded to an aromatic (benzene) ring

Pheromones attractor hormones of insects and animals

Photosensitivity when ingredients or drugs cause a chemically induced change in the skin that makes an individual unusually sensitive to light

Polar Covalent Bonds a covalent bond in which the electrons are shared unequally

Polarity an attraction determined by the distribution of electrical charges within a molecule

Primary Metabolism the manufacture in plants of substances necessary for energy, the building of raw material and oxygen, or those materials necessary for day to day survival

Proton a subatomic particle with a positive charge within the nucleus of the atom

Psycho-Aromatherapy the term coined by Robert Tisserand that describes the use of essential oils to achieve and maintain emotional balance

R

Racemic Mix the term used to describe a 50:50 mix of two, one right-handed and one left-handed, enantiomers

Rancid the partial decomposition of a fatty acid

Receptors cell components that interact with hormones, drugs, and chemical mediators in the body that trigger a response in the cell

Redistilled (Rectified) The repeated, or redistillation, of essential oils already extracted from the plant material. This is used to remove colors and unwanted compounds from the essential oil.

Redox Reaction the process of an atom or molecule losing (oxidation) or gaining (reduction) an electron

Reduced a molecule that has gained an electron

Reduction the word used to describe an atom, molecule or ion gaining an electron

Reductionist a scientific philosophy that believes that the properties of the whole can be reduced to the effects of single components

Retention Hyperkeratosis when keratinized cells, the corneocytes, of the stratum corneum do not exfoliate properly

S

Scarification The process used to extract the essential oil from citrus peels. Also called cold expression or cold pressed.

Secondary Metabolism A process in plants that developed to aid survival and propagation of the species. These are summarized as secondary metabolites and include essential oils and portions of the plant that are useful as drugs and medicines.

Sensitization the development of an allergic reaction that occurs over a period of time

Serotonin an important neurotransmitter related to sleep-wake cycles, is a vasoconstrictor and is related to depression

Sesquiterpene Alcohols a compound defined by a hydroxy functional group (-OH) bonded to a sesquiterpene (C-15) hydrocarbon

Sesquiterpene Hydrocarbon 15-carbon (C-15) hydrocarbon compounds that, in general, make up about 10 to 20 percent of the total composition of the essential oils that contain them

Slip ability to glide along the skin

Specific Effects Essential oil effects defined by the interaction with receptors and the interaction many oils have with physiological systems. Specific effects are often noted at lower rather than higher concentrations.

Steam Distillation a process of distillation using steam only

Structural Isomers a special case of isomers, in which they have a variation in the covalent arrangement of the atoms, called enantiomers

Structure-Effect Diagram A chart designed to connect essential oil components to pharmacological effects based on the electronegative, electropositive and polarity of the essential oil compounds. The diagram offers guidance to the therapeutic selection of essential oils by visually sorting benefits, activity, and functions of the chemical families, or groupings, of essential oil components.

Surface Tension the molecules at the surface of water liquids that are pulled inward rather than in equal directions

Surfactant a surface-active ingredient used in cleansers to lift debris and cleanse skin and also act as foam boosters and emulsifiers

Synergy when two or more agents, organs, or organisms work and cooperate with each other to produce a sum, or result, greater than the whole

T

Terpene Hydrocarbons The most abundant component in essential oil chemical composition. Terpene hydrocarbons are made up of multiples of a five-carbon atom unit called isoprene units.

Terpenoid Compounds hydrocarbon compounds made up of multiples of a five-carbon atom unit called isoprene units

Therapy a healing and curative treatment intended to remedy a disorder or undesirable condition

Tonic strengthening, or toning, the body or a specific organ or area

Triglyceride a saturated structure comprising three fatty acid chains attached to a glycerol molecule

Triple Bond occurs when two atoms bond by sharing three electrons

U

Unpaired Electron the result of an atom or molecule that loses an electron, as they do in chemical reactions or when weak bonds are split

V

Valence Electrons electrons that occupy the outermost energy level

Vitamin C Ester when ascorbic acid (vitamin C) is reacted with fatty acids from palm or an alternate oil, the vitamin is esterfied and becomes a fat-soluble form of vitamin C

Volatile a substance that evaporates easily

Volatility the evaporation rate

Vomeronasal Organ (VNO) an organ just behind the opening of the nose on the human septum whose function is mysterious but is thought to be the detection mechanism for pheromones

W

Water Distillation Plant material is placed in a still completely immersed in water that is heated, causing the evaporation of the oils without the use of steam. Also called hydrodistillation.

Water/Steam Distillation The process of distillation placing the plant material in a still filled with heated water. Steam is injected from a separate apparatus.

Index

R

S